A Ring Without End

Reflections on Classical Chinese Medicine

Mind/Body Mapping

Also by Z'ev Rosenberg & Stephen Cowan

Fire Child, Water Child
How Understanding the Five Types of ADHD Can Help You Improve Your Child's Self-Esteem and Attention
Stephen Cowan
ISBN 978 1 60882 090 0

Vessel of Promises:
A Bookish Fable
Stephen Cowan
Illustrations by Ed Young
ISBN 978 0 52551 387 2

The Weather's Bet
Ed Young
Words by Stephen Cowan
ISBN 978 0 52551 3827

Afterglow
Ministerial Fire and Chinese Ecological Medicine
Z'ev Rosenberg
Foreword by Stephen Cowan
ISBN 978 1 78775 412 6

Ripples in the Flow
Reflections on Vessel Dynamics in the Nàn Jing
Z'ev Rosenberg
Foreword by Lonny S. Jarrett, M.Ac.
ISBN 978 0 85701 391 0

Returning to the Source
Han Dynasty Medical Classics in Modern Clinical Practice
Z'ev Rosenberg
Foreword by Dr. Sabine Wilms
ISBN 978 1 84819 348 2

A Ring Without End

Reflections on Classical Chinese Medicine

Mind/Body Mapping

CW01500915

Z'ev Rosenberg & Stephen Cowan

Foreword by David White

Afterword and Contributions by Brian Kirbis

Edited and Contributions by Daniel Schrier

Contributions by Anne Shelton Crute

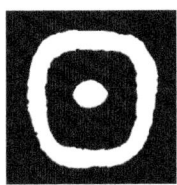

Ring Press Collective

Published by Ring Press Collective

Softcover ISBN - 979-8-9926868-0-7
Hardcover ISBN - 979-8-9926868-1-4

Cover Artwork: *Landscape of the Four Seasons in the Styles of Old Masters. Wèi Zhīkè* 魏之克 *(1635) - Metropolitan Museum of Art - Object Number: 68.195*
Cover Design: Emily Do
Book Layout and Design: Daniel Schrier

Disclaimer:

This book is designed to provide useful information on the subject matter covered and should not be considered a substitute for advice from a medical professional, whom the reader should consult before beginning any diet or exercise regime and before taking any Chinese herbal formulas, dietary supplements or other medications.

This text is sold with the understanding that this information is scholarly in nature and is in no way meant to be a practical hands-on guide to prescriptive medicine by non Traditional Chinese Medicine (TCM) practitioners. All readers seeking such guidance are directed to seek professional education, including Chinese medical diagnosis techniques, which are not included in this text. As with any form of medicine, preventative or curative, herbal chemical, ingested or performed readers should NOT self-medicate or administer these treatments to others without appropriate education from licensed professionals. The author, publisher, and editor, shall have neither liability nor responsibility to any person or entity with respect to any loss, injury, or damage caused, directly or indirectly, by the information contained in this book. It is imperative that you consult a licensed physician or other licensed healthcare provider before considering any of the measures discussed in this publication.

Dedication

Z'ev:

This book is dedicated to all of our ancestors who contributed to the wisdom of humanity, selfless observing life, nature, and the universe.

Stephen:

To all my teachers: the wind, mountain streams, trees and clouds.

The Ring Press Collective:
Publisher's Mission Statement

Ring Press Collective was established to provide a platform for a collective group of Chinese Medicine practitioners who propose that the practice of "Ecological Medicine" is desperately needed in the 21st Century world at large. Application of the principles of *yīnyáng* 陰陽, *wǔxíng* 五行/five phases, channel theory, and seasonal *qì*, emphasize the importance of living in coherence with Change. Such change is governed by solar, lunar, sidereal, diurnal, seasonal and yearly cycles that inform and guide our practice of Chinese medicine in lifestyle as well as therapeutics. Our work encourages deep study and reflection on the classics, living in accordance with the processes of *Dào* 道, in order to reduce the current stresses on our planet caused by strains on resources, ecological damage, and loss of connection to heavenly and earthly *qì*. Our aim is to provide texts, media and resources that inspire our fellow human beings to walk with grace upon our planet, in harmony with all sentient beings. The clinical tools at our disposal include acupuncture/moxibustion, herbal medicine, counseling, dietetics, *qìgōng* 氣功, *tàijí* 太極, yoga, and meditation practices. We at *Ring Press Collective* wish to make these tools and texts available to as many people as possible, in order to build a better world and ensure a future for our children, grandchildren and beyond, while honoring the ecological, medical and philosophical teachings bestowed upon us by our ancestors.

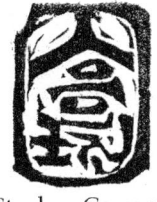

Stephen Cowan

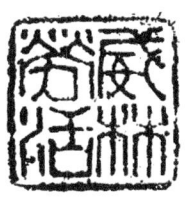

Z'ev Rosenberg

Testimonies

The traditional transmission of knowledge in East Asian Medicine relied on apprenticeships and, especially for literate and elite physicians, on meticulous reading of canonical texts, commentaries and commentaries on the commentaries. It was understood and demonstrated through East Asian Medicine's history that scrupulous examination of canonical texts — no matter how impenetrable and obscure — can reveal a constant source of new wisdom, innovative knowledge, and creative clinical strategies. Our canonical texts beckoned physicians to embrace, clarify, discover, and reveal. The vibrance of the elite traditional was embedded in the back and forth between text and scholar. The text and the scholar were one; they sustained each other. In modernity, this rigorous method of uncovering insights in ancient wisdom has been mostly lost. The ancient knowledge has been frozen. In modern times, we mostly learn in licensed schools that prepare us for national accreditation examination. We learn the "factoids" not wisdom. Progress and innovation in Chinese medicine seems too often come from our interactions with biomedicine or other complementary medicines. Science has more sway than the *Nèi Jīng* 內經. We depend on innovation from the outside; not enough from the inside. Z'ev Rosenberg and Stephen Cowan, two of leading scholars and teachers of Chinese medicine the West, have been exemplary scholars who have consistently drawn the inspiration from ancient wisdom. Their new volume, *A Ring Without End*, is a wonderful addition to their many efforts to contemplate the old to enlighten the present. They reacquaint us with the timeless sources.

Ted Kaptchuk
Author, *The Web That Has No Weaver: Understanding Chinese Medicine*

The *Nàn Jīng* 難經 is replete not only with original and empirical insights, but with explicit recommendations. Still relevant in our time, through their engaging, innovative, dialogical exegesis, Cowan and Rosenberg bring the *Nàn Jīng* 難經 to life!

Efrem Korngold, L.Ac., OMD
After Spring Snow Moon
Author, *Between Heaven and Earth: A Guide to Chinese Medicine*

This book is the opposite of a "how to" manual. Instead, it's a thoughtful conversation on the dynamic of "how things are." *A Ring Without End* is not a veneration of the history of Chinese medicine, it's an invitation to kindle it within yourself. Engage it as you would a fine tea.

Michael Max, L.Ac.
Founder/Host of Qiological

Medicine is not a fixed system but a perpetually emergent process. In *A Ring Without End*, Z'ev Rosenberg and Stephen Cowan explore the dynamic, interconnected nature of health through the lens of classical Chinese medicine, modern complexity theory, and systems thinking. Drawing from the *Nèi Jīng* 內 經, *Nàn Jīng* 難經, and Daoist philosophy, they reveal how the body's circulation reflects the fluidity of rivers, the cyclical turning of seasons, and the rhythms of the cosmos. Far from static anatomical structures, the body's channels are continually unfolding systems shaped by time, space, and reciprocal influence. This book challenges the rigidity of modern biomedicine by offering a vision of healing centered on harmonizing flows rather than merely fixing parts—an essential read for those who see medicine as an art of timing, adaptation, and resonance.

Justin Penoyer, DACM, L.Ac.
Owner of Su Wu Herbs

Throughout *A Ring Without End*, the central concern as I see it is a reckoning with the tension between form and function and between static locations and structures and dynamic movement both as they are expressed in classical Chinese medical texts and how this tension has been interpreted and translated into practice since then in the East and later on in the West.

Rosenberg and Cowan are calling us to reconnect with the "hidden landscape" of the body, to look beyond function, two dimensional maps, container spaces and "junctions" to see the ever-present flux, the flow of qi and blood through these spaces which interpenetrates and connects the organism as a whole, and whose impediment is the ultimate source of disease. They note that what distinguishes eastern maps from western ones, whether it be a hexagram or a landscape painting, is the ability to depict change and flux, to wed form and function 體 and 用.

It is my hope that through this book, others may join in this vital conversation and work together to restore a vision of acupuncture that embodies the spirit and boundless vitality of the classics.

Will Ceurvels
Author, *An Archaeology of the Qiao Vessels*

Table of Contents

List of Figures

Acknowledgements

As with all creative projects, this book began as a series of non-linear conversations during the great pandemic of 2020, while Z'ev was working on his previous book, Afterglow. Over the years, like many open-ended conversations that spin off into daily life, colleagues, friends and family brought ideas to the table that helped inspire the development of this book. We'd like to thank Brian Kirbis for his steady supply of articles, books, pu'er, and thoughts from the world of Tea, Anne Shelton Crute for her expertise in cosmic medicine, Christoph Wiesendanger for his constant encouragement, Daniel Schrier for his unflagging support and effort in editing and refining the form this book has taken and Emily Do for her cover design, which seamlessly and beautifully captures the natural elements emphasized in this book. Several other important people whose expertise in the field of Chinese medicine has inspired the thoughts gathered in this book include: Paul Unschuld, Efrem Korngold, Ed Young, Volker Scheid, Michael Max, Ken Rose, Shigahisa Kuriyama, Lán Fènglì, Liú Lìhóng, Heiner Fruehauf, David White, Moshe Heller, and of course Zhuāngzǐ, and Lǎozǐ.

This book would in no way have been possible without the nourishing support of our life-companions, Susan and Edith, who encouraged us to roam in this wild world of the classics amidst our busy lives.

Foreword

David White

Studying and expanding on the complexities of classical, Han-era, channel (*jīngluò* 經絡) theory is no easy undertaking. The varying perspectives and lenses that are required, enabled, and hermeneutically cultivated, lead to fascinating endeavours of historical, clinical, and philosophical findings. Z'ev Rosenberg and Stephen Cowan have achieved this in their pivotal text "*A Ring Without End,*" where they take the reader into a wonderfully rich and deep conversation on the intricate architecture of classical Chinese anatomy and physiology, blending it with concise ecological metaphor.

This metaphor is of utmost importance to any scholar-physicians approach to the medical classics of the *Huángdì Nèijīng* (黃帝內經) or *Nàn Jīng* (難經). To be able to draw on the ancients ability to abide by patterned change (*biàn* 變), principle (*lǐ* 理), method (*fāng* 方) and image (*xiàng* 象), among others, when encountering the described body and its manifestations, allows us to truly appreciate Paul Unschuld's take on these texts as a "medicine of systematic correspondence." When we are in our practices palpating the vessels (*mài* 脈) and listening to the movements, we are simultaneously embodying the ecological terrain of vessel and river, tissue and soil, qi and gas, or even assessing bone as bathymetry. To evaluate and treat one is to treat the whole, and this rings true throughout the entire text corpora - something that seems to be lost in the modern study of the *jīngluò*, where they are often segmented as individual entities of patho-physiological activity, where "points" reign supreme, and the inner gaze of the physician is diluted to a two-dimensional process.

However, the "classical renaissance" as it were, is well and truly in its stride in the continuous global inquiry into Chinese medicine. Today we are finding scholars young and old, investigating the primary sources with an intense knowledge base and vigour. As more of the ancient texts and their commentaries are translated, studied, argued, and clinically tested, we start to find that the above diluted process is suddenly looked upon through a different lens altogether. What was a seemingly flat prairie with defined start and finish is now that of deep valleys and mountainous terrain nourished by watersheds and structured movements on longitudinal and latitudinal patterned pathways where beginnings become ends and ends become beginnings. This in turn takes us closer to the mindset of our medical ancestors, to envision their world, their outlook, their medicine. Approaching the *Nèijīng*, and especially the foundational chapters of the *Língshū Jīng* (靈樞經), requires a distinct ability to read what is not written when it comes to channel theory. On some occasions this requires foreknowledge of adjunct texts; and on other occasions it calls for a deep meditation on meaning, etymological study, dialogue, and always, clinical consideration. *A Ring Without End* continues a two-millenia-old conversation of this material and helps us refine and define not only the place of the texts and theories for the current Chinese medical landscape, but for the individual as scholar or practitioner for generations to come.

It is truly wonderful to see such work continue to be developed in our field, and more so, to see the work published by long-standing and original practitioners of this medicine in the west. I have no doubt this text, and future works of Z'ev Rosenberg and Stephen Cowan, will be a sustained source of support and reference for those seeking clarity in this medicine.

David White
Director, Institute of Neijing Research Sydney, Australia
April 08, 2024

The Fields of Flow: *Context is Everything in Medicine*

Z'ev Rosenberg

Field and context are everything. Our perception of the human entity depends on what the physician's 'clinical gaze' focuses on. Dr. Shigahisa Kuriyama is right on target with his observations when he write about the contrast between Western and traditional Chinese perspectives on anatomy in his article *The Imagination of the Body and the History of Embodied Experience*.[1] He suggests that perception is shaped by context. The Western anatomical study is influenced by the voyeuristic setting of the dissection theater, which isolates the body for scrutiny. Whereas the Chinese medical illustrations depict the body as part of the natural world, seamlessly integrated into the cosmic flow of the natural landscape encompassing mountains, rivers, and winds. This difference in perspective reflects broader cultural understandings of the human body's relationship to nature and the universe.

Chinese medicine, based in classical Chinese texts such as the *Yìjīng* 易經 / *Classic of Change*, and the *Lǎozǐ* 老子 / *Book of Venerable Masters*[2] has a very specific worldview beginning with the *Dào* 道 / universal whole. From there it moves to find resonating functions and structures in the human being, reading the textures of movement, color, motion, emotion, along with striations in skin, muscle and organ tissues. The origin in the universal source is never abandoned, it is always guiding the mind of the Chinese scholar / physician. From this perspective, the human being is a multi-layered energetic field of flow and dynamics, with structural interfaces along the path of the channel system.

We can approach anatomy and physiology from this perspective as well, nothing needs to be rejected out of hand. It is all about the context! The Chinese scholar / physician looks at structures, tissues and substances as sublimations of the dynamic flows of cosmic and earthly rivers in constant movement and transformation. Just as the author(s) of the *Nàn Jīng* 難經 observed how some

---

[1] Kuriyama, *"The Imagination of the Body and the History of Embodied Experience,"* pg. 25.

[2] Usually known and referred to with its honorific title *Dàodé Jīng* 道德經 / *Scripture on the Dào and Inner Power*.

organs would float in water, others sink,[3] and other early anatomists in China observed the striations and visual manifestations of *qì* 氣 / *xuè* 血 flowing, a unified vision of health as flow and illness as blockages to flow emerged in the Han dynasty and beyond.[4]

The scholar/physician, like a mariner at sea, consulted the different maps offered to him by the medical tradition, and read the pulse, nails, tongue, and palpated the vessels to perceive disharmonies in the flow, trace them back in time, and predict their future course. Each needle and herb was applied to gently/subtly alter the flow and unblock the channels to activate the *yuán qì* 原 氣 / original source *qì*, and along with it the self-correcting intelligence of the body/mind.

The scholar/physician also consulted the maps of the heavens, the seasons, the movements of *wèi* 衛 / *yíng* 營 with the breath, five movements and six qi (*wǔ yùn liù qì* 五運六氣) theory, lunar and solar cycles, winds, humidity, unseasonable weather, guest *qì* (*kè qì* 客氣) and host *qì* (*zhǔ qì* 主氣). Just as today we see how the movement of the great dragons, the atmospheric rivers as they clash with the California mountains and drop their rain and snow, understand high and low atmospheric pressure systems, wind flows, and how they affect human health, epidemics and tendencies to illness. The scholar/physician examined the environment in which medicinal herbs grew, the soil, water sources, patterns of growth, medicinal qualities of root, branch, leaves and flowers.

In *Nàn Jīng* 16 the commentators make the point that diagnosis is corroborated by both internal and external evidence. This begins with the complexion, bodily shape, and tone voice and extends internally to the tongue and finally the three sections and nine indicators of the pulse, depth and pressure, and palpation of abdominal locations which provide additional "evidence." These locations later became the basis of abdominal palpation in Japanese medicine, and combined with front/*mù xué* 募穴 points and *yuán* 原 points (as described in the commentaries on *Nàn Jīng* 16) were adapted as treatment systems in their own right.

It is important to emphasize, however, that without a strong grounding in classical medicine and its source texts, one will easily lose the thread and oversimplify one's work and limit one's discoveries.

---

[3] See *Nàn Jīng* 難經 33.

[4] This is an important statement that highlights the fundamental unity of blood and *qì*. Where blood is the material form of the body that defines circulation beyond just red blood, to include plasma, lymph, membranes and other bodily fluids. Later in the book we will discuss the various implications of this.

This can be illustrated in our chapter *The Sinew Channels in Língshū* 靈樞 and *Nàn Jīng* 難經[5]. Many acupuncturists feel challenged by the sudden appearance of "dry needling" that has been adapted by many therapists in the biomedical system as if it were an original discovery taken from the work of Dr. Janet Travell and Karel Lewit. However, these strong techniques, needling tendino-muscular structures were already described in the *Língshū* two thousand years ago!

The problem arises from the tendency towards an inferiority complex by practitioners of Asian medicine who, being immersed in a Western culture, feel that biomedicine with its specific anatomy, biological and cellular dynamics is "real," and Asian medicine is "metaphorical" and somehow less accurate and scientific. Without immersing oneself in the world view of the *Língshū* and *Nàn Jīng,* understanding Chinese medicine and how it works is literally impossible. A textbook course in TCM may teach points, locations, "meridian lines" and associated illnesses that can usually be treated with biomedical descriptions.Without an understanding of the channels, points/holes, and the entire dynamic of the human organism as viewed through a Han dynasty mindset, it is impossible to fully understand or practice Chinese medicine to it's full potential.

Historically, we have seen how Chinese medicine was adapted in its journeys to Japan, Korea, Taiwan, Tibet and Mongolia, and then back to China for cross-fertilization. It then connected and cross fertilized with other traditional medical systems along the Silk Road, through India (Ayurveda आयुर्वेद and Unani طب یونانی), Persia and Greece (Greco-Arabic Medicine), and Egypt.[6] And then in the modern era, Chinese medicine has been informed by the technology research and practicum of biomedicine, a potential source of richness. However, this is dependent on not losing the thread that runs all the way back to the Han dynasty classics that provide the foundation.

In summation, Chinese medicine reads the visible and invisible aspects of the universe as maps that decode the territory of human life. As scholar/physicians, we are like mariners riding the seas, directing our rudders, and setting our compasses towards the goal of human health, happiness, long life and peace.

---

[5] See *The Sinew Channels in Língshū* 靈樞 and *Nàn Jīng* 難經 pg.197-204.

[6] See *Arabic Medicine in China* (2021), translated by Eugene Anderson and Paul Buell, Brill Press, and *Ben Cao Gang Mu* (2021-2024), translated by Paul Unschuld, UC Press which contain multiple "foreign medicinals" that were incorporated into the body of Chinese medicine.

The Art & Science of Seal Form Characters

Stephen Cowan

"Chinese is phenomenological, it pictures what is."
- Schatz, Larre & Rochat de la Vallée [7]

Over 25 years ago, my late teacher Ed Young, renowned children's author/illustrator and *Tàijí* 太極 master opened my world to the seal-forms of Chinese characters to help me understand the hidden meanings in Chinese language. He had learned from Cheng Man-Ching 郑曼青 (1902-1975) how to use the seal-forms to better explain the multilayered meanings of *Tàijí* terms. He recognized that because I am a visual learner (like him), that I needed to "see" the meaning with my own eyes. And so, he systematically deconstructed the various etymological elements of ideograms which became, as he said they would, "old familiar friends" to me. Over the years I've used the seal-form characters to help students bring to life subtle concepts in Chinese medicine. I have also used them in my practice, drawing the characters on my prescription pad for patients to use as a kind of talisman to promote healing through their special power of visualization.

The earliest forms of writing in China were hieroglyphic carvings, dating back to Neolithic shamanic times that then evolved into the so-called "oracle bone script" (*jiǎ gǔ wén* 甲骨文). According to Dr. L. Wieger [8], the so called "greater seal forms" (*dà zhuàn* 大篆), date back to approximately 800 BCE, during the Zhòu 籀 dynasty (1046 – 256 BCE), when the grand recorder drew up a catalogue of the existing characters of the time, known as the *zhòu wén* 籀文, and standardized them for the scribes to use as official seals. By the time of the Qín 秦 dynasty (221-206 BCE), much of the greater seals were lost and a newer form of approximately 3,300 characters known as the "lesser seal forms" (*xiǎo zhuàn* 小篆) appeared. In the process, mistakes were made in interpreting the etymological meanings of the characters. By the time of the Han dynasty, numerous etymological dictionaries arose to study the roots of meaning embedded in these images. One of the most famous of these was the *Shuōwén*

---

[7] Schatz, Larre & Rochat de la Vallée, *"Survey of Traditional Chinese Medicine,"* pg. 31.

[8] Wieger & Davrout, *"Chinese Characters: Their Origin, Etymology, History, Classification and Signification."*

Jiězì 说文解字 which literally means "discussing writing and explaining characters." This dictionary containing over 9000 characters has survived the rise and fall of many dynasties and serves as a basis for getting a glimpse of how the ancients conceived the world around them. In contrast to Western alphabetic languages, Chinese language (and culture) based in images is essentially relational by nature. There are no absolutes. Meanings change with the context and relationships they find themselves in. Indeed if one contrasts the four element philosophy developed by Aristotle with the Five phase maps that evolved in China, there is no center in the greek element philosophy whereas for the Chinese, Soil (earth phase) was always the central field in which the four directions, four seasons, four movements relate. In health and medicine this is the basis of harmony as an active process rather than a static absolute state.

As a cultivation practice, I find that this soil/earth based focus can help develop empathy and tolerance for our common ground and our uniqueness. When we clear our mind of our own biases and conceptual judgments, an image (*xiàng* 象) takes form that brings the character to life, revealing hidden depths of meaning. This practice requires trust in your innate powers to process visual information the way one does when looking at a landscape. Each ideogram is a kind of map in itself that unfolds worlds of metaphoric meanings that guide our multidimensional understanding of what is being communicated.

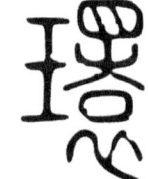

Figure 1 - Huán 環

Take for example the ideogram *huán* 環 (*fig. 1*), the character for "ring" in the title of this book, *A Ring Without End*, which is a quote mentioned prominently in *Nàn Jīng* 難經 texts.

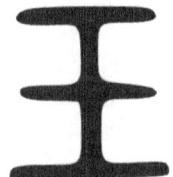

Figure 2 - Wáng 王

The ideogram *huán* 環 *(fig. 1)* shows, on the left, three horizontal lines joined by a single vertical *(fig. 2)*. It has been commonly taken to mean the precious stone jade (*yù* 玉). If one looks back at the oracle bone carvings, it simultaneously has a deeper meaning of the heaven-earth-human unity that the emperor was supposed to be the embodiment of and so, *wáng* 王 means emperor or king, who wore a jade medallion representing that triune unity. A fundamental principle in Chinese medicine is that we each are an embodiment the Heavens descending to meet the ascending Earth. This radical *wáng* 王, therefore gives the feeling and movement of the character *huán* 環.

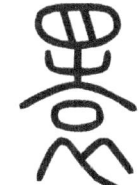

Figure 3 - Huán 睘

On the right we see an image of *huán* 睘 *(fig. 3)*, said to be an image of long flowing robes, meaning "around" or "encompassing."

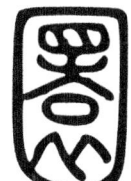

Figure 4 - Huán 圜

When placed in a circle, *huán* 圜 *(fig. 4)* pronounced the same way, means "to encircle" or "surround."

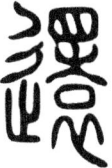

Figure 5 - Huán 還

When the heaven-earth-human radical is replaced by the image of a foot traveling the character 還 *(fig. 5)* also pronounced *huán*, means "returning." These three homophones of *huán* together give the reader a holographic map of the feeling of something actively flowing around and around.

Put together *huán* 環 / ring (*fig. 1*) becomes a metaphor for the feeling of the heavens and earth circulating around, cycling and recycling as in the water cycle in Nature or the circulatory system in our body (as radically defined in *Nàn Jīng* medicine). From a Daoist perspective, this *huán* 環, encircling ring might be considered a metaphor for the microcosmic orbit.[9]

By enabling us to see hidden relationships, the metaphoric imagery of seal script characters enables us to relate to the world of the classics and bring them to life in the world around us. Such relational understanding is no less a science than our western reductionist way of studying the world. As Lán Fènglì 蘭鳳利 says:

"Metaphors in Chinese medicine reveal relationships and metaphor thinking is an exact thinking."[10]

Mapping relationships is fundamental to Chinese medicine. When we ask a patient "what does it feel *like?*" we're asking them to relate their experience to something we might understand (e.g. "it burns *like* fire," "it's pounding *like* a hammer" so that we may better get the feel for what's alive in them and know how to relieve their suffering. The art of pulse-taking in Chinese medicine is loaded with such Nature-based metaphors.

When we look, for example, at the names that have been passed down for acu-points, I have found that these seal-forms and their earlier bronze and oracle bone images deepen our metaphoric understanding of what the sages were really thinking and feeling when they chose these names on their body maps.

For example, the ideogram *huán* 環 / ring appears in the name for acu-point *huán tiào* 環跳 (GB 30), translated as "jumping around" which is particularly effective in treating conditions like Sciatica where the gluteal muscles have tightened around the sciatic nerve causing intense pain; the pain being a signal of blocked circulation (whether we think of it as blocked blood or *qì* or nerve conduction or all three at once for that matter!) Moxibustion, massage, or needling this point serves to release the obstruction and promote circulation, enabling one to move about more freely.

The examination of characters as it was taught to me over the last 25 years is a meditative process of ongoing "interpretation" which must not be confused with the art of "translation" for which I have the utmost respect for the work of such eminent scholars as Paul Unschuld and Sabine Wilms, who have given us

---

[9] See Daniel Schrier's chapter *"Charting the Inner Ecosystem Through Chinese Medical and Daoist Alchemical Body Maps,"* pg. 159- 180.

[10] Lan & Wallner, *"Metaphor The Weaver of Chinese Medicine."*

essential access to the classics both technically and authoritatively. I am also keenly aware of a long history dating back to the Han Dynasty of debate between Confucian and Daoist scholars about the skillful use of language. The Confucian scholar Xúnzi 荀子 (298-238 BCE) author of the classic *Zhèngmíng* 正名/*Rectification of Names* showed great concern for the inaccurate use of words leading to confusion: *"Men are careless in abiding by established names, strange words come into use, names and realities become confused and the distinction between right and wrong has become unclear. Even officials who guard the laws or the scholars who recite the classics have all become confused."*[11] In contrast, the *Lǎozi* 老子 (*Dàodé Jīng* 道德經), from the very first chapter, cautions us that *"the name named is not a forever name"*[12] and *Zhuāngzi* 莊子 adds: *"The Way has never known boundaries; speech has never known constancy. But because of 'this' and 'that,' there arise boundaries."*[13] Roger Ames has written extensively about this debate of correct naming, stating:

> *"Daoist literature is preoccupied with the possible fragmenting and ossifying effect of language functioning as precedent. The application of language and concept arrests the fluidity of an ever novel flow of events. When our experience is mediated through language, we in varying degrees deny the uniqueness of particular phenomena by imposing a given structure and patterned regularity upon the world around us. The alternative is to reflect events as they are in our dynamic relationship to them, without distortion."*[14]

Ideogram study in general and the study of *huán*, in particular, with reference to this book, reflects the kind of lively free-flowing conversation that Z'ev Rosenberg and I have had over the years in exploring the *Nàn Jīng* texts that has allowed them to come alive. It is what Krishnamurti calls *"the freedom to inquire,"* to look deeply without the biases and prejudgments we have been conditioned to see the world with. Throughout this book, I've included various seal-form characters based on the *Nàn Jīng* texts to serve as metaphoric maps to bring to life the deep meanings of the ideas we are discussing. It's that same poetic/scientific freedom, I hope we will inspire in you, to see with fresh eyes what the ancients had to say in order to discover their relevance to our modern day practice.

As they say, *"A picture is worth a thousand words."*

---

[11] Watson, *"Basic Writings of Mo Tzu, Hsün Tzu, and Han Fei Tzu."* Hsün Tzu Chapter 22. Rectifying Names

[12] *Lǎozi* 老子 1 translation/interpretation S. Cowan 名可名非常名.

[13] Watson, *"The Complete Works of Chuang Tzu,"* pg. 37.

[14] Hall & Ames, *"Thinking from the Han: Self, Truth, and Transcendence in Chinese and Western Culture"* pg. 51.

How to Read and Utilize This Text

A Ring Without End: Reflections on Classical Chinese Medicine Mind/Body Mapping embodies an innovative approach to studying Classical Chinese Medicine, one in line with the modern digital age and tendencies to absorb information in a non linear fashion. It is designed as a deep and reflective exploration of Classical Chinese Medicine enriched with many concepts and references. To make the most of its contents, a thoughtful approach to reading is encouraged. Below are some guidelines to help you navigate and utilize this text effectively.

The Four-Part Structure & Reading in Chunks

The book is divided into four parts (Ecologies; Maps, Circulation & Channels, Ring), each covering a specific dialog and contemplation pertaining the subject. Within these four parts, there are individual chapters which explore nuanced topics that interconnect and can also be appreciated independently.

Due to the depth of discussion and complexity of ideas presented, the best way to engage with this book is in sections. Treat each section as an opportunity for contemplation rather than rushing to the next. While reading from cover to cover is certainly possible, each chapter is structured to function as a standalone discussion, similar to enjoying a cup of tea with a friend. Dialog among friends/colleagues allows one to absorb the insights being presented without becoming overwhelmed.

Discussion, Reflection, and Application

Since *A Ring Without End* is structured as a series of conversations between Z'ev and Stephen, it invites dialogue and discussions with others who are also exploring these ideas. Conversations enhance comprehension and reveal new relationships and perspectives. While reading, you may notice thoughts and ideas repeated in various chapters. This repetition is intentional, serving to reinforce circular learning and deepen your understanding of key themes over time.

A Journey

This book is not meant to be rushed through. Take your time as you would, a stroll in Nature, enjoy the process, and allow the material to unfold naturally. Bring it with you one a hike in the woods or mountains. Whether you read a chapter a day, or a week, the goal is to cultivate a meaningful and enriching reading experience. By approaching this book with patience and intention, you will find that its wisdom resonates more deeply. Dao is process. The journey begins when you open these pages.

Resources for Further Learning

For those seeking further exploration and deeper historical context, the following texts provide valuable insights into the classical foundations of the material discussed in this book. These offer detailed translations, and footnotes, serving as essential references for anyone looking to deepen their understanding of the historical and theoretical underpinnings of this book's discussions.

A large portion of this text is based on the *Nàn Jīng* 難經 and other classics of Chinese medicine such as the *Língshū* 靈樞 and *Sùwèn* 素問. While one does not need to have these texts nearby while reading this text, utilizing the footnote references and exploring the various chapters will assist in further insight. We suggest the following translations by Paul U. Unschuld.

- *Nan Jing: The Classic of Difficult Issues*
- *Huang Di Nei Jing Su Wen: An Annotated Translation of Huang Di's Inner Classic - Basic Questions, 2 Volumes.*
- *Huang Di Nei Jing Ling Shu: The Ancient Classic on Needle Therapy*

Pleco Chinese Dictionary (*for Apple iOS devices and Android devices*): Provides comprehensive translations, definitions, and detailed information about Chinese words, phrases, and characters. The program includes various free and paid dictionaries and add-ons, such as Wiseman and Ye's *A Practical Dictionary of Chinese Medicine*, Kroll's *A Student's Dictionary of Classical and Medieval Chinese* along with document readers, and optical character recognizer (OCR) to look up unknown Chinese words "live" or from still image. With the **Outlier Dictionary of Chinese Character** (*Pleco add-on*) providing a detailed historical and etymological information for 2,000 characters.

Chinese Etymology: https://hanziyuan.net: Created by Richard Sears, this website is dedicated to providing historical information on the origins, evolution and meanings of Chinese characters through detailed etymological analysis and ancient script references in a easy searchable format.

Chinese Characters: Their Origin, Etymology, History, Classification, and Signification by L.Wieger, breaks down thousands of characters and traces their historical evolution and explains their meaning through etymology and classification.

Part I:
Ecologies

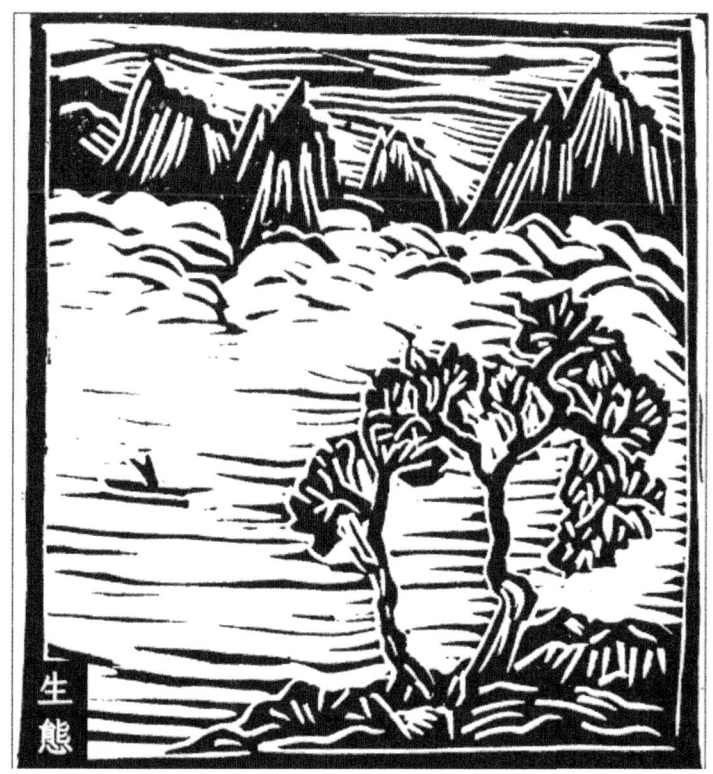

15

---

¹⁵ S. Cowan Woodcut: Ecologies / *Shēngtài* 生態.

Ecological Passages: *Qualities of Life, Longevity and Death*

Stephen Cowan & Z'ev Rosenberg

Stephen: The *Nàn Jīng* 難經, like its forerunner, the *Nèijīng* 內經, is concerned with predicting qualities of life, illness, longevity and death. Indeed, all forms of medicine have some aspect of this desire to predict the course of an illness in order to be prepared to treat it. The difficulties presented in the *Nàn Jīng* are an attempt to correlate the conceptual body maps (*shēntú* 身圖) put forth in *Nèijīng* while confronting real life situations. The human brain, like that of other animals, has the capacity to construct "cognitive maps" that create a unified representation of the spatial-temporal environment to support memory and guide future action. These maps are influenced by context, cultural traditions, local resources, experience, economic power structure and most of all language.

Z'ev: While Chinese medicine is replete with militaristic metaphors, these are not as predominant as in modern biomedicine. After Virchow, Pasteur and the development of germ theory, applied medicine was basically envisioned as a war against germs that attacked a host body, and the weapons used were what the famous chemist Paul Erlich (1854-1915) called "chemotherapy." To these harsh substances, including unrefined mercury, were added antibiotics and ever broadening categories of pharmaceutical drugs. These drugs were largely the result of manipulation of coal tar chemistry, producing molecules that were the basis of multiple chemical compounds that could be manipulated for therapeutic use.

In Chinese medicine, militaristic metaphors were designed to eliminate exterior *xié* 邪/evils/pathogens/perverse *qì* that disturbed the orderly balance of *yīnyáng* 陰陽 in the organism and created chaos. They were often guided by philosophical directives from such texts as Sūnzǐ 孫子's (771–256 BCE) *Sūnzi Bīngfǎ* 孫子兵法/*Art of War*.[16]

However, the ecological model of Chinese medicine that I've discussed in my previous book, *Afterglow: Ministerial Fire and Ecological Chinese Medicine* is more

---

[16] See Wu, She, and Wang. *Sun Zi's "Art of War" and Health Care: Military Science and Medical Science.*

predominant, and the *Nàn Jīng* clearly emphasizes these metaphorical relationships in its description of medicine.

Stephen: Maps are metaphors for reality. They are not reality themselves. They function as a means of deepening our understanding of context. The noted anthropologist and linguist Gregory Bateson (1904-1980) stated that:

"The relation between the report and the mysterious thing reported tends to have the nature of classification, an assignment of the thing to a class. Naming is always classifying and mapping is essentially the same as naming."[17]

Thus the map of the thing is not the thing itself because, in reality, the "thing" can never be isolated but can only exist relationally.

Z'ev: In *A Ring Without End*, we have included MindNode™ "maps" and translated several of Zhāng Shìxián 張世賢's maps that he designed as visual tools for engaging with the text of the *Nàn Jīng*. We think that "visual learners" specifically will find these maps excellent tools for not only deciphering the text, but providing mandalas that can be memorized and used in the clinical setting as a way to enhance one's diagnosis and practice.

Stephen: Chinese language is distinctive in being based in pictograms and ideograms that carry multiple meanings, existing as both noun and verb, adjective and adverb, and each character's meaning depends on the context within which it is found. Whereas alphabetic languages like ancient Greek (or English for that matter,) tend to carry fixed ideas regardless of the context which leads to more linear-logic thinking in contrast to the more circular Chinese perspective. This linguistic difference greatly shaped the kind of medicine practiced in the East and West.

In *What is Medicine? Western and Eastern Approaches to Healing*, Paul Unschuld questions how the idea of a complete circulatory system could evolve in China by the Han dynasty but did not arise in Greek medicine and suggests that it is the result of the economic political structure based on the power (health) of a unified China.

While there is certainly evidence of this, it is clearly not the *only* reason! One has only to look at the twelve branches astrological map dating back to the time of the *Yìjīng* 易經/*Classic of Changes* (1000–750 BCE) to see a deep understanding of a complete circulatory system. This natural cyclic thinking laid out in the *Book of Changes* predates the unification of China and clearly influenced the writings of *Nàn Jīng* authors. Rather than a supernatural

---

[17] See Bateson,*"Mind and Nature: A Necessary Unity."*

influence, the succession of *yīnyáng* 陰陽, four seasons and *wǔxíng* 五行/five phases influenced all aspects of life.

This idea of a continuous cyclic circulation is given throughout the *Lǎozǐ* 老子 written during the Warring States period before China was unified and certainly must have had an influence on much of Han dynasty thought. For example, *Lǎozǐ* 40 states..

反者道之動

Returning is how the Dao-process moves.
-*Lǎozǐ* 老子 40[18]

It is perhaps reasonable to consider that the idea of cyclic circulation laid the foundation for a unified Qin Dynasty (221-206 BCE) rather than the other way around.

Z'ev: Astronomy developed both in ancient China and ancient Greece. While both cultures developed maps/charts of the heavens, the Chinese saw the constellations as moving, flowing heavenly rivers that corresponded to the earthly landscape of flowing waters. In contrast to the West, astro-cartography was not a science isolated from other disciplines. In modern investigations of complexity theory at the Santa Fe Institute, scientists have come to believe that the specialization of particular sciences is no longer a position that can be useful as the vast informational nature of the physical universe is unfolded by research in various disciplines. This reflects the need of a unifying principle that would be the Western equivalent of the *Yìjīng* and its *yīnyáng* 陰陽 theory. Niels Bohr (1885-1962) was so impressed with Chinese science and philosophy that he adapted the *yīnyáng* symbol in his coat of arms (*fig. 1.1*).

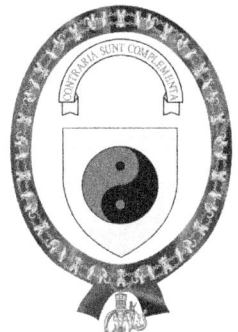

Figure 1.1 - Niels Bohr Coat of Arms

---

[18] *Lǎozǐ* 老子 40 translation/interpretation S. Cowan.

Stephen: Even the Chinese ideogram for map *tú* 圖, has *huí* 回 (*fig. 1.2*), the image of a circle within a circle: meaning to circulate/revolve embedded within it.

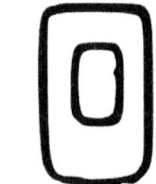

Figure 1.2 - Huí 回[19]

This circular timekeeping in Han Dynasty China was linked to the twelve lunar month cycle, and the twelve earthly branches (*shí'èrzhī* 十二支) starting with *chǒu* 丑 hour, (1:00 AM - 3:00 AM) and became a metaphor for the human body's circulation, as *Língshū* 靈樞 34 states *"the twelve vessels correspond to the twelve months."*[20] Indeed, this concept of a 12 month lunar cycle is why the *Nàn Jīng* authors were so keen on resolving the twelve channels/eleven organ problem as stated in the *Nèijīng* 內經. By conceiving the pericardium & *sānjiāo* 三膲 couple as the missing link they were able to map a complete circulatory system of flowing-irrigating *xuèqì* 血氣 that was consistent with the 12 Earthly branches to ensure that human life properly resonates with the heaven-earth macrocosm.[21]

In *Nàn Jīng* 30 we're given a clear picture of this single unified cycle within the body, a *"ring without end"* which Zhāng Shìxián 張世賢 [22] later illustrated with his own innovative map (*fig. 1.3*). Here we see the central importance of the middle burner as the fuel to keep circulation of *xuèqì* (in the form of *yíngwèi* 營衛) flowing through the day and night.

---

[19] *Huí* 回 to circulate, revolve, return, time (ideogram of a circle within a circle). this idea of circulating is found embedded in the Chinese idea of *tú* 圖 map; diagram; chart.

[20] Unschuld, *"Huang Di Nei Jing Ling Shu: The Ancient Classic on Needle Therapy,"* pg. 262-271 & 331-33.

[21] See *Nàn Jīng* 25 & 38.

[22] Also known by his style name Zhāng Tiānchéng 張天成. His maps and commentary on the *Nàn Jīng* published in 1510 as *Tú Zhù Bāshíyī Nàn Jīng* 圖註八十一難經.

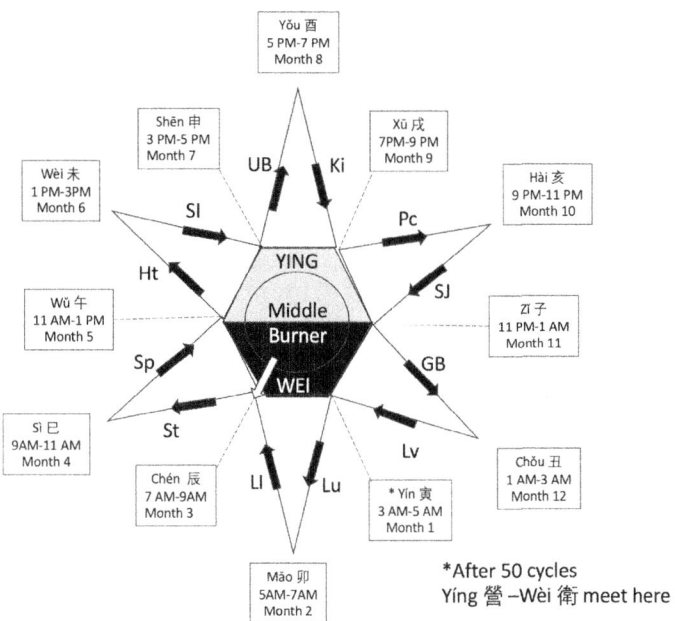

Figure 1.3 - Nàn Jīng 30 Map

No such twelve branch ten stem system unifying heaven and earth existed in Greek philosophy. The Greeks did have a 12-month numerical calendar by the 2nd century BCE, but it was not perceived of as a microcosmic metaphor for our body and therein lies a fundamental difference between East and West.

It was this microcosmic thinking, the idea that we live as an ecological resonance with the forces and rhythms of Nature that would invariably lead to conceiving a complete circulatory system where irrigation and warm flow (*xuèqì*) or blood-breath were recognized as the key to life and that therefore anything that disrupted the continuous ring threatened health.

Z'ev: In my second book, *Ripples in the Flow: Reflections on Vessel Dynamics in the Nàn Jing*, the first chapter comments on how the author(s) of the *Nàn Jīng* conceptualized the *cùn kǒu* 寸口 vessel position as a place where this circular flow in the channels met at *tài yuān* 太淵/supreme abyss (LU 9), the location of the beginning and end of the flow of *wèi qì* 衛氣/*yíng qì* 營氣 through the channels, moving with the breath fifty times per day. Already at this point of development in Han dynasty medicine the circular nature of the medicine, channel flow, vessel diagnosis and treatment was fully developed and canonized. Zhāng Shìxián's chart is consistent with many great physician's perspectives on Chinese medicine, from Lǐ Dōngyuán 李東垣's Spleen/Stomach

(Supplement Earth) School to Péng Ziyì 彭子益's (1871-1949) *Circular Dynamics of Ancient Chinese Medicine*. The earth phase is the "hub of the wheel" on which the other phases turn, ascend and descend.

Stephen: This "fifth element," the Earth-Phase center is a primary contrast to the Greek four element concept on which Western medicine is based. Earth/soil is where we meet, relate and converse. It is where harmonizing takes place, the very basis of Chinese acupuncture and herbal recipes. The microbiome is a perfect example of Earth/soil phase dynamics. Western medicine continues to resist the central place of digestion in health and wellness and only recently is beginning to consider the importance of the microbiome to all aspects of our health.

Ditches and Reservoirs

Stephen Cowan

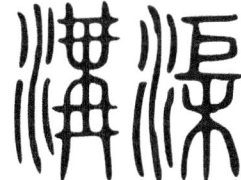

Figure 1.4 - Gōuqú 溝渠[23]

One of the most distinctive characteristics of Chinese medicine's holographic model of the world is the use of metaphor and analogy to explain the human resonance with the cosmos, as Lán Fènglì 蘭鳳利 has so eloquently noted.[24] Concerned as they were with creating a complete map of the circulatory system, it is the *Nàn Jīng* 難經 writers, who first grouped and named the eight extraordinary vessels (*qí jīng bā mài* 奇經八脈) as surplus vessels and questioned how they are functionally related to the twelve channels as part of this circulation.

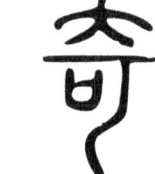

Figure 1.5 - Qí 奇[25]

---

[23] *Gōuqú* 溝渠 together is translated as a "channel, moat or irrigation canal." *Gōu*: ideogram has a wooden gateway + water as in locks in a canal system. It means a drain or ditch. *Qú* 渠: ideogram has a wooden trough +water = canal, gutter, channel, ditch. Paul Unschuld uses the interesting term "ditches and reservoirs" which carries a wider meaning related to the *qí jīng bā mài* 奇經八脈.

[24] See Lan & Wallner, *"Metaphor the Weaver of Chinese Medicine."*

[25] *Qí* 奇 has two meanings. First: "Strange, unusual, out of the ordinary." Second: means "surplus, remainder" (see Wieger, *"Chinese Characters,"* phonetic series 328 Wieger, pg. 469) the ideogram contains the image of a breath *Kě* 可 below - an exhale as in "ah" as in the sound of satisfaction , meaning to consent or "I can." Above it the pictogram of a person with arms held wide *dà* 大 meaning big, great, vast) – together the implied meaning "to utter an exclamation of surprise as in "oh wow""

聖人圖 設溝渠 通利水道 以備不然

"The sage's map (shèngrén tú 聖人圖) devised and constructed drainage ditches and irrigation canals to keep the waterways flowing in case of extraordinary circumstances."
- Nàn Jīng 27[26]

Three consecutive *Nàn Jīng* Difficult Issues 27, 28, 29 discuss the extraordinary vessels (*qí jīng bā mài*) which lead up to the Difficulty 30, where the phrase *"the ring without end."*[27] is described. Here we find the *Nàn Jīng* writers' radical resolution to the dilemma of how these "odd" outlier vessels mentioned in the *Sùwèn* and *Língshū* relate to the 12 primary channel circulation. Using the metaphor of draining ditches and reservoirs that form in nature (or were manually constructed by the Han) during times of great flooding, they saw a metaphoric resonance within the human body.

天雨降下，溝渠溢滿。

"When rain poured down from the heavens, the ditches and reservoirs became filled."
- Nàn Jīng 27[28]

As in nature, the body has reservoir spaces that take off the surplus of fluid and hold it there where it can stagnate or get resorbed depending on the condition of health. In Western medical terminology, this occurs in pathological conditions when hydrostatic forces between intravascular and extracellular compartments are out of balance, and fluid seeps into these potential spaces. When the extra fluid is in the interstitial spaces (now known as "the interstitium,"[29]) it's called "edema." When the extravascular fluid accumulates within a body cavities it's called "third spacing" as in ascites, for example. This overflow can be caused by several conditions:

1. Increased hydrostatic pressure
2. Reduced osmotic pressure
3. Lymphatic obstruction
4. Sodium retention
5. Inflammation with increased vascular permeability.

---

[26] *Nàn Jīng* 難經 27 translation/interpretation S. Cowan.

[27] See MindNode in *Appendix II: Blueprints and Charts from Z'ev's Notebook* pg. 290.

[28] *Nàn Jīng* 難經 27 translation/interpretation S. Cowan.

[29] Bert, & Pearce, *"The Interstitium and Microvascular Exchange. In: Renkin EM, Michel CC (eds) Handbook of physiology, section 2: cardiovascular, vol IV: microcirculation,"* pg. 52-547.

All of these conditions are potentially life-threatening signs. "The interstitium" was only recently identified in western medicine as a true organ network with its own circulation running through the fascia. This bears a striking resemblance to descriptions of the *sānjiāo* 三焦, governor of the waterways.[30] In extraordinary circumstances, when the *sānjiāo*/interstitium (and the *luò* 絡 networks) can no longer contain the excess fluids, it overflows into the potential spaces throughout the body that act as ditches and reservoirs collectively called the *qí jīng bā mài*.

In *Nàn Jīng* 28 it's further stated that when this overflow occurs, these vessel-spaces hold the fluid there and it's no longer part of the general circulation. Whenever this extra-vascular fluid is stagnant (not part of the circulation) it is at risk of invasion by pathogens that will result in swelling and heat that require drainage. This radical observation occurred centuries before Western physicians recognized the pathological risks of edema and third spacing ascites.

Nàn Jīng 29 then goes on to describe the pathological manifestations of this circulatory fluid overflow in each of the eight reservoirs:

- When *yīn wéi* 陰維 and *yáng wéi* 陽維 cannot maintain their ties: there is discomfort, weakness, inability to stand and madness (*diān kuáng* 癲狂) (possibly correlated with brain swelling or perhaps meningitis.)
- When *yáng wéi* is diseased there are fits of cold and heat (possibly *shàoyáng* 少陽, syndromes), (perhaps correlated with sepsis)
- When *yīn wéi* is diseased there is heart pain (perhaps correlated with angina, pericarditis, pleural effusion or heart failure with secondary pulmonary edema),
- When *yīn qiāo* 陰蹻 is diseased there is weakness in the *yīn qiāo* and tightness in the *yáng qiāo* 陽蹻 and vice versa
- When *yáng qiāo* is diseased there is weakness in the *yáng* and tightness in the *yīn qiāo* resulting in difficulty ambulating (one possible correlation might be postural pitting edema related to end stage kidney or heart failure, deep vein thrombosis or extravasation following trauma).
- When there is disease in the *chōng* 衝 vessel there is abdominal distention and bloating (corresponding to ascites)
- When there is disease in the *dū* 督 vessel, there is back rigidity, and "internal knots." (possibly corresponding to meningitis, or stroke)
- When there is disease in the *rèn* 任 vessel, one suffers from "internal knots" (possible correspondence with hernias, torsions, or tumors).

All of these presentations are considered medical emergencies e.g. extraordinary conditions. Furthermore *Nàn Jīng* 29 states that from a gender

---

[30] See *"The Secret Circulation,"* pg. 249-256.

perspective in males, disease in *rèn* causes the "seven elevation-illnesses" and in females "conglomeration-illness-collections." Unschuld makes a note of describing *"seven elevation illness"* (*qī shàn* 七疝)[31] as swelling in various parts of the body though it's not totally clear. In terms of swelling in the genitals I wonder if this might possibly relate to specific conditions such as testicular torsion, a true medical emergency, or perhaps varicocele, orchitis, and epididymitis, all of which would have been extraordinary conditions of concern to Han physicians.

Unschuld then states that female conglomeration-illness-collections refers to various swellings in the female reproductive tract. We may speculate that this genital swelling might refer to uterine fibromas, Gartners duct cysts, Bartholin cysts, cellulitis, or even possibly yeast infections, sexually transmitted disease and sexual assault, all conditions that would have been extraordinary conditions observed by doctors during the Han Dynasty.

All of these extreme pathological conditions occur when fluid accumulates outside the normal circulatory system and becomes inflamed and/or secondarily infected.

當此之時，霧霈妄行，聖人不能復圖也。

"In times like that when flooding rushed wildly even the sages could not manage them without being prepared"
- Nàn Jīng 27[32]

In ancient China, the engineering geniuses of the time devised manmade versions of these natural ditches to prepare for and manage the extraordinary floods that occurred from time to time.

Again we can see how carefully the *Nàn Jīng* writers are using their understanding of fluid dynamics to map out the metaphoric-anatomical locations of these potential extravascular drainage areas in the body, tracking their individual paths and noting the specific acupuncture holes through which we have access to influencing them when extraordinary conditions of fluid accumulation occur. Thus, we see how important an understanding of a complete circulatory system was to the *Nàn Jīng* authors, that anything which disrupts the circulatory system *the "ring without end"* will lead to potential life-threatening pathologies. This once again drives home the point that the Chinese systemic metaphoric maps have profound scientific value, that led to conceptualizing physiologic fluid mechanics and a deep understanding and

---

[31] Unschuld (2016), *"Nan Jing: The Classic of Difficult Issues,"* pg. 281

[32] *Nàn Jīng* 難經 27 translation/interpretation S. Cowan.

treatment of pathological conditions long before the West conceived of a complete circulatory system. As we will discuss throughout this book, this ecological perspective has practical applications for today's extraordinary conditions of chronic inflammation.

Mapping the Flow: *Channel Dynamics*

Stephen Cowan & Z'ev Rosenberg

Stephen: In *Língshū* 靈樞 2, Huáng Dì 黃帝 asks Qíbó 歧伯 about the beginnings and endings of the vessels, where the five transport openings are, where the connections between the five *zàng* 臟 organs (*wǔ zàng* 五臟) with the six *fǔ*/bowels (*liù fǔ* 六腑) take place and where the five *zàng*/viscera, have their flow *liū* 溜. This concern for "where" and "how" in Chinese medical classics is all about mapping the flow. I find it interesting that this character *liū* 溜 which appears in the *Nèijīng* 內經 doesn't exactly mean "flow" and ends up being replaced by *liú* 流 by the *Nàn Jīng* 難經 authors.

Figure 1.6 - Liū 溜

Liū 溜 (*fig. 1.6*) means to stay, slide, glide, slip away, escape. The character shows the water radical on the left, which give the sense of water nature to the meaning, and on the right is a kind of large container or vase. In *Língshū* 2, Huáng Dì asks where/how are things *Liū* 溜, are contained, connected, where do they stay, slip away. For me, this "staying and slipping away" has a tactile quality of feeling akin to feeling a pulse in the *mài* 脈.

Z'ev: Shigehisa Kuriyama, like Paul Unschuld, looks at *mài* 脈 in terms of flows rather than fixed nouns/positions/structures. Whether used in terms of specific channel flows, or reading the *cùn kǒu* 吋口 position on the vessels, the emphasis is much less on fixing a marker in space than tracking a flow in time.

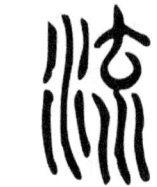

Figure 1.7 - Liú 流

Stephen: *Liú* 流 (*fig 1.7*) is the character used more frequently in the *Nàn Jīng*, on the other hand, has a broader meaning: to flow, circulate, spread, disseminate. The ideogram implies the capacity to change. In the ideogram, once again on the left is the water radical and on the right *liú* 㐬 is the image said to be a baby being born head first with the amniotic fluid pouring out before it. If you've ever been present at a birth, typically once the water's broken, everything begins to flow, labor takes on a much greater dynamic force of transformation, until the head and shoulders of the baby comes "flowing" out.

Z'ev: This image of a "breaking through" speaks a lot to the force of channel flow. This is perfectly depicted in the *Língshū* and *Nàn Jīng* in terms of the *wǔ shū xué* 五输穴 / five transporting holes, which are designated as progressively increasing flows of water / fluid from wells to springs to streams to rivers to seas. As the channel fluids travel from its origins at the extremities, it "picks up" speed, depth and flow widens, and this is mapped and reflected in the specific indications for each position and its associated phase. This is explained by Dīng Déyòng 丁德用's commentary on *Nàn Jīng 65*:

> *"Man's yang qi appear and disappear in accordance with the four seasons. Hence, in spring the qi are in the wells, in summer they are in the creeks, in autumn they are in the streams, and in winter they are in the confluences."* [33]

Stephen: For me, this distinction between *liū* 溜 location and *liú* 流 circulation captures the revolutionary ideas described in the *Nàn Jīng* about a unified flowing circulatory system that grew out of the earlier *Nèijīng* 內經 classic where the movement contained in the *mài* 脈 pulses (*liū* 溜) reflected separate independent channels. One of the unique qualities of Chinese thought is that we can hold *both* contrasting ideas at once: container AND flow. This quality of simultaneously being noun and verb (as in particle / wave concepts in quantum mechanics) is likewise a way to conceive all couples as a single dynamic entity: *yīn* 陰 / *yáng* 陽, *yíng* 營 / *wèi* 衛, *xuè* 血 / *qì* 氣 or *jīng* 精 / *shén* 神 for that matter. The *Nàn Jīng* authors hold this idea of a unified system of

---

[33] Unschuld (2016), *"Nan Jing: The Classic of Difficult Issues,"* pg. 471

flowing circulation to be the key to health. Thus like a stream, what is contained *must* flow and what flows must be contained.

Z'ev: This revolutionary conception of channels as container/flow simultaneously should come as no surprise to those who investigate the Uncertainty Principle and quantum physics. These modern scientific theories that continue to confound human beings almost one hundred years after their conception by Niels Bohr, Einstein, and Godel are directly related to the mode of thought and philosophy covered in detail in such texts as the *Yìjīng* 易 經, *Lǎozǐ* 老子 and *Zhuāngzǐ* 莊子. The ability to see location in space and movement in time simultaneously is the key to understanding how the channels were "mapped." They were experienced as flows in specific directions based on heaven and earth resonance, and as locations where *qì* could be influenced, directed dynamic equilibrium to the human being by bringing the body/mind in tune with the universal flow.

Stephen: *Nàn Jīng 37* goes on to ask *"where do the five zàng originate (fāqǐ 發起) and where do they pass through (tōng 通)?"* This concern for beginnings and passages, *fāqǐ* 發起 and *tōng* 通, expresses a fundamental understanding that any block to circulation will result in dis-ease.

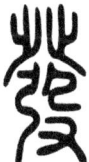

Figure 1.8 - Fā 發

Fā 發 *(fig. 1.8)* means "to send out, emit, dispatch, issue forth." In the ideogram we see two feet, implying a way of moving forward, placed above the image of a bow and arrow being pulled. When combined, we get the spirit of the movement of releasing an arrow.

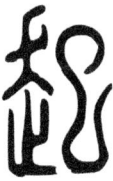

Figure 1.9 - Qǐ 起

Qǐ 起 *(fig. 1.9)* means "to rise up, stand up, to begin." On the left of the ideogram there is a foot below a person, giving the sense of moving upward and out. On the right is the image of a newborn baby. For me, as a pediatrician, the *xiàng* 象 / visual impression, of this character has that sense of a baby getting up and taking first steps to walk!

Translating *fāqǐ* 發起 as "originate" does not quite give enough of the developmental spirit of rising up and getting going (as in circulation through the *wǔ shū xué* 五输穴 / five transporting holes).

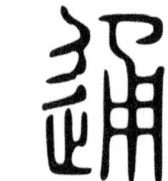

Figure 1.10 - Tōng 通

Tōng 通 *(fig. 1.10)* carries several meanings depending on its context: to communicate, to connect, to know well, to flow, (see discussion of *biàntōng* 變通 – flux and flow, change and continuity in later chapter.) *Tōng* 通 is a central concept in Chinese medicine. To treat the aches and sorrows of suffering (*tòng* 痛 – the related character now with the sick bed radical next to it, which implies a blockage to flow) is exactly what practitioners using moxa-acupuncture and herbs are trying to promote to enable free-flowing circulation between the organ-networks, and healthy communication with the flowing world around us.

Z'ev: As it states in *Nàn Jīng* 37, "*Nobody knows its break; it ends and begins anew.*"[34] There is no place where the flow is interrupted. Acupuncture students are often misled (and anatomists who attempt to dissect acupuncture channels as if they were fixed nerves or blood vessels) to think that acupuncture channels are straight lines drawn on a map in two dimensions; therefore the early translation of *jīng* 經 as "meridians," like lines drawn on a map. The channel system is actually multi-dimensional with variations of width, depth, flow, circumference, and quality much more ecologically akin to streams / streaming than artificially constructed roads.

Stephen: *Nàn Jīng* 難經 37 asks "*where do the five zang originate (fā qǐ 發起) and where do they pass through (tōng 通)?*" It is in this chapter that we're told that our connection to the circulation of the cosmos is literally where / how we (and our channels) originate. The so-called "nine orifices" are the "upper gates" later explained by Zhāng Yuánsù 张元素 (1151–1234) and beautifully illustrated by Zhāng Shìxián 張世賢 *(fig. 1.11)* as two eyes, two ears, two nostrils, one mouth,

---

[34] Unschuld (2016), "*Nan Jing: The Classic of Difficult Issues,*" pg. 325.

one tongue and one throat. I get the sense that the *Nàn Jīng* authors are answering this difficult question of where the channels begin by implying that the circulation in our organs have their origins within the environment that we have direct access to through our orifices and senses.

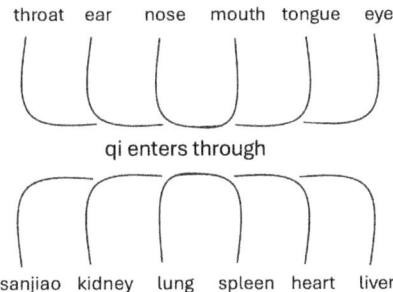

Figure 1.11 - Nàn Jīng 37 Map

Stephen: Even though European Medicine did not conceptualize a unified circulatory system for another 1000 years, when they did, they still conceived it as a *closed system* within the body in contrast with the *Nàn Jīng*'s radical idea of an open circulation connected with the cosmos. We flow because we are a microcosmic reflection/resonance of the universe. This intimate open-ended connection did not exist in western thought until the early 20th century when Gödel shook up the world of physics by presenting his "theorem of incompleteness."[35] He asked us to look beyond pure conceptual logic and empirical science, to comprehend the universe through open-ended direct experience. This idea of direct experience, for me, is a very Daoist way of understanding our relational existence.

Nàn Jīng 37 goes on to make an even more radical statement about healthy circulation *"When at ease then you will know."*[36] As practitioners of medicine, when we are centered enough to use this direct experience (without judgement, bias or preconceived ideas) we are open to receiving much greater information about what's going on with our patient. This is what advanced Chinese medical practitioners (particularly the *shén* 神 doctors) cultivate in order to

---

[35] See Theise, *"Notes on Complexity: A Scientific Theory of Connection, Consciousness, and Being."*

[36] Unschuld (2016), *"Nan Jing: The Classic of Difficult Issues,"* 和則知 *hézé zhī* " *Hé* 和 – I find it interesting that in his translation of the *Nàn Jīng* 37, Paul Unschuld, translates *hé* 和 as "at ease" when typically it is translated as *"in harmony or harmonized."* e.g. "The qi of the liver passes through the eyes. when the eyes are at ease, (or in harmony with the world) one knows the difference between black and white." "The qi of the spleen passes through the mouth. When the mouth is at ease one knows the difference between grains." And so on.

connect more deeply with their patients. One must be "at ease" and "in harmony" within ourselves and with the person we are treating in order to experience oneself as a microcosm resonating with the whole that is greater than the sum of the parts. *Tàijí* practice teaches us to use "soft focus" to be able to take in greater awareness of our surroundings and that any tension will block the flow, cutting us off from the Whole. And this is exactly what the "dissectors" in the West have missed and why it took hundreds of years for them to see what was right before their eyes.

Z'ev: *Hézé* 和則 "at ease" implies the normal, balanced functioning of *yīnyáng* 陰陽 in each of the five yin viscera covered in *Nàn Jīng* 37, and their connection to the outer world through the nine orifices / sense organs. The text then goes on to map the flow of the six fu / bowels. The *yīn* vessels must flow into the *yáng* vessels, they must be in constant pulsation of potential, pulsing back and forth, like rocking a baby in one's arms back and forth.

Modern illnesses can be reframed as various "degrees of disconnection" through closures and barriers, when substances, blood and *qì* accumulate within the vast flowing system of channels, viscera, bowels, and sense organs, only then can disease take root in a human being. Of course, as Chinese medicine does not distinguish between body and consciousness, being of one entity, a blockage in thought or emotion (so well mapped in the *wǔ zhì* 五志 / five minds associated with the yin viscera) can lead to physical "blocks," and vise-versa.

Stephen: During my days working in the busy pediatric practice I ran for 25 years, I had a powerful experience that illustrates this idea. If I was preoccupied with a previous sick child, or feeling rushed because of the number of patients still waiting during flu season, when I abruptly entered a treatment room where a little sick baby was sitting on her mother's lap, the baby would instantly cry. That was my signal to step back out of the room, do some *qìgōng* 氣功 centered breathing, clear my mind ("mind in the *dāntián* 丹田" as *tàijí* 太極 practice says) and reenter the room. Instantly, the baby though still sick, offers me a broad smile allowing me to gain an accurate take on what was going on. That baby was my teacher in that moment, demonstrating the efficacious nature of resonance, flow and interconnectedness.

The Goodness of Water: *A Developmental Perspective*

Stephen Cowan

The highest goodness[37] is like Water.
It benefits everything
yet goes to the lowly places most people loathe.
It always knows the right place to settle.
Its heart goes so deep,
In sharing, it is so kind,
In communicating, it is so reliable,
In healing, it is so effective,
In serving, it is so capable,
In moving, it is so well-timed.
- Lǎozǐ 老子 8[38]

The idea that we are resonant reflections of the mountains and rivers landscape (*shānshuǐ* 山水) is deeply embedded in Chinese thought and the Han Dynasty medical classics express this in terms of the metaphoric-anatomic maps they made of human physiology. Observing the water cycle that rains down from the skies/heavens (*tiān* 天), filling the streams and rivers and nourishing life on Earth (*dì* 地), then eventually rising up as mist and clouds again, the *Nèijīng* 內經 and *Nàn Jīng* 難經 medical practitioners recognized an ecological image of how human beings exist within the heavens-and-earth cycle. The circulation within these waterways was a core concept in the *Nèi Jīng* that was further elaborated in the *Nàn Jīng*. As stated above, it was this very notion that led to the mapping of a complete circulatory system. Understanding the nature of water, its capacity to flow, to nourish, to go deep, to stagnate, to be blocked, became a guiding principle for promoting human health, growth and development. Water's capacity to circulate between heaven and earth was, as Lǎozǐ says, the highest goodness/skillfulness reflecting the *yīn* and *yáng* flow into each other that generates life.

---

[37] *Shàn* 善 "goodness" in the sense of being "well-disposed, good at, kind, benevolent." The ideogram shows a goat flanked by two mouths speaking. The goat or sheep is a symbol for goodness or benevolence in Chinese culture.

[38] *Lǎozǐ* 老子 8 translation/interpretation S. Cowan.

Língshū 靈樞 2 and 10 offer a detailed map of the *shū* 輸-transport system that give doctors access to ways of influencing the flow of this circulation. *Nàn Jīng* 68 furthers the discussion of how to use this five *shū*-point system (*wǔ shū xué* 五輸穴) in treating pathological conditions.[39] Throughout the *Nèijīng*, there is a common concern for how / where the channels begin and end. As we stated in the previous chapter, the *Nàn Jīng* resolves this question by recognizing a unified circulatory system as a ring having no beginning or end that is integrated with the space-time integrity of the cosmos.

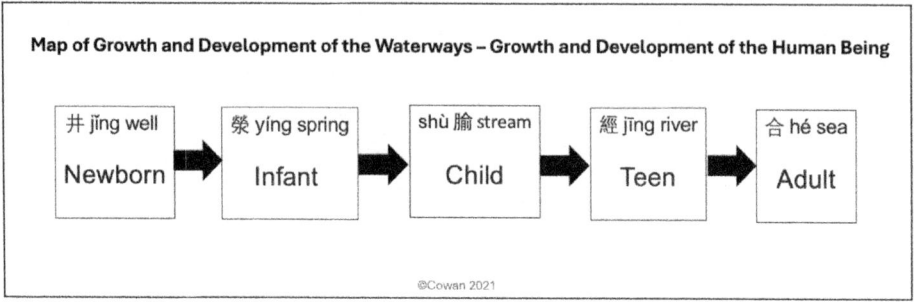

Figure 1.12 - Growth and Development Map

I have spent the last 35 years as a developmental pediatrician observing the growth and development of children through the lens of Chinese medicine. The *shū*-transport system maps out the growth and development of the *xuèqì* 血氣 flow in the channels and I find that this map serves as a space-time model for understanding the path of human growth and development (*fig. 1.12*).

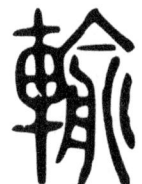

Figure 1.13 - Shū 輸[40]

Shū 輸 (*fig. 1.13*) is the image of a boat transporting "stuff" on the waterways. This "stuff" is the information that a child needs to grow and develop into an adult. Just as a stream "begins" as the condensation of moisture high in the mountains where heaven and earth converge, so too is a child born from the spark of *yīn*-mother and *yáng*-father meeting. The *shū*-transport system tells us

---

[39] See MindNode in *Appendix II: Blueprints and Charts from Z'ev's Notebook* pg. 294.

[40] *Shū* 輸 to transport, carry, the ideogram shows a wheel indicating movement, on the right is a boat traveling on water.

that the fingertips and toes are this very place where *yīn* and *yáng* channels meet at the *jǐng*-well (井) points, ensuring the *"ring without end."*

At the tips of the fingers and toes, where capillaries are quite small, blood *qì* (*xuèqì*) circulation moves very slowly and is prone to stasis. Just so, *jǐng*-well points are often indicated in acute painful situations, to ensure that circulation is unbroken in its flow, that *yīn* and *yáng* remain connected. Likewise, the first few minutes in a newborn's life depend on this spark to get things going. I have often been called to delivery rooms for emergencies where a baby fails to take that first breath or the heartbeat is too slow and these *jǐng*-well points (along with *yǒng quán* 湧 泉/bubbling well (KI 1) work like magic to bring the baby to life.[41] The first three months of life are commonly referred to as the "fourth trimester," a transition period when the infant's physiology is still tenuous, and the so-called neuro-gastro-immune complex (*sānjiāo* 三膲/triple burner responsible for *yuán qì* 原氣) is not yet fully coordinated. Common challenges such as newborn feeding problems, weight gain, colic, sleep/wake dysregulation and risk of infection often require close attention and support. I have found that teaching parents gentle *tuīná* 推拿 massage techniques using these *jǐng*-well and *yuán*-source points to wake up the flow and integrate their channels often works quite effectively. It is no accident that the *yīn jǐng*-well points are associated with the wood phase and the *yáng jǐng*-well points are associated with the metal phase. Coordinating blood/*qì* reflects this wood-metal relationship, critical for healthy circulation of nutritive/defensive (*yíng* 營/*wèi* 衛) through the infant's body. The water phase serves as a critical bridge between metal and wood phases, highlighting the transition from prenatal to postnatal life. Is this not the highest goodness of water? I have often conceptualized the *sānjiāo* 三膲/triple burner, the official in charge of the waterways, as having a key developmental function in the transition from prenatal to postnatal life by way of its capacity to integrate communication between all the channels.

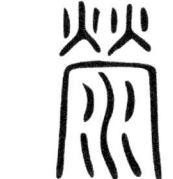

Figure 1.14 - Yíng 滎

Just as the channels begin to take on more volume and movement at the *yíng*-spring (滎) point, so too the infant beyond the fourth trimester begins to reach,

---

[41] Indeed pressing sharply on the *jǐng*-well points in a newborn can dramatically shift a newborn's APGAR scores from low to high.

grasp, roll, sit, etc. as it moves out into the world. The ideogram *yíng* 滎 (*fig. 1.14*) shows the image of water within a shelter on top of which are two flames. This ideogram has a relationship to its homophone *yíng* 營/nutrient *qì*, part of the couple with *wèi*/defensive *qì*, that is the key to healthy growth and immunity. Both *yíng* 滎 and *yíng* 營 have the two fires on the rooftop indicating warmth. In the pediatric chapter of the *Bèi Jí Qiānjīn Yào Fāng* 備急千金要方/ *Prescriptions Worth a Thousand Gold Coins for Emergency Use*, Sūn Sīmiǎo 孫思邈 (581-682) describes the physiologic heat generated in the young child as "steaming and transforming" (*biàn zhēng* 變蒸) necessary for growth and development.[42] It is no accident then that the *yíng* 滎-spring points are "fire phase" points on the yin channels and are often used to clear heat. The combined water radical coupled with the two fires above can create the steam needed to fuel growth. However, Sūn Sīmiǎo cautions us, that unless this heat goes on too long, we should *not* view this as pathological and suppress it in the growing child but rather understand it as a necessary warmth that generates growth. *Tuīná* at these *yíng*-spring points is a gentle way to support a child during these steamings. Sūn Sīmiǎo did not have to manage the artificial inflammation stemming from hyper-stimulation we deal with in the modern world. For example, rather than using anti-fever pharmaceuticals, I will frequently suggest to parents that they massage these *yíng*-spring points before and after vaccination to help clear heat generated by the inflammatory response caused by artificial stimulation of the immune system.

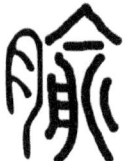

Figure 1.15 - Shù 腧

As the flow in the channels gathers more speed, volume and depth, likewise the developing child grows bigger, from toddler to child, picking up more information about the world, learning to talk, play, share. This development is reflected in the nature of the *shù*-stream 腧. Like *shū*-transport 輸 this ideogram *shù* 腧 (*fig. 1.15*) has the same image of a boat traveling on water but now instead of a wheel axle, it has the flesh radical giving both the more literal reference to a physical part of the body and the metaphoric idea of a boat carrying cargo. It is said that at this point in the channels, the streams are wide enough to be navigable. Developmentally, a child is now able to carry themselves forward, having more physical strength, entering school, putting

---

[42] Wilms, "*Venerating the Root: Sūn Sīmiǎo's Bèi Jí Qiān Jīn Yào Fāng Volume 5: Pediatrics: Part 1*," pg. 15.

more effort into learning without the constant help of parents, sharing their ideas with others and their own constitutional style becomes more pronounced in the world. It is no accident then that these *shù*-stream points are also the *yuán* 原-original source *qì* points on the yin channels, just as the child's primary nature makes itself known in the world. *Nàn Jīng* 68 describes the flow of *xuèqì* 血氣 at these stream locations as *zhù* 注/pouring through. *Zhù* 注 is a term also used for describing focused attention. I use *shù*-stream/*yuán*-source points as key components in my treatment of children with attention deficit hyperactivity disorder (ADHD) which typically manifests once they enter institutionalized education system.

As the child continues on their journey of maturation past their 10th birthday, their lives take on greater momentum. They gain deeper knowledge of the world. The waterway nature of the channels now widens into a river, behaving more like a true channel *jīng* 經 for which the *jīng*-river 經 points carry the same name. These *jīng*-river points are typically located in areas of deeper flesh than previous points. *Nàn Jīng* 68 recommends using these points to release exterior pathogens. The ideogram *jīng* 經 carried the image of an underground aquifer, but there is an additional meaning of *jīng* 經, that of the sacred book, (or "classic" as in *Nèijīng* 內經, or *Dàodé Jīng* 道德經 (*Lǎozǐ* 老子) reflecting the deeper enduring wisdom that the maturing child gains. The "classic" represents sacred information passed down through the ages. Likewise, as a child enters puberty, the body begin to dramatically transform, with all the metabolic changes this entails, readying to be able to create the next generation. It is no coincidence that *jīng* 經 is also one of the medical terms used for menstruation! I find these points extremely useful for teens experiencing physical and emotional problems, from acne to anxiety as they contend with the host of stressors our modern world bombards them with, in particular the pressure to grow up fast.

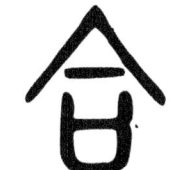

Figure 1.16 - Hé 合

All rivers and streams will eventually empty into the sea. Just so, as the child enters adulthood, they are ready to be a part of the wide world. The *hé*-sea points characterize this confluence. The ideogram *hé* 合 (*fig 1.16*) shows a triangle above a mouth. The triangle represents unity in all cultures around the world. *Hé* 合 has many meanings: to join, to fit in, to be equal to, to be whole. *Nàn Jīng* 68 advises the use of *hé*-sea points to regulate organ *qì* transformation and treat counter-flow (*zhì nì qì* 治逆氣). This greater depth reflects the level of a grown child's maturity. They are ready to deepen their relationships in the world, to be an active member of the wider community, to play a role in the procreation of the next generation, thus fulfilling their destiny and taking part in the *"ring without end."*

Thus our own human development is like a journey down a river. Before the modern era began numbering acupuncture points (making them thus devoid of their original metaphoric meanings), the ancient names given to the five *shū*-points (*wǔ shū xué* 五輸穴) are akin to the way indigenous peoples name the qualities of landscape. To give but one of many examples of this eco-logical flavor embedded in our medicine, we can look at the names along the Kidney channel:

- *Jǐng*-well - Wood - *Yǒng Quán* 涌泉 /Bubbling Spring (Ki 1)
- *Yíng*-spring - Fire - *Rán Gǔ* 然谷 / Blazing Valley (Ki 2)
- *Shù*-stream - Earth - *Tài Xī* 太溪 /Supreme Stream (Ki 3)
- *Jīng*-river - Metal - *Fù Liū* 復溜 /Returning Current (Ki 7)
- *Hé*-sea - Water - *Yīn Gǔ* 阴谷 / Yin Valley (Ki 10)

Starting from a tiny Bubbling Spring, through the Blazing Valley into the Blazing Valley, then the Returning Current, we eventually join the Yin Valley. This watery adventure might as well be describing a trip down the Colorado River, though these days, with climate change, diversions of rivers to irrigation troughs and dams, we can readily see how deficient the "kidneys of the planet" are.

The *shū* 輸-transport system is one way of mapping the resonance between the way channel *qì* develops and the way we develop as human beings. As Roger Ames says:

"In the human experience we are radically contextualized, constituted by the roles and relationships that locate us within our social, natural, and cultural environments. Proper Way-making is getting the most out of these relationships as we make our way in the world: it is making this life significant."[43]

Like our mother Earth, we are made up of roughly the same 70-80 percent water. From a Daoist perspective, *what* water knows is not the question but *how* water knows. The way water knows how to travel down a mountainside without fighting the mountain or take on the shape of any container it happens to find itself in will teach you how to live your life well. This is truly the goodness of water.

---

[43] Ames and Hall, *"Dao De Jing: Making This Life Significant: A Philosophical Translation,"* pg. 87.

Stream Waters (*Jīng Shuǐ* 經水)

Stephen Cowan & Z'ev Rosenberg

"Walking by the banks of Yellow Flower Brook
I chase a blue stream
Turning, twisting down the mountain
The path is not long
Water splashes from one stone to another
Coursing through the still green
Deep inside a pine forest
Ripples radiate from water-chestnut weeds
Reeds reflect in clear water
My heart is quiet like a still pond
I want to stay on this flat stone
And cast my fishing line forever"
- Wángwéi 王維 (699-761)[44]

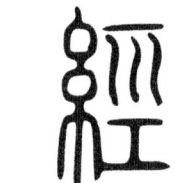
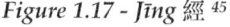

Figure 1.17 - Jīng 經 [45]

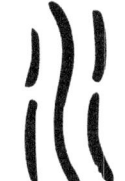

Figure 1.18 - Shuǐ 水

Stephen: When we enter a particular place in nature, say an old growth forest, looking, listening, sensing its relative health or risk of disease, fire, flood, we join in a conversation with Nature. And doing so it speaks volumes. How rich is the soil? How well does it support plant and animal-life? Are the stream beds full or empty? Is the water stagnant or moving? What is the relative moisture and air exchange?

---

[44] Wang, Graham-Storer, White, & Wang, *"Walking to Where the River Ends,"* pg. 24
Wángwéi 王維 was a Chinese musician, painter, poet, & politician of the Tang dynasty.

[45] *Jīng* 經 ideogram of silk thread next to image of an underground stream: meaning a conduit, aquifer or channel, also used for a book or classic as in information bound by thread & passed down through the ages as in *Dàodé Jīng* 道德經 (*Lǎozǐ* 老子) or *Nàn Jīng*.

經脈十二者，外合於十二經水，而內屬於五藏六府。

"The twelve conduit/stream vessels (jīngmài) link up with the twelve stream waters outside, and they are connected with the five long term depots (zàng) and six short term repositories (fǔ) inside"
- *Língshū* 靈樞 12[46]

For Han dynasty doctors, Chinese medicine is akin to observing a landscape. Everything resonates with a larger meaning found in the relationships in Nature. These ideas discussed in *Língshū* 12 are the primary elements that make up the maps for the channel system.

- **Coloring:** red-fire yellow-soil etc.
- **Shapes:** big-small, round, branching, paired
- **Position:** above or below
- **Quality:** clarity or turbidity
- **Texture:** firm or brittle
- **Volume:** solid or hollow

"The [vessel on the] earth[-side] of the great thoroughfare is called minor yin [vessel]. [The vessel] above the minor yin [vessel] is called major yang [vessel]. {The major yang [vessel] originates from the extreme yin [hole], and ends in the gate of life. It is called yang in the yin.}

The [region from the] center of the body upwards is called broad brilliance. [The vessel] below the broad brilliance is called major yin [vessel]. The [vessel in] front of the major yin [vessel] is called yang brilliance [vessel]."
-*Sùwèn* 素問 6[47]

Just as in every landscape, it is the relationships between various components that allow one to understand the feel and function of the whole. The clinician's purpose is to understand the deeper meanings that reveal themselves through their relative patterns and resonances.

經水者，受水而行之；五藏者，合神氣魂魄而藏之；六府者，受穀而行之，受氣而揚之；經脈者，受血而管之。

"Now, the stream waters receive water and transmit it.
The five long-term depots unite the spirit qi with the hun and po souls and store them.

---

[46]Unschuld, "*Huang Di Nei Jing Ling Shu: The Ancient Classic on Needle Therapy,*" pg. 215.

[47] Unschuld, Tessenow, and Zheng, "*Huang Di Nei Jing Su Wen: An Annotated Translation of Huang Di's Inner Classic - Basic Questions, 2 Volumes,*" pg. 130.

The six short-term repositories receive grain and transmit it; they receive the qi and
disperse them.
The conduit/stream vessels receive the blood and circulated it."
- *Língshū* 12[48]

As a young medical student at the University of Padua, the very place where Andreas Vesalius (1514-1564) the great anatomist, once taught, we were required to attend fifty autopsies held in one of the amphitheaters designed after the same one he attended. There, in hushed silence, we saw a corpse laid out before us, heard its medical history, and were asked to observe first its outer form: pale, cold, still, looking for telltale evidence of abnormalities. Then, with typical Italian dramatics, the professor and his assistant would take their sharpened blades and carefully peal back the layers of flesh and fascia, muscle and bone, to open the inner cavities that held the secrets that once belonged to a human life. Each organ was removed and weighed, each tendon carefully dissected and measured, noting any irregularities. A history, pieced together from the parts (*fig. 1.19*).

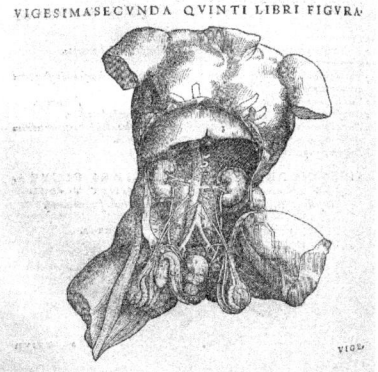

VIGESIMASECVNDA QVINTI LIBRI FIGVRA·

Figure 1.19 - De Humani Corporis Fabrica - Human Torso[49]

Now imagine, instead, opening up a corpse and examining it with the eyes of a poet-painter gazing at a landscape *shānshuǐ* 山水 (*fig. 1.20*). Carefully measuring and mapping the terrain, naming the qualities and character of the place, looking for meanings hidden in the metaphors that all landscapes offer if

---

[48] Unschuld, *"Huang Di Nei Jing Ling Shu: The Ancient Classic on Needle Therapy"* pg. 216.

A literal translation says *"the shén 神/spirit of each zàng-organ receives the hún 魂 and pò 魄"* which is an interesting statement - *hún* 魂 associated with liver/blood flow that follows the *shén* 神 and *pò* 魄 associated with lung - air/breathing that enters and exits (see also *Língshū* 8)

[49] Vesalius, *"De Humani Corporis Fabrica,"* pg. 372 - Wellcome Collection. Source: Wellcome Collection.

one knows how to look, remaining ever-mindful that the whole is always greater than the sum of the parts.

What would you see with eyes like these?

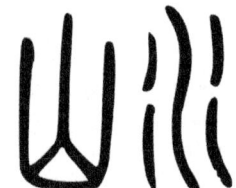

Figure 1.20 - Shānshuǐ 山水 [50]

In *Língshū* 12 we see clear evidence that the Han Dynasty physicians practiced dissection:

若夫 八尺之士，皮肉在此，外可度量切循而得之，其死可解剖而視之。其藏之堅脆，府之 大小，穀之多少，脈之長短，血之清濁，氣之多少，十二經之多血少氣，與其少血多 氣，與其皆多血氣，與其皆少血氣，皆有大數。其治以鍼艾，各調其經氣，固其常有 合乎。

"Now, [let us take] a male person of eight feet height [as an example]. He has skin and he has flesh. His outer [appearance] can be measured. [His structures] can be followed and pressed [with the fingers] so as to locate them. Once he has died, he may be dissected to observe his [interior appearance]. Whether the long-term depots are firm or brittle, and whether the short term repositories are large or small, how much grain [they have in them] and what length the vessels are, whether the blood is clear or turbid, and whether the qi is many or few, whether the twelve conduits transmit much blood and a little qi or little blood and much qi and whether overall they contain much blood and much qi or little blood and little qi , all this can be quantified."[51]

The *Nàn Jīng* 難經 also contains examples of these careful anatomic observations and measurements, for example 41 and 42.

Z'ev: Here's where we get into a conundrum. Shigehisa Kuriyama in *The Expressiveness of the Body and the Divergence of Greek and Chinese Medicine* and his articles, claims that there is only a historical record of one official dissection of a criminal by Wáng Chōng 王充 (27-100) a critical thinker of the Later Han dynasty, best known for his book *Lùnhéng* 論衡. Since clearly there is a

---

[50] *Shānshuǐ* 山水 literally mountain-waters or "mountains-and-rivers" the term used for "landscape," often applied to landscape painting and poetry.

[51] Unschuld, *"Huang Di Nei Jing Ling Shu: The Ancient Classic on Needle Therapy,"* pg. 217.

description in both *Língshū*, and *Nàn Jīng* of dissection and measurement of organs, what historical evidence do we draw on?

Stephen: There is no doubt in reading *Língshū* and *Nàn Jīng* that the authors were grappling with how to correlate what they were seeing anatomically with the *Huáng-Lǎo* 黃老 nature-based philosophy of *yīnyáng wǔxíng* 陰陽五行 (fig. 1.21) as an example from Zhāng Shìxián.

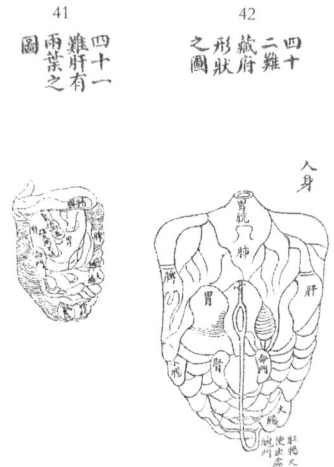

Figure 1.21 - Nàn Jīng 41/42 Map [52]

However, the medical mapmakers of the Han dynasty did not just stop at the calculation of size and form as the Italian renaissance anatomists did. Numbers, like colors, shapes, textures and volumes have correlated meanings. They recognized that the flow of blood resonated with the flow of streams and aquifers, and it was this flowing irrigation that determined the health of the human landscape.

氣主呴之, 血主濡之

The qi are responsible for providing the [body] with a warm flow; the blood is responsible for providing the [body] with moisture.
- *Nàn Jīng* 22 [53]

Mapping the dynamic body-landscape, these two qualities, the warming breath and the moistening irrigation, were understood to provide the basis of vitality. But what exactly did the *Nàn Jīng* anatomists see when they looked with the poet-artist eyes? Stream-like forms enwrapped in sheaths like silk that

---

[52] Unschuld (1986), "*Nan-ching: The Classic of Difficult Issues,*" pg. 703.

[53] Unschuld (2016), "*Nan Jing: The Classic of Difficult Issues,*" pg. 235.

connected to each other creating a vast communication network just as the life-giving stream waters do in a landscape.

Z'ev: It is important as well to address the "physics," alongside the biology of the channel system. My understanding has been that the neurological/vascular/lymphatic pathways followed the "invisible blueprint" of the body/mind imprinted by the relationship of heaven and earth. Pattern first, visual manifestations second.

Neil Shubin in *The Universe Within*[54], discusses the effects of Jupiter's gravitational pull on the form of human beings. If Jupiter's orbit was farther away from the Sun (and, as a result, the earth) it would have a less powerful gravitational pull on the earth. As a result, human beings would be much shorter than the present average of five foot. If Jupiter orbited closer to the sun, it's stronger gravitational pull would increase the average height of a human being to seven feet tall. While these "difficult issues" are discussed and delineated in modern science, they are not often paid attention to in medicine. There are numerous gravitational, celestial/planetary forces at work that in a seemingly miraculous manner maintain equilibrium in the dynamic systems of the body. The *Sùwèn* 素問 and *Nàn Jīng* 難經 provide an extrapolation on dynamic cosmology that informs the structure and function of the human organism. As the *Nèijīng* 內經 points out, *shùn* 順 and *nì* 逆, going with and against the flow is one of the foundations of channel theory and its expression in the human organism. However, there are also "chaotic forces" that can intercede, that Chinese medicine defines as *xié qì* 邪氣 or chaotic/evil *qì*.

脈為營

"The vessels enable circulation"
- *Língshū* 10 [55]

Stephen: From the very first difficulty in the *Nàn Jīng*, the authors seem to be obsessed with the movement within these conduit-vessels. They called it *dòngmài* 動脈, the pulsing aspect of arteries, and the quieter aspect of veins. On dissection, however, there were also silk-like threads (nerves, lymphatics, fascia) that follow these streams (*fig. 1.22*).

Z'ev: Do you feel that the Han dynasty Chinese scientist/physician/poets perceived the nerves? There are some modern scholars who claimed that Chinese medicine classically does not recognize a nervous system. I don't think that is true, but how was it addressed? How do we address it today? I never got

---

[54] Shubin, "*The Universe Within: Discovering the Common History of Rocks, Planets, and People,*" pgs.51-53.

[55] Unschuld, "*Huang Di Nei Jing Ling Shu: The Ancient Classic on Needle Therapy,*" pg. 176.

to dissect corpses in acupuncture school, your experience is very valuable, especially in such an "old school" as the University of Padua.

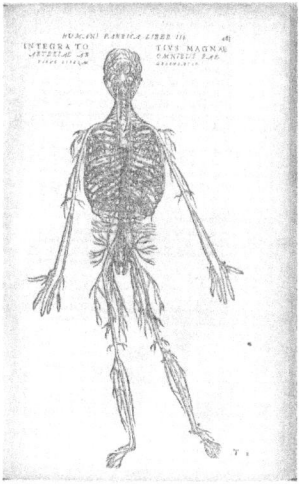

Figure 1.22 - De Humani Corporis Fabrica - The Array of Nerves[56]

Stephen: It seems to me that what the Han Dynasty physicians were concerned with was flow/communication (*tōng* 通). Any silk-like threads, whether arteries, veins, nerve bundles , lymphatics or fascia and tendons for that matter, all represent communication pathways. So, whether Chinese medicine recognized nerves is not the question. It is how does the dynamic flow within the body terrain communicate vital information.

The difficulty the *Nàn Jīng* 難經 authors seem to be grappling with is how one can assess the nature of a human living landscape from a dead person? There are certainly traces left from life, in the same way perhaps that archeologists search for traces of human life buried in shards of pottery. Perhaps it's more akin to the way astrophysicists search for traces of water (life) in the canals of Mars. Unlike the western anatomists, the *Nàn Jīng* authors recognized that to truly understand a living breathing life, one must naturally look for evidence of "the warm flow of air and moisture" in a living being. A corpse can only tell you so much.

Z'ev: I appreciate your point here and this gets to the heart of the issue. How do dead bodies illuminate living qi? We see how Wáng Qīngrèn 王清任 (1768-1831) completely erred in his attempts to "reform" Chinese medicine during the Qing dynasty *Yī Lín Gǎi Cuò* 醫林改錯/*Correcting the Errors in the*

---

[56] Vesalius, "*De Humani Corporis Fabrica,*"pg. 483 - Metropolitan Museum of Art OA - Object Number: 53.682.

Medical Forest.[57] He concluded that *qì* flowed through "*qì* pipes," solid structures! By examining with the eyes of an artist, one sees two sets of underground thread-like conduits (*jīng mài* 經脈) connecting and nourishing the organs: one hollow, carrying blood and the other (nerves) carrying "the *shén* 神/ spirit."

I'm trying to stand in the shoes of a Han Doctor viewing all these channel like structures in the body (blood vessels, capillaries, nerves,) that clearly function as some kind of channels of "something" I think you're right, this paragraph goes too far in suggesting one carries blood the other *qì* - that's exactly the trap I myself am trying to avoid here....we must be careful NOT to dissect *qì* from blood! So, to see *jīng* 經 as responsible for *tōng*/ flowing communication between organ networks...lets' just keep it at that!

To infer the health of a landscape from traces is perhaps why after dissection revealed the structure, pulses and tongues became a more important method of inferring the state of movement circulating in a living person. As we see in *Nàn Jīng* 23, it was this examination of the movement of these streams that enabled them to infer a complete circulatory system, a *"ring without end."*[58]

皆因其原, 如環無端, 轉相灌溉

"Returning to its origin (yuán) like a ring without end, circulating in order to irrigate the body."
-*Nàn Jīng* 23[59]

Stephen: It is a different kind of science, a science of geomancy rather than geometry, that sees with the metaphoric eyes of a poet-artist, who does not separate the substance from the function, the inside from the outside, the human form from the patterns in Nature and thus is able to map the mysteries of a whole living landscape in order to predict health and treat disease.

---

[57] See Shoja, et.al. *"Wang Qingren and the 19th Century Chinese Doctrine of the Bloodless Heart."* International Journal of Cardiology 145, no. 2 (November 2010): 305–6. https://doi.org/10.1016/j.ijcard.2009.10.042.

[58] This is also confirmed in several *Sùwèn* chapters such as: 17 *"Essentials of Vessels and the Subtleties of the Essence,"* and 19 *"Discourse on the Jade Mechanism and the True of the Depots."*

[59] Unschuld (2016), *"Nan Jing: The Classic of Difficult Issues,"* pg. 242.

Streams, Branches and Unity of Patterns: *Understanding the Absolute Unity of Channel Theory*

Z'ev Rosenberg

"Bodies, Earthly and Human"
"Leonardo mapped the human body. He charted its skeletal rocks, the course of its
'rivers' and its fleshly soil both within and without. He dissected the world, teasing out
its boney rocks, its earthy flesh and its watery veins."
- Martin Kemp [60]

While discussing *"Tree Theory, Biogeography and Branching"* with my co-author Stephen, we talked about Brian J. Enquist's recent article, where he points out that there are principles of branching that allow us to predict how entire forests, plants and trees function, from the fluxing of carbon dioxide, to the deep ecology of the forest. He explains that Da Vinci understood these rules that the patterns of *"daughter branches and twigs"* contain the same combined cross-sectional area as the trunk from which they originated. These "branching networks" provide maximum efficiency - for transportation of nutrients (fluids and sugars) to the whole organism. This is what Benoit Mandelbrot revealed in his studies of fractals, which infinitely recreate the original pattern of a whole system in fractional parts. Forests, mushroom mycelia, distribution of soils by composition, sunlight exposure and climate all contribute to whole systems that are greater than the sum of its parts. This also explains why "industrial forests," where trees are mono cropped and grown for profit, like tea plantations that eliminate wild trees, forest canopies and the wide range of wild and often medicinal plants that surround the trees often are prone to disease and the need for "nutritional additives" (fertilizers) and chemical attacks on invasive pathogens (herbicides, pesticides).

Língshū 靈樞 11 "the conduits and their diverging vessels" (branchings) recognizes the same ecological principles fundamental to the coherent whole.

---

[60] Kemp"*Leonard Da Vinci: Experience, Experiment and Design,*"pg. 132.

內有五藏，以應五音、五色、五時、五味、五位也；外有六府，以應六律。
六律建陰陽，諸經而合之十二月、十二辰、十二節、十二經 水、十二時、十二
經脈者，此五藏六府之所以應天道。

Internally [man] has the five long-term depots and they correspond to the five musical notes, the five colors, the five seasons, the five flavors and the five cardinal directions.

Externally [man] has the six short-term repositories and they correspond to the six pairs of flutes. The six pairs of flutes are categorized as yin and yang. They are one with all conduits, as well as with the twelve months, and the twelve stars, the twelve seasonal sections, and the twelve streams, the twelve double-hours and the twelve conduit vessels. This is how the five long-term depots and the six short-term repositories correspond to the WAY of heaven.
- Língshū 11[61]

The WAY of heaven refers to the patterned processes we find everywhere in Nature. The internal "five" and the external "six" refer to the ten heavenly stems (*tiān gān*天干) and twelve earthly branches (*dìzhī* 地支). To understand circulation in such a manner allow the clinician to observe the uniqueness of each patient as an embodiment of the universe and treat them with the same reverence and understanding of space-timing as one would promote growth in a landscape.

Língshū 12, *"The Conduit/Stream Waters"* is built on the same foundation, acknowledging that Han dynasty philosopher/scientist/physicians perceived these branching patterns 2000 years ago, long before Da Vinci. They shared his eye for the human landscape. As Huáng Dì黃帝 notes: *"The twelve conduit/stream vessels link up with the twelve stream waters outside."* Paul Unschuld translates:

"The parallelism between the significance of the major rivers for the well-being of the country, and the conduit streams for the well-being of the individual body is emphasized."[62]

This is exactly the same principle that Da Vinci describes above, and is the basis of mapping out of the channel system. Like Da Vinci's anatomical and topographical studies of landscapes and streams, there is an underlying mathematical logic that unifies the information, and allows a consistent and concise reading of the human entity that leaves nothing out and compromises nothing, from the smallest cell to the most complex structures and functions. Or as *Língshū* 12 states:

[61] Unschuld, *"Huang Di Nei Jing Ling Shu: The Ancient Classic on Needle Therapy,"* pg. 209.
[62] ibid, pg. 215.

凡此五藏六府十二經水者、外有源泉、而內有所稟、此皆內外相貫、如環無端、人經 亦然。

"To all the five long-term and six short-term repositories as well as the waters of the twelve streams the following applies: externally they have a source [to supply them] and internally they have [locations] supplied by them. All these [units] in the interior and exterior penetrate each other. This is like a ring without beginning. The same is true for the streams/conduits in man."[63]

Nàn Jīng 難經 23 refers to this same unified circulatory process (*yíng qì* 營氣) through the channels as *"[the movement through] all of them returns [again and again] to its origin, as a ring without end, with [the qi and blood] pouring from one [conduit] into the next, thus revolving [through the entire organism].* [64]

On a recent Torrey Pines hike, my wife and I were discussing how essential it is to be in tune with what the great scholar/physicians are describing in *Língshū* 12, to constantly meditate on these essential chapters in order to understand the absolute unifying principle that unfolds in the *Língshū* and *Nàn Jīng*. I noted that I could sense while in clinic when I felt more "tuned in"/resonant with the patient's channel system, and when I was not. Being "tuned in" allowed me as a practitioner to give the treatment that was absolutely required in that particular space/time location.

After weeks of suffering with a stubborn *shānghán* 傷寒/upper respiratory tract/sinus disorder that kept "recycling" itself, from *tàiyáng* 太陽 to *yángmíng* 陽明 to *shàoyáng* 少陽 and back, I finally was able to break the cycle with the help of a naso-probiotic, which helped restore the normal flora of my nasal mucosa. After that was relieved, however, I still had chill, stiffness in the neck, shoulders and joints, and a deep blocked sensation at *qū chí* 曲池/pool at the crook (LI 11) on the right arm and *yáng líng quán* 陽陵泉/yang mound spring (GB 34) on the left leg. I decided to give myself an acupuncture treatment on these two points, with moxa, along with *wài guān* 外關/outer pass (TB 5) on the right hand and *qiū xū* 丘墟/mound of ruins (GB 40) on the left foot, adding moxa with needle to *tiān shū* 天樞/heaven's pivot (ST 25) as well. After I treated these points immediately, it was like a cloud lifted; all the achiness, and stiffness left my body and I felt normal for the first time in weeks.

The physician of Chinese medicine always needs to keep this pattern that is described in *Língshū* 12 in one's mind and heart, and study it over and over again, and get out into nature to experience these natural cycles around and the sun, the moon, the tides, the changes of light, the responses of plants and trees

---

[63] ibid., pg. 219.

[64] Unschuld (2016), "*Nan Jing: The Classic of Difficult Issues,*"pg. 242.

to the seasonal changes. With this internal awareness, one, like Biǎn Què 扁鹊, we can potentially create the essential healing resonance with the acupuncture needles. In this context, study of the medical classics becomes a form of meditation, tuning one's mind to a world view that allows one to engage in human health and illness in an all-encompassing manner.

When we observe our patients (and ourselves) with the eye of an artist-scientist like Leonardo (or the Han clinicians) we realize that we are all branches and streams linked to the same natural trunk, and we each carry a proportionate distribution of heaven-and-earth cycles within us.

Navigating the Four Seas of Healing

Stephen Cowan & Z'ev Rosenberg

"Jo of the North Sea said, "You can't discuss the ocean with a well frog - he's limited by the space he lives in. You can't discuss ice with a summer insect - he's bound to a single season. You can't discuss the Way with a cramped scholar - he's shackled by his doctrines. Now you have come out beyond your banks and borders and have seen the great sea - so you realize your own pettiness. From now on it will be possible to talk to you about the Great Principle."
- Zhuāngzǐ 莊子 (Autumn Floods)[65]

Stephen: As we have been discussing in previous chapters, the Han dynasty doctors held a deep interest in mapping the body in accordance with the patterns found in Nature. This is evidenced in the *Nèijīng* 內經 and is further conceptualized in the *Nàn Jīng* 難經 as forming a continuous circulatory system. The focus on open communication and flow dynamics (*tōng* 通 and *liú* 流) essential to health was deeply influenced by the understanding of landscape in China. As Unschuld points out, the rivers and streams became metaphors for understanding health. The construction of canals designed to manage floods and provide ongoing communication and exchange of goods influenced the mapping of the channels of the human body.

The Han dynasty also saw a significant expansion of oceanic exploration that would open up alternate trade routes (beyond the silk roads) to southeast Asia, India, Africa and the Middle East. It would take European explorers more than a thousand years later to discover the continuity of the oceans and the roundness of the Earth. Perhaps this is another reason why the Europeans took so long to conceive of a unified continuously flowing circulatory system, a *"ring without end."* Their concept of the world was flat!

On land, the geomancy of tracking the rivers, choosing a path through the mountains and plains by reading the natural elements of the land takes a certain highly-developed skill. All streams and rivers eventually empty into the great seas. Navigating the sea is an entirely different matter. There are no fixed

---

[65] Watson,"*The Complete Works of Chuang Tzu,*"pg. 175.

landmarks to guide the sailor. Only the currents, the stars and the distant horizons serve as guides. The vastness of the ocean hides deep mysteries.

Navigation of the seas closely mirrors the early Daoist self-cultivation techniques linked to the *dāntián* 丹田 (the sea of *qì*) and the microcosmic circulation beyond the peripheral channels.

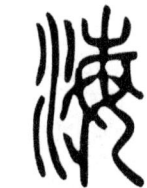

Figure 1.23 - Hǎi 海

Hǎi 海 (*fig. 1.23*) is a powerful ideogram loaded with meanings. It shows the water radical on the left signifying its water-nature. On the right is the great mother figure so important to feminine power / mystery for *Lǎozǐ* 老子 and *Zhuāngzǐ* 莊子.

Língshū 靈樞 33, entitled *"On the Seas"* begins with an interesting question regarding the four seas where Qíbó states,

歧伯答曰：人亦有四海，十二經水。經水者，皆注于海，海有東西南北，命曰
四海。

Man, too, has four seas and twelve conduit/stream waters. All these conduit/stream waters pour into the seas. There is an East, a West, a South, and a North Sea. Hence one speaks of the four seas.

必先明知陰陽表裏滎輸所在，四海定矣。

"First of all, it is essential to be familiar with the locations of the yin and yang [regions], the exterior and interior sections (biǎolǐ 表裡) and the creek (ying-stream 滎) and transport (shu-transport 輸) [openings]. Then the four seas can be identified."
- Língshū 33[66]

---

[66] Unschuld, *"Huang Di Nei Jing Ling Shu: The Ancient Classic on Needle Therapy,"* pg. 361-362.

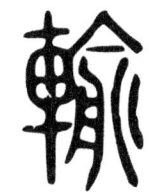

Figure 1.24 - Shū 輸[67]

The etymology of *shū* 輸 (*fig. 1.24*) previously discussed in the *The Goodness of Water*[68] chapter, is also one of a number of Chinese ideograms that references sailing. On the left we see the wheel axle indicating movement/traveling. On the right is the image of a boat in water (turned sideways with its stern pointing up). The vessel represents the power to move across the waters. This is a common metaphor for healing. Indeed, we see the same boat imagery in *shù* 腧 referring to any acu-point and *yù* 愈 meaning to recover from an illness.

Joseph Needham gives us incredible details on the elaborate advancements in shipping by the time of the Han Dynasty, advancements that enabled far-off exploration, transportation and exchange of information across the seas to distant lands.[69]

Access to the four seas in Chinese medicine is one of the keys to deeper understanding of the continuity and circulation within the human landscape.

- The stomach *wèi* 胃 is the sea of fluids and grains (food).
- The *chōng mài* 衝脈 is the sea of the twelve channels/streams (blood system).
- The *dàn zhōng* 膻中 is the sea of *qì*/breaths.
- The brain *nǎo* 腦 is the sea of marrow/essence (*suǐ* 髓).

Língshū 33 tells us that we have access to each of these seas at specific locations on the body.

---

[67] Wieger & Davrout, "*Chinese Characters: Their Origin, Etymology, History, Classification and Signification*" lesson 14, pgs. 45-49.

[68] See Stephen Cowan's "*The Goodness of Water*," pgs. 53-58.

[69] Needham, "*Science and Civilisation in China: Vol. Physics and Physical Technology: Part III: Civil Engineering and Nautics*," pg. 379.

Sea of Qì	Sea of Fluids & Grains
rén yíng 人迎 (ST 9) above shān zhōng 膻中 (Ren 17) below	qì chōng 氣沖 (ST 30) above zú sān lǐ 足三里 (ST 36) below
Sea of Blood Vessels	**The Sea of Marrow**
dà zhù 大杼 (BL 11) above shàng jù xū 上巨虛 (ST 37) below	bǎi huì 百會 (Du 20) above fēng fǔ 風府 (Du 16) below

Língshū 33 indicates that conditions where there is long-standing *xūshí* 虛實 (depletion/excess) treating the deep seas may be warranted in order to restore the proper *"movement in accordance with the norms"* as Qíbó says, to achieve recovery.

Here are two clinical examples of Four Seas treatment in my pediatric practice:

1. An eight year old boy is brought to me with a longstanding history of chronic eczema that appears thick, dry and itchy. His complexion is pale and his tongue is red with a white coat. His eyes are dull and glassy. His mother says he's always fidgeting but has no stamina. His diet consists of excessive processed foods and he eats at irregular times, often filling up on snacks while plugged in to screens. The itching disrupts his sleep. He has recently had bouts of wheezing asthma particularly in Spring and Autumn when the seasons change. He's been tested for allergies but nothing specific has come up. Having been treated off and on for years with topical steroids nothing has helped. Indeed, each time he comes off the steroids the eczema flares back worse then ever. The lack of sleep and discomfort during the day have caused him constant distraction and restlessness (ADHD symptoms.) No one can figure out what the triggers are because they appear to be constantly changing as if he has multiple sensitivities. This presenting picture of mixed excess/deficiency, to me, is a red flag that in order to influence the circulation of blood/*qì* (*xuèqì* 血氣) we may need access to the four seas.

In addition to advising dietary and lifestyle changes, I incorporated acupuncture/moxa and *tuīná* 推拿 massage of the Blood and Qì Seas points *shàng jù xū* 上巨虛/upper great void (ST 37), *shān zhōng* 膻中/chest center (Ren 17) into my treatments and taught his mother how to massage these points each night before bed. Within 1 month, his parents already saw subtle signs of improvement in his skin. I then included *zú sān lǐ* 足三里/leg three miles (St 36) treatment of the Sea of Grains and fluids to promote proper hydration and digestion which are essential for healthy skin, immune regulation and cognition. Addition of treatment of the Sea of Marrow point *fēng fǔ* 風府/palace of wind (Du 16) improved his attention in school.

2. A 3 ½ year old girl diagnosed with Autism came to see me for possible treatment. She exhibited mixed signs of excess/deficiency: alternating intense/wild and withdrawn/spacey behaviors red tongue with yellow coating, poor digestion with undigested food in her unformed stools. She was reported to be an extremely picky eater, her diet consisting only of sugars and carbs. Past history was significant. She was conceived by IVF and born by C-section due to failure to progress following prolonged Pitocin induction. As an infant, she developed multiple ear infections requiring repeated antibiotics. Around 16 months she began losing the language she seemed to have developed, began exhibiting repetitive behaviors and lost interest in her toys. She underwent tympanostomy procedure for her chronic middle ear effusions though her language has remained significantly delayed. In the treatment room, the child seemed literally "lost at sea," a metaphor that did not go unnoticed by her parents. She held her hands over her ears, her mother explaining that she was extremely sensitive to sounds. She showed no interest in the many toys in my office. Her eye contact was inconsistent and she did not respond to her name nor was she able to follow any requests.

When confronted with such a case, it is good to follow Qíbó's advice. First orient to the four directions (above/below/left/right). Then examine the *yīnyáng* parts of the body and recognize the *biǎolǐ* 表裡 (outside/inside) relationships. I often think of a child manifesting regressive autistic features as "the inside-out child"(hypersensitive to outside influences, particularly challenged by transitions, and underdeveloped "inside" (immature cognitive and digestive system.) Once she felt safe in my office space, the first treatment simply involved applying a low frequency tuning fork on *bǎi huì* 百會/hundred meetings (Du 20) and *fēng fǔ* 風府/palace of wind (Du 16), the Sea of Marrow points and right before her parents eyes, the child appeared to wake up, look at me and smile. Indeed later in that first visit she spontaneously came over to me and pointed her head in my direction indicating she wished for more treatment.

We discussed dietary changes, to support a more diverse microbiome, clear dysbiosis and introduce a low dose herbal formula (*bǔ zhōng yì qì tāng* 補中益氣湯) to bring some balance to her center. At the next visit again once she felt safe in my presence, I repeated the tuning fork treatment and added *zú sān lǐ* 足三里/leg three mile (St 36) acupuncture and these three points became the basis of later treatments with additions based on her presentation. Eventually I added the sea of blood and sea of *qì* points to round out her treatment. Over time, with many adjustments to her treatment, she began making slow progress back into our world, language gradually emerged with the help of a gifted speech therapist that saw the inner intelligence within her rather than just seeing the labels that the western medical system had trapped this girl in.

As Zhuāngzǐ 莊子 advises us in confronting complex conditions:

"There is no end to the weighing of things, no stop to time, no constancy to the division of lots, no fixed rule to beginning and end. Therefore great wisdom observes both far and near, and for that reason recognizes small without considering it paltry, recognizes large without considering it unwieldy, for it knows that there is no end to the weighing of things."[70]

Z'ev: In *Língshū* 34, Qíbó defines health and disorder in terms of the dynamics of the five phases and clear divisions of the four seasons. He notes that *"when camp [qi](yíng qì 營氣) and guard [qi](wèi qì 衛氣) follow each other, when yin [qi] and yang [qi] harmonize and when the clear (qīng 清) and the/turbid [qi] (zhuó 濁) do not attack each other, this then is a movement in accordance with the norms, and hence there is order."*[71] Here we have a clear definition of health, and an implied definition of acupuncture / moxibustion in restoring this delineated equilibrium.

---

[70] Watson, *"The Complete Works of Chuang Tzu,"* pg. 177.

[71] Unschuld, *"Huang Di Nei Jing Ling Shu: The Ancient Classic on Needle Therapy,"* pg. 368.

Part II:
Maps

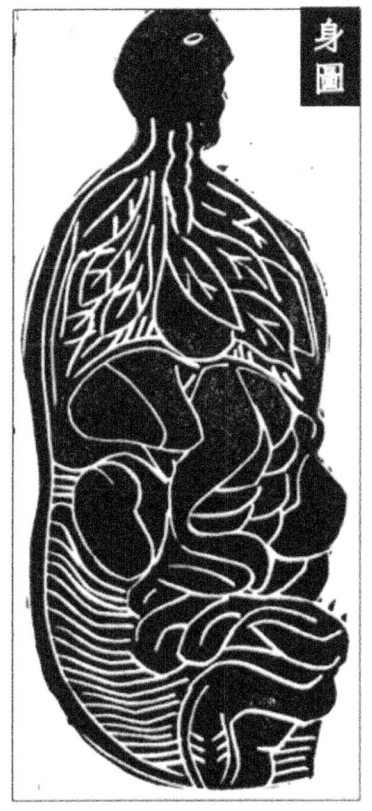

72

A Word about Zhāng Shìxián's 張世賢 Maps (*Tú* 圖) of the *Nàn Jīng* 難經

Stephen Cowan & Z'ev Rosenberg

"[T]he meaning(fulness) of one single tú 圖 can not be exhausted by millions of words."
- Wángbó 王柏 (1197-1274)[73]

Stephen: Throughout this book, I have added a number of the 81 maps created by Zhāng Shìxián 張世賢 that I am particularly drawn to for several reasons:

1. Maps as a way of illustrating *relational* understanding are a central theme to our book.
2. Most of Zhāng's maps are "word maps," a distinctive form of map-making that began during the Song Dynasty and continues to the present day.
3. Both Z'ev and I are visual learners. Z'ev creates what he calls "mind maps" using Mindnode™ program as a way of collecting ideas in one picture to help organize and guide to his writing. Being a visual artist, I, too, have a long history of creating visual maps to gain deeper insights into the meaning of whatever I am studying.

During my medical studies, both Western and Chinese, I created extensive visual maps for myself to illustrate ideas in order to better retain them. During my clinical rotations, these enabled me to "picture" vast swaths of information at once, a form of systems-thinking that I have found extremely useful both in practice and in teaching.

Zhāng's maps appear at the end of Paul Unschuld's translation of the *Nàn Jīng* 難經 without translation or explanation. They derive from a text entitled *Tú*

---

[73] Adler, "*Reconstructing the Confucian Dao: Zhu Xi's appropriation of Zhou Dunyi*,"pg. 3. from Wángbó's 王柏 (1197–1274) preface to his *Yánjǐ Tú* 研幾圖/*Diagrams on the Fathoming of Incipience*, translated by Michael Lackner, "*Diagrams as an Architecture by Means of Words*" in Bray, Dorofeeva-Lichtmann, and Métailie, "*Graphics and text in the Production of Technical Knowledge in China: The Warp and the Weft.*"

Zhù Bāshíyī Nàn Jīng 圖註八十一難經 / *The 81 Maps of the Nàn Jīng* written in 1510 during the Ming Dynasty. According to Joseph Adler, "*One of the distinctive aspects of the Song dynasty revival of Confucianism (so called Neo-Confucianism) was a surge of interest in the use of tú* 圖 *maps as a means of conveying the subtler meanings of the Way (Dào* 道*) that can elude discursive expression.*"[74] This map-making trend, both representational (as in anatomic illustrations) and word-based (as in charts and schematics) were designed to communicate ideas beyond the text the way a collage creates an emergent property that the parts cannot. This is what Roger Ames calls an "*aesthetic composition*"[75] to differentiate it from the linear-logic ordering of information we often find in scientific books. This aesthetic composition allows for the emergence of novel ideas through the relational qualities between various concepts. I have been very drawn to Zhāng's maps ever since they were first published in Unschuld's first edition of the *Nàn Jīng* and was inspired by Z'ev to translate them and reproduce some of them in our book as a way of "walking the talk" so to speak, that is, illustrating the radical ideas of mandalic circulation expounded in *Nàn Jīng* thinking.

Here's an example of one of Zhāng's wonderful *tú* 圖 maps that demonstrates how he organized a summary of concepts in such a way as to allow interesting relationships to emerge. In *Nàn Jīng* 27, a discussion of the function of the eight extraordinary vessels is given.[76]

In this map (*fig. 2.1*), the typical relationships between the paired vessels is not given but rather, Zhāng offers a new pairing, that follows hand to foot to hand etc. For example, *yīn qiāo mài* 陰蹺脈 is placed next to *chòng mài* 衝脈 which in turn is placed next to *dū mài* 督脈. Zhāng arranges these vessels in this way because he has overlayed the 12 channels onto the schema, adding a time element to the sequence. This is his own idea, not mentioned in *Nàn Jīng* 27. He then adds a note in the center, stating that "*the eight vessels fill not adhering rigidly to the channels.*" If we look at this mandala[77] like a double cycling clock, we can see the body (hand-foot-hand-foot) circulation rotating in accordance with the 12 channels plus the eight extraordinary vessels having a relative relationship rotating on the outer ring. Like the planetary orbits, Zhāng's (literally) revolutionary map of *Nàn Jīng* 27 offers us a powerful way to understand space - time movement within our body.

---

[74] Adler, "*Reconstructing the Confucian dao: Zhu Xi's appropriation of Zhou Dunyi,*" pg. 151.

[75] Ames, "*Putting the Te Back into Taoism,*" pg. 117.

[76] See MindNode in *Appendix II: Blueprints and Charts from Z'ev's Notebook* pg. 290.

[77] The word / concept of Mandala मण्डल derives from the Sanskrit meaning of relationship gathered into a circular design.

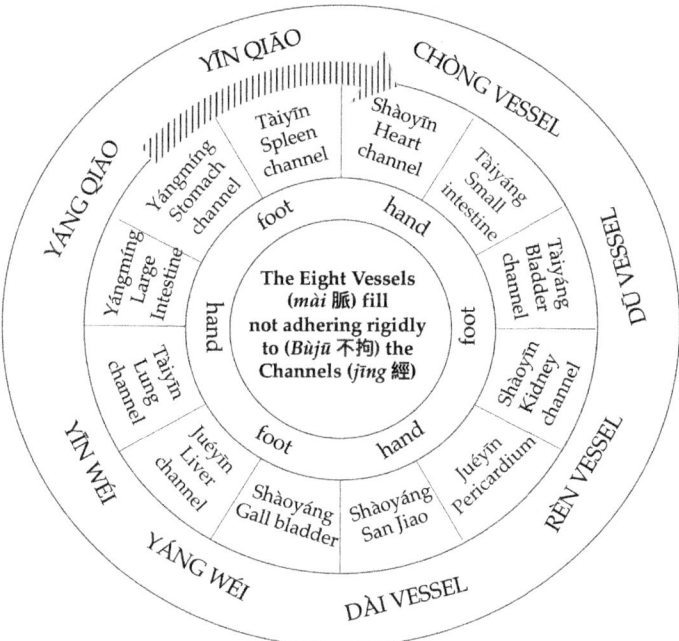

Figure 2.1 - Nàn Jīng 27 Map

I have attempted to translate some of Zhāng's wonderful maps when they seem particularly appropriate to illustrate a point we are making in this book. What strikes me about all of these maps is how they unwittingly illustrate the fundamental concept of ecological circulation, the *"ring without end."*

Z'ev: It is uncommon to find such examples of mandalic visual tools used to illustrate classical medical texts anywhere else in Chinese medical history. Here, the entire text of the *Nàn Jīng* is covered, chapter by chapter, making this perhaps the most clinically useful text in the entire classical acupuncture corpus. The use of mandalas to organize diagnostic principles is an extraordinary tool for preparing practitioners for clinical practice.

The Trap in the Map: *Transcending Limitations*

Stephen Cowan & Z'ev Rosenberg

*"A map is not the territory it represents, but if correct,
it has a similar structure to the territory, which accounts for its usefulness."*
- Alfred Korzybski [78]

Stephen: Our hunter-gatherer ancestors located themselves through a direct experience in living territories, the mountains-and-rivers landscape, shaped by natural borders, within which the procession of seasons promote local plant and animal life. It was this direct living context of space-time that shaped their experience and their world view.

By the time of the Warring states period in China (480-221 BCE), Lǎozi recognized the dangers of deception that names, labels and maps (in any language) can create. Naming is inherent to human nature. It begins as an expedient means for sorting and navigating space and time and communicating ideas to others, but over time names can create artificial fixed boundaries that harden into their own kind of absolute and unchanging reality that runs counter to the way life exists in nature.

The state of confusion (*luàn* 亂)[79] that occurs when the labels and maps no longer serve to enlighten our experience but rather cut us off from our direct connection to the changes that occur in our surroundings is evident today in the many chronic disorders (autoimmune diseases, chronic allergies, Autism, ADHD, Alzheimer's, etc.) that share a common quality of alienation, that is, being cut off from healthy relationships to Nature. Even these diagnostic labels give the impression that they are written in stone leaving little room for change that the uniqueness and complexity of each individual possesses. The

---

[78] Korzybski,"*Science and sanity: An Introduction to Non-Aristotelian Systems and General Semantics,*" pg. 747–761.

[79] *Luàn* 亂 "state of confusion" "revolt" break in connection see *Língshū* 34 the five states of confusion or disturbance. The ideogram shows a silk thread being cut or blocked.

pharmaceutical industry often takes advantage of this *fixed mind* language to offer one-size-fits-all relief rather than customized treatment.

The Han Dynasty Chinese anatomists were aware of this danger and attempted to capture the living ever-changing landscape of a human being, through a deeper understanding of the flow of *xuè* 血 / *qì* 氣 in the midst of transformation. As stated above, Zhāng Shìxián 張世賢 created a series of amazing mandala-like maps, one for each chapter of the *Nàn Jīng* 難經, examples of which appear throughout our book. These maps attempt to capture qualities of changing relationships (seasonal cycles, daily cycles, lunar cycles) that reflect the flow of circulation within the body and contrast starkly with the rather fixed anatomic maps made by Europeans that were derived from cadaver models.

Z'ev: These are important arguments. My response would be that "circular" or "mandalic" maps are different than "flat earth" maps that have only two dimensions. While multidimensional simulations that are available to us today through computer technology can provide more accurate tools, just as we are finding in biomedical diagnostics. Today we have a plethora of virtual reality tools that allow us to illuminate a living landscape of viscera, vessels, tissue planes and a multi-dimensional body, but this opportunity seems to have not been taken advantage of in terms of shifting our perceptions of the human landscape. Recently there was a multimedia presentation, *Fluid Matters: Flow and Transformation in the History of the Body* by Natalie Köhle and Shigahisa Kuriyama which points to a more sophisticated approach to viewing human anatomy and physiology from different cultural perspectives, East and West.[80] Hopefully this will offer physicians of all persuasions and disciplines a chance to rethink the "old maps" that the *Lǎozi* speaks about and create fluid, multi-dimensional maps that actually "move" with the flow of life. In summation, mapping the states of change is a sophisticated form of understanding complexity theory that can be applied to human physiology as in all phenomena being investigated at the cutting edges of modern science.[81]

Stephen: In the classics of Chinese medicine we find many overlapping maps available that offer a holographic perspective of reality that illustrate both space *and* time: the classic 12 channels map, the *wǔ shū xué* 五输穴 / five transport map, the *wǔxíng* 五行 / five phases, maps of *shēng* 生 / *kè* 剋 relationships, the *qí jīng bā mài* 奇經八脈 maps of eight extraordinary vessels, the maps of divergent channels, the maps of the 12 earthly branches and 10 heavenly stems map, the *Shānghán Lùn* 傷寒論 and *wēn bìng* 溫病 maps, maps of

---

[80] see Köhle, and Kuriyama,"*Fluid Matter(s): Flow and Transformation in the History of the Body.*"

[81] A institution involved in this kind of research is The Santa Fe Institute (https://www.santafe.edu/).

the *shén* 神 / spirit, and of course the oldest maps of all, *Yìjīng* 易經's map of the 64 hexagrams (*fig. 2.2*).

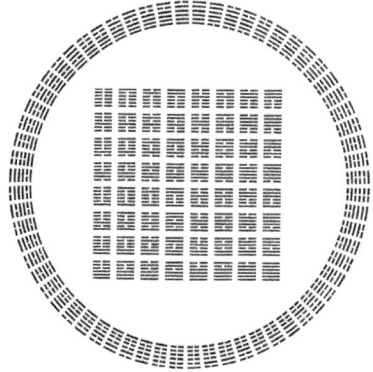

Figure 2.2 - 64 Hexagrams of the Yìjīng 易經

What these Chinese body maps have in common is their attempt to illustrate *change* rather than delineate fixed borders of forms. Change is a core principle of China's understanding of Nature. The Great Commentary on the *Yìjīng* by Confucius states:

"The ongoing alternation of openings and closings is called flux/change (biàn 變), and the inexhaustibility of the comings and goings is called continuity (tōng 通)."[82]

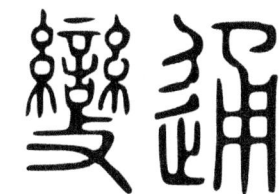

Figure 2.3 - Biàntōng 變通[83]

---

[82] Ames, *"The Great Commentary (Dazhuan 大傳) and Chinese Natural Cosmology."*

[83] *Biàntōng* 變通 變通 – Roger Ames defines this term as "change and continuity or flux and flow." *International Communication of Chinese Culture* (2015) 2(1): 1–18. The ideogram *biàn* 變 shows two silk threads with speech between them. Alone this can mean a kind of entangled chaotic confusion that can occur during change. Below it is a hand holding a stick, like a conductor. *Biàn* can mean transitional change. The ideogram *tōng* shows the foot traveling with a kind of plant form or bell meaning to channel or communicate. In Chinese medicine *tōng* is a central idea of health when there is free flowing communication through the channels.

Biàntōng 變通 (*fig. 2.3*) implies that relationships are the source of change, each part is related to the others and that the body-mind only exists as an ever-changing contextual form. *Biàntōng* is embodied in all relative pairs: *yīn* 陰 / *yáng* 陽, *xuè* 血 / *qì* 氣, *yíng* 營 / *wèi* 衛 etc. Therefore, all patterns and diagnoses only exist in the context of specific instances and are subject to change at any given instance as relationships and contexts change. This is what makes each patient that comes through the door a unique opportunity to embrace the spirit of the sages, understanding that the level of theory is always moderated by the level of practice.

Western medicine of course is just another map. Like any map, it has its utility in terms of detailed structure and mechanical function. There is no reason to fear the Western mechanical map. However, Chinese medical practitioners, must be careful not to fall into the trap of the Western diagnostic labels that exert a powerful influence on our perceptions. When we recognize the limitations of artificial fixed labels and use them when necessary but always remember to see whatever information being presented through the eyes of a Chinese landscape artist, we are better able to communicate with our patients living in a Western culture and treat them effectively.

Cheng Man-ching 郑曼青 (1902-1975), the great *tàijí* 太極 master of my lineage, was a renowned painter as well as a physician. I have had the privilege of being involved in translating his medical notes[84] and one of the amazing observations I have had was his open-hearted curiosity and his ability to interpret Western medical data through the eyes of a Chinese medical practitioner. Here is an example from his medical book.

"Qíbó 岐伯 says, "*When tendons and blood vessels are in harmony, bone and marrow dense and firm, the qi and blood will follow each other.*"[85]

Lǎozǐ 老子 10 says:

老子: 專氣致柔能嬰兒乎

"*if one concentrates his qi, he will be as resilient as a young child.*"[86]

---

[84] In the process of being published under the title, *The Sage Principles*, translated by Ed Young and Stephen Cowan.

[85] *Huáng Dì Nèijīng* 黃帝內經 3 translation/interpretation S. Cowan from *The Sage Principles*, which is in the process of being published.

[86] *Lǎozǐ* 老子 10 translation/interpretation S. Cowan from *The Sage Principles*, which is in the process of being published.

Professor Cheng's commentary: "*I can explain these words of the sages by physiological evidence. By examining the X-ray of the hand, one will notice the difference between the skeleton of a child and that of an adult. The bones of a child appear to be separated far apart at every joint. What holds them together at these junctures is the network of tendons and blood vessels, which act as links that facilitate movement.*[87] *Thus we can see that harmony of tendons and blood vessels gives utmost benefit to movement. When qi and blood are full (and flowing), the entire body is like a rubber ball. A young child may fall to the ground, yet no harm is done to its body because the bones and marrow are firm and strong. This is what Lǎozǐ meant by "concentrate qi to attain resilience." It is hopeful that even for the elderly if they learn how to circulate qi they will regain this resilience and rejuvenation.*"[88]

Professor Cheng demonstrates how to use Western technology without losing the spirit of Chinese medicine's principles. It is important however to note here that Chinese medicine can be just as dangerous when its ideas and labels become too narrowly fixed and loses its spirit of *biàntōng*.

Z'ev: This cautions us not to rely on *xíng* 型/type casting (simplistic *biàn zhèng* 辨證/pattern differentiation) and *bā gāng* 八綱/snapshot diagnostics which are designed to create "subtypes" to biomedical disease entities to make it easier to practice "*integrative medicine*" as in modern static TCM *bā gāng* 八綱/eight principle (more accurately viscera/bowel) pattern differentiation, which is often a "snap shot view" and quite rigid in boxing in a patient. Unfortunately, this is also the basis of many Western schools of Chinese medicine, which tries to simplify diagnosis in order to best fit biomedical disease patterns. While this can be useful, and is practiced at a more sophisticated level in mainland China, the problem is when we label the patient as having a static pattern, we lose the sense of complexity and systems theory view of the entire body/mind constellation. For example, *gān qì yù* 肝氣鬱/liver *qì* depression is often present in modern patients, and treated with such formulas as *xiāo yáo sǎn* 逍遙散/free wanderer powder and acupuncture holes such as *tài chōng* 太沖/great rushing (Liv 3), *yáng líng quán* 陽陵泉/yang mound spring (GB 34), *qí mén* 期門/cycle gate (Liv 14), *nèi guān* 內關/inner pass (PC 6), and *zhōng wǎn* 中脘/middle cavity (Ren 12).

While both of these strategies can be useful and effective, the pigeonholing of the *zàngfǔ* 臟腑 pattern "box" does not allow for the how and why this pattern developed, it just treats the manifestation of pre-existing disharmonies. This diagnosis also is not fluid enough to recognize subtle changes in the pattern

---

[87] Radiologic imaging does not pick up cartilage, tendons and blood vessels yet this is where the vital activity of nourishment and growth take place.

[88] *The Sage Principle*s, translated by Ed Young and Stephen Cowan which is in the process of being published.

over time, or reflect seasonal, circadian, or lunar cycles. Potentially we may "lock in" treatment, and not reflect changes over time. There are multiple methods of pattern differentiation in Chinese medicine, and acupuncture/ moxibustion and herbal medicine have different methodologies that are often necessary to engage. True Chinese medical diagnosis is a flowing, changing dynamic, reflecting the ever changing nature of the universe reflected in clinical time and space. This is often misunderstood by modern practitioners as a lack of focus or certainty about one's diagnosis.

Stephen: A patient coming in with a fixed diagnosis given by a Western doctor can be a dilemma for a Chinese medical doctor trained in the West. We always run the risk of treating these diagnostic labels; "asthma" or "migraines" or "colitis" or "Parkinson's disease" instead of treating the *biàntōng* change-and-continuity of relationships. To treat relationships rather than fixed parts is the true spirit of Chinese medicine. Just as the skies and seas are always changing so must we honor the ever-changing relationship between the heavens and earth within our patients. This is how the *Yìjīng* has been used for centuries as a foundation for the many maps used in Chinese medicine.

Z'ev: We approach these biomedically defined illnesses as damage to the *qì* dynamic, and repair it accordingly. One "antidote" to this problem of a "pre-diagnosis" is when a patient first comes in. Instead, I focus on restoring balance and repairing the disruptions in the *qì* dynamic, focusing on the terrains of the channel system or three *yáng*/three *yīn* progressions as defined in the *Shānghán Lùn* 傷寒論. For example, I do not have them tell me their problem or disease. I read the pulse, look at the tongue, observe, and then give them a diagnostic preliminary reading. This significantly allows the patient to reframe their condition even before I take a detailed history. I strongly feel that my patients do not want yet another bio-medical therapy approach, but a new, fresh perspective to their condition that also increases their self-awareness without playing on their fears, as biomedicine often does.

Stephen: The point here is to always remember that the map is not the territory. To treat change is the great challenge of the Chinese Medicine practice. Change is the fundamental expression of relationships, and these relationships define the uniqueness of who we are at any given moment in a particular context. Our human habit of conceptual thinking can impede successful treatment if it becomes fixed or absolute.

The Emergent Whole

Stephen Cowan & Z'ev Rosenberg

"Here 'emergence' does not mean mysteries popping out of the undergrowth; it means that with a sufficient understanding of interactive processes, we should come to understand why a complex whole has properties its parts lack on their own, and how the parts are modified by the context in which they lie."
- Richard L. Gregory [89]

Stephen: The *Nàn Jīng* 難經 authors are grappling with success and failure in treating living relational beings. When the treatment is successful it reinforces the veracity of the map that has guided us and we pride ourselves on our medical tradition. When the treatment is unsuccessful, doubt is cast on the skill of the practitioner rather than on the map. Perhaps the failure resides in failing to adapt the map to the living circumstances.

Z'ev: This is very important. As one studies and restudies these classics (*jīng* 經), one uncovers new layers of understanding. Failure and reconsideration is a part of that process. The characters *jī* 機 mechanism or (preferably in this context) dynamic and *yì* 意 intention or attentiveness are two antipodes of a dynamic pendulum between practitioner and patient. The practitioner discovers the *jī* in reading the patients' channel system, by focusing in one's *yì*. This is more than a "meeting of the minds," it is a "meeting of the *qì*."

Stephen: Yes, a fixed map is antithetical to the spirit of treating ever-changing relationships. It treats form as if it's a fixed entity rather than a unique convergence of events. This dichotomous perspective is a very Western approach that has influenced westerners practicing Chinese medicine. Is the problem *yīn* or *yáng*? blood *or qì*? *yíng* 營 *or wèi* 衛? This is not truly nourishing life (*yǎngshēng* 養生). Inner patterns *lǐ* 理 reveal themselves through their changing relationships. They are never fixed patterns but rather emergent properties of relationships over time. Many Chinese medical practitioners have fallen into this trap by the very nature of non-imagistic alphabetic languages that are the root of the Western diagnostic label system. However, it is human

---

[89] Camazine, et.al., *"Self-Organization in Biological Systems,"* pg. 91 & Gregory, *"DNA in the Mind's Eye,"* pg. 359-360.

nature to categorize what we perceive. We see this tendency in China even before the influence of Western medicine existed, in the differing commentaries Unschuld has given us in the *Nàn Jīng*.

Z'ev: This again, is the failure of textbook TCM, relying on *xíng* 型/type casting (over simplistic *biàn zhèng* 辨證/pattern differentiation) and *bā gāng* 八綱 snapshot, one dimensional diagnostics which are designed to create "subtypes" to biomedical disease entities. This in order to make it easier to practice "integrative medicine." This of course favors a disease-oriented approach over a terrain-based, field dynamics approach.

Chip Chace (1958-2018) described this as *shì* 勢/propensity, reading the ground of the clinical encounter as a whole, a moving dynamic. Propensity is also the translation chosen by François Jullien, who wrote a book on this topic.[90] D.C. Lau and Roger Ames translate *shì* 勢 as *"strategic advantage."*[91] In the book Sūnbìn 孫臏's (382-316 BCE) *Sūnbìn Bīngfǎ* 孫臏兵法/*Art of Warfare*[92], writes *"morning and night we wear a sword, but we don't necessarily use it."*[93]

Stephen: The *Nàn Jīng* tells us that the skill in treating changing relationships requires constant discipline and vigilance. Ultimately *"the ring that has no end"* is *biàntōng* 變通 (change and continuity), a term used repeatedly in the *Yìjīng* 易經, the basis of Chinese thinking and perceiving. The ring is you as a practitioner in constant relationship with your changing context, always being mindful that the map is *not* the ever-changing territory of being who is sitting before you in the treatment room. I am constantly reminded of this emergent reality in my treatment of children who are in a constant state of change and transformation by their very nature. Indeed, my role is to help promote that transformation each time they come in the door. This, for me, is treating the Whole, of which I cannot help be a part.

Z'ev: This failure is reflected not only in modern Westernized TCM textbooks, but in biomedical practice. I have countless numbers of patients who are given powerful pharmaceutical medications, and years later they are on the same dosage and drug, even as their bodies and minds have changed in that period. The result is that their symptom patterns become frozen in time and space. I had a recent patient with pain spreading down her gall bladder channel from side flanks at hip to knees, treated with prednisone and muscle relaxants with no effect. She was on an abnormally high dosage of Wellbutrin (450 gm)

---

[90] Jullien,*"The Propensity of Things: Toward a History of Efficacy in China."*

[91] Sun, Lau, and Ames,*"Sun Pin: The Art of Warfare,"* pg. 163-5.

[92] While Sūnbìn 孫臏's *Art of War* and Sūnzǐ 孫子 (Sun Tzu)'s *The Art of War* share a similar name, they are distinct works by different authors.

[93] ibid., pg. 163.

for four years running because of her inability to overcome grief at the death of her brother. I asked her to go back to her physician and suggest reducing the dosage of the Wellbutrin, as I felt she was "frozen" in her tendino-muscular channels. This particular type of pain is also listed a s a potential side effect of the medication. Her tongue body was very stiff, dark red and shiny surface, her pulses felt sticky like molasses, with embedded roughness. Her complexion was shiny as well. I treated her with a 50/50 combination of *dāng guī sháo yào sǎn* 當歸芍藥散/angelica and peony powder and *guì zhī fú líng wán* 桂枝茯苓丸/cinnamon twig and poria pill, and acupuncture on *wài guān* 外關/outer pass (TB 5)/*zú lín qì* 足臨泣/foot governor of tears (GB 41) (opposite limbs unilaterally), points along the GB channel, *hòu xī* 後谿/back stream (SI 3), *shēn mài* 申脈/extended vessel (BL 62) (opposite limbs unilaterally) and moxa to the lower abdomen. The condition was resolved in two treatments.

Nàn Jīng 難經 **34:** *Constructing a Clinical Mandala*

Stephen Cowan & Z'ev Rosenberg

"The 'enclosure' or 'circumambulation' is expressed by the idea of a circulation. The circulation is not merely motion in a circle, but means on the one hand, the marking off of a sacred precinct, and on the other, fixed concentration."
- Carl Jung, *The Secret of the Golden Flower* [94]

Stephen: Because the circle has no beginning or ending, it is a symbol of immortality. In Paleolithic cultures around the world, the circle has always held special spiritual meaning, the power of gathering (e.g. drumming circles, medicine wheels, ceremonial structures, such as Stonehenge). In ancient Greece around 300 BCE, Euclid stated the properties of a circle as *"a plane bounded by one curved line, such that all straight lines drawn from a certain point within it to the bounding line are equal. This bounding line is called its circumference and the point, its center."*[95] It would take over 2000 years for a German mathematician, Ferdinand Von Lindemann (1852-1939), to solve the mystery of the area of a circle with *pi* π's value and proved that *pi* π is a "transcendental number" meaning that which is not a root of any polynomial with rational coefficients.

Z'ev: This is as always with your work fascinating, but I want to be careful not to "cast our nets" too wide. I have to admit my biases with the history of Western thought, I don't personally like drawing too much on these resources.

Stephen: I agree. In fact the whole idea of *transcendence*, the concept of disembodied ideals and out-of-context absolutes that lies at the root of Greek philosophy, is absent from Chinese thought. Roger Ames has argued that *"the concept of strict transcendence has seriously distorted aspects of Confucian and Daoist understanding."*[96] However, the fact that Euclid was investigating the nature of a

---

[94] Wilhelm, Jung, and Liu, *"The Secret of the Golden Flower: A Chinese Book of Life,"* pg. 103.

[95] See Euclid's Elements Book 1 definitions 15, 16 Clark University https://mathcs.clarku.edu/~djoyce/elements/bookI/defI15.html.

[96] Hall and Ames, *"Thinking from the Han: Self, Truth, and Transcendence in Chinese and Western Culture."*

circle from a mathematical perspective at around the same time as the *Nàn Jīng* writers were describing a *"ring without end."* I find very interesting. What is it about the circle that sent the Greeks in one direction and the Chinese in another? I think this illustrates how far ahead the *Nàn Jīng* writers were in working out one continuous circulation in ways that I believe the Western world still has not.

In ancient China, Tibet, and India, the spiritual aspects of the circle was called mandala मण्डल, which in Sanskrit means any circle or disc-like object (e.g. sun, moon) that contains natural power.[97] In India the term mandala initially referred to a sacred space where the oral verses of the Vedas, the sacred words of the gods, could be transmitted but during the first millennium, as the world expanded with Silk Road multicultural exchanges, a more humanistic understanding of mind-consciousness as a sacred mandala space began developing: consciousness as the way the cosmos makes itself known.

The Mandala principle refers to a coherent system of spiritual relationships, what Chögyam Trungpa (1939-1987) calls a map of *"orderly chaos."*[98] Bob Thurman defines mandala as a "mystic diagram" consisting of a square within a circle that defines a sacred space.

Z'ev: We can see this in the various Islamic motifs in madrassas and tombs, Navajo and Tibetan sand paintings. One can view mandalas as a way to organize a virtual cloud of information, as in MindNode™ charts. It is a way of thinking/perception, arranging thoughts and ideas in a continuum that allows access to them and makes room for new connections and interpretations.

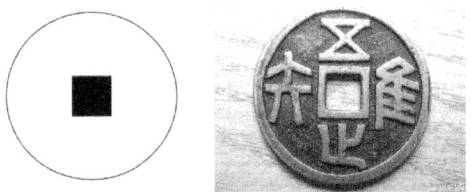

Figure 2.4 - Chinese Coins[99]

---

[97] Etymologically maṇḍa मण्ड meaning the highest point and la ल implies a sign of completion.

[98] Trungpa and Chödzin, *"Orderly Chaos: The Mandala Principle."*

[99] Typical of Chinese love of hidden meanings, my teacher, Ed Young, loved the humor in this coin's message about money: the square in the center takes part in the making of four characters starting from the top and moving counterclockwise around the coin *wú* 吾, *zhī* 知, *zú* 足, *wěi* 唯, meaning "I know I have enough."

Stephen: Exactly! Likewise, in traditional Chinese symbology, the spirit of the circle represents the Heavenly expanse while the Earth is represented by the square with its four equally measured sides, four corners, four directions, four seasons. We can still see hints of this mystic diagram in the old Chinese coins with the square cutout (*fig. 2.4*).

In the first part of *Nàn Jīng* 34, the clinical space-time map described in *Nàn Jīng* 33 is further expanded upon.The physical manifestations of the five *zàng* 臟/organs are mapped in accordance with five phase *wǔxíng* 五行 principle to include complexion, sound, odor, taste and bodily fluid. Each yin organ has its corresponding designated expressions. This map enables the clinician to identify the health or disease in living organs without requiring cutting the patient open. As Elizabeth Rochat de la Vallée says, *"the impression given by the appearance to a practiced eye is very important for diagnosis."*[100] Indeed one of the characteristics of the so-called *Shén* 神 doctor is the uncanny ability to "see" and "hear" the organ networks.

Z'ev: I think here we have reached a critical point in the book. Translating and transmitting the concept of *jīng* 經/classic/warp correctly is the crux of what we are trying to communicate. How were the *Nàn Jīng* and *Língshū* organized, compiled and transmitted? I see these texts as an attempt to produce a multi-dimensional grid that contains the essential laws of the universe in an accessible form for physicians to draw upon. We, in essence, must "unpack" the text and apply the teachings of *gǎnyīng* 感應/resonance in a real time manner. The charts of Zhāng Shìxián 張世賢 are important tools in that respect.

Stephen: Yes this multi-dimensional grid is what I think of as "mandala-thinking" that enabled these ancients to comprehend complexity in all its non-linear ways. I see this same multidimensionality in the oracle bone and seal-form characters that simultaneously contain multiple perspectives. The "whole" speaks in imagistic and analogic language, while the parts speak in linear alphabetic logic.

Z'ev: This is a clear antithesis to "flatlands" thinking. We must be careful not to view the acupuncture channels as lines connecting points on a flat surface like a piece of paper. The channels have different depths, thicknesses, expand and contract with the seasons, lunar cycles and daily rhythms. The mandalic views revealed in Zhāng Shìxián's charts provide visualization tools to enter the complexity of human life and health, and find tools to work on multiple levels of our patients' health. Once this is done, we can apply acupuncture/ moxibustion and herbal medicines with maximum efficiency, in other words avoiding over treatment with too many needles, moxa cones or herbs.

---

[100] Larre, Rochat de la Vallée, and Root, *"Essence, Spirit, Blood and Qi,"* pg. 21.

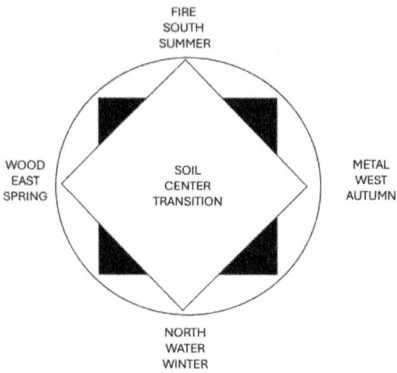

Figure 2.5 - Mandalic Map Directions & Seasons

Stephen: The clinical map described in *Nàn Jīng* 34 is constructed to give us a sense of how the body-mind functions within the context of the cycles of Nature. As previously stated in our chapter on the Four Seas, Qíbó 岐伯 advises that first the practitioner must orient themselves to the four directions. At the center of this mandala structure is the ground we stand on (*fig. 2.5*). The four directions and four seasons represent how the Heavenly cycles influence the Earth. As a clinical guide, *Nàn Jīng* 34 demonstrates how physical appearances inform us of the specific context, that is, what environmental influences are resonating with which *zàng* 臟 organs (*fig. 2.6*).

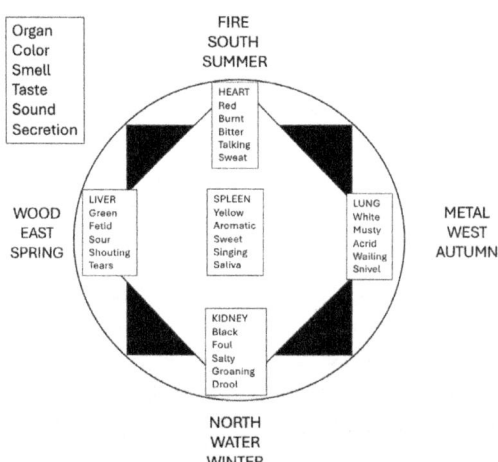

Figure 2.6 - Mandalic Map Elemental Resonances

Then, in order to complete the clinical mandalic map of a human being, the spiritual aspects that enliven our consciousness are added. This, by itself, distinguishes Chinese medicine's anatomy from the mind-body split pervasive in Western medicine. Here *Nàn Jīng* 34 raises an interesting "difficulty." If each of the *wǔ zàng* 五臟/five *zàng* organs has its complementary color, sound etc. Why/how then are there said to be seven spirit-*qì* (*shénqì* 神氣) in the *Nèijīng* 內 經?

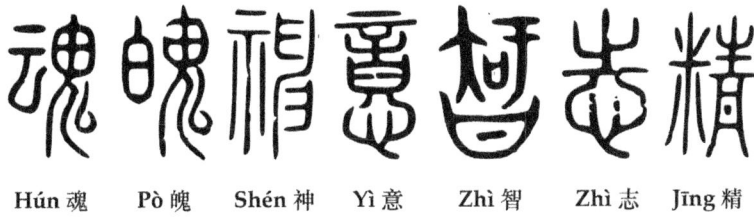

Hún 魂   **Pò** 魄   **Shén** 神   **Yì** 意   **Zhì** 智   **Zhì** 志   **Jīng** 精

Figure 2.7 - The Seven Shén

To solve the problem of five organs and seven spirits (*fig. 2.7*), the *Nàn Jīng* states that the Spleen and Kidney each house an additional "spirit-*qì*"; *yì* 意/ intention and *zhì* 志/knowledge in the spleen and *jīng* 精/essence and *zhì* 志/ will in the kidneys.

藏者，人之神氣所舍藏也

"The human zàng 臟 *store and house shénqì* 神氣*"*

The *Nàn Jīng* authors seem to be emphasizing the special importance of spleen and kidney as containing two aspects of spirit, mapping what defines human intelligence, the spirits that animate such qualities as attention, information processing, memory, planning and conceptual understanding. For the Han dynasty doctors, these aspects of spirit-consciousness reflect the influences of the celestial circle and are key aspects of the circulation of the cosmos within us.

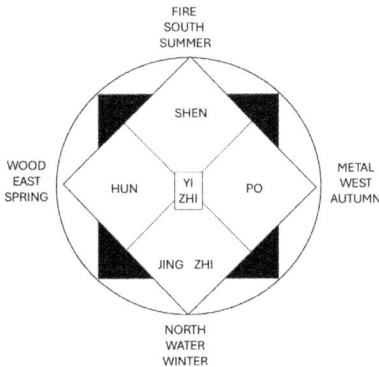

Figure 2.8 - Storage of the Seven Shén According to Nàn Jīng 34 Map

One way to consider these seven spirit-consciousness is as aspects of our own cognitive development as humans. From this perspective,

Hún 魂 - Represents "spiritual vigor." It is housed in the Liver and is associated with a kind of spirit-consciousness associated with forward thinking planning ahead. The ideogram shows an image of a cloud-ghost-spirit often referred to as "ethereal soul" that comes and goes depending on our level of wakefulness. *Hún* being associated with the liver has a relationship to the movement of blood circulation. It was this cognitive development that enabled the neolithic peoples to visualize the future, put food away in their caves in order to survive the last ice age!

Pò 魄 - Represents "physical vigor." It is housed in the lung. The ideogram shows a white-ghost-spirit often referred to as the "corporeal soul." It is said to open and close in accordance with breath. Like *yīn/yáng* or *xuè/qì*, *Hún/Pò* make a coupled unit whose whole is greater than the sum of the parts. When breath and blood circulate together we have a felt sense of physical and mental vigor.

Shén 神 - Represents "divine inspiration," the lively expansive expression of awe in our consciousness. It is housed in the heart. On the left, the ideogram shows the bright lights of the heavens (sun, moon, constellations) and on the right, two hands extending and grasping what some say is an image of lightning, meaning grasping the "divine power." *Shén* housed in the heart is one aspect of the seven *shénqì* 神氣 spoken about in *Nàn Jīng*. As with *Hún/Pò*, the *Shén* of the heart forms a couple with *jīng*, housed in the kidney.

Jīng 精 - Essence as a "spirit" is an interesting concept. We normally think about *jīng* as the essential material form necessary for life, something akin to our DNA, sperm and ovum. As an aspect of cognition, *jīng* has the "spirit of arousal/vitality," that quality that *Lǎozǐ* 老子 55 notes is "*the extreme jīng of the newborn. Who has tender bones and muscles yet their grasp is so strong and though they have no concept of sex,*"[101] the newborn males have spontaneous erections! I think of this quality of arousal/vitality-consciousness as what the Zen masters call "beginner's mind." *Jīng* is the spirit of tremendous potential within us. In the *jīng* ideogram, there is the image of a single grain of rice that carries the feeling of life ready to burst open. This is what Thoreau calls "the faith in a seed." It is this faith in our own seed-potential that has a sense of time and patience: the knowledge that fruit takes time to grow from a seed. It's the same spirit-consciousness that a mother senses when the fetus firsts kicks. *Jīng*

---

[101] *Lǎozǐ* 老子 55 translation/interpretation S. Cowan.

consciousness is small and subtle, as *Lǎozǐ* 52 advises us: *"perceiving the small is clear-sightedness, safeguarding the tender is strength."*[102]

This same seed consciousness is released when something complex has been broken down to its smallest microcosmic form, like splitting an atom or more to the point, the way we digest food from Nature in order to release its essences. *Jīng* refers to the quality of food that is invigorating, nourishing life. Sometimes you can taste the love in food prepared for you. That is *jīng* - spirit consciousness. From a cognitive perspective *jīng* - intelligence is what a master chef manifests when adding a pinch of salt to the food being prepared to bring out the flavors (salt of course being one association with the water phase (kidneys). It's interesting to note that specific phytochemicals exhibit biphasic dose-response on cellular function: low doses activating signaling pathways that result in expression of genes encoding cyto-protective proteins, whereas high dose block it. Mindless eating leads to over-eating which misses this subtle awareness completely (so do most western trained doctors!). However from a cognitive perspective *jīng*-spirit corresponds to how one processes information, breaks it down in order to release the deeper meanings hidden within it. I tend to think that from a Chinese perspective, these *jīng spirits engender analogic meanings* rather than analytic.

Z'ev: This idea of "potential" is really a key to the unfolding of the channels that are the scaffolding of the human entity. This understanding is key to how to treat disharmonies and illnesses, by recognizing essential patterning, along with the *xié qì* 邪氣 / pathogenic influences that distort these essential patterns that form the human being. Within this is the secret of the 'magic' of acumoxa-therapy and how it is able to correct so many conditions.

The *Língshū* 靈樞 and *Sùwèn* 素問 discuss in terms of how illnesses progress through the channel system, navigating the body / mind 'landscape' and settling into vacuous areas and hiding there. These are usually seen as pockets of cold that must be "excavated" and expressed outwards by relieving blockages in the channels. When one palpates the vessels, blockages are revealed. For example, it is very common in my practice to find that the *guān* 關 / gate and *cùn* 寸 / inch pulses on either or both wrists are crowded up against each other, leaving the *chǐ* 尺 / foot pulse below empty. This usually indicates a blockage in the diaphragm, or counterflow *qì*. I will usually find that breathing is inhibited, or that there is emotional blockage encumbering the heart and liver from their full expression. In those cases, one may needle the *juéyīn* 厥陰, *shàoyáng* 少陽, *shàoyīn* 少陰 or *tàiyáng* 太陽 channels to open these areas. If there is spleen / central *qì* involvement, one raises the clear *yáng* and descends turbid *yīn* by

---

[102] *Lǎozǐ* 老子 52 translation / interpretation S. Cowan.

employing methods developed by Lǐ Dōngyuán 李東垣' in his *Pí Wèi Lùn* 脾胃論 / *Treatise on the Spleen and Stomach.*[103]

Over the centuries of Chinese medicine, strategies have been developed to access *jīng* 精 / essence in practice. I often will treat, for example, paired *yuán xué* 原穴 points such as *yáng chí* 陽池 / yang pool (TB 4) and *qiū xū* 丘墟 / mound of ruins (GB 40) on opposite limbs to access and facilitate *shàoyáng yuán qì* 少陽原氣 circulation, or *tài xī* 太谿 / supreme stream (Kid 3) with *shén mén* 神門 / spirit gate (Ht 7) for *shàoyīn* 少陰, *tài chōng* 太沖 / great rushing (Liv 3) with *dà líng* 大陵 / great mound (PC 7) for *juéyīn* 厥陰. Combined with associated back *shù* (*bèi shù xué* 背俞穴) and front *mù* points (*mù xué* 募穴), these treatment strategies invoke the *yuán qì* 原氣 to circulate and heal from deep within the body. We can also access *yuán qì* via the *bié* 別 / branching (diverging) channels, which tap directly into *yuán qì*.

I see many cases of exhaustion, i.e. *láosǔn* 勞損 / taxation detriment in practice, as we live in a culture that runs our patients "through the mill" of emotional, physical and mental exhaustion. Paradoxically, such patients find themselves unable to sleep properly, and often attach themselves to unhealthy lifestyles or emotional strategies to keep going. Just today I saw a patient who is vegan (not really appropriate for her, as she is thin, nervous with tremors, and cold natured), and works 60 hour weeks managing business seminars. She is fifty years old, single, no children, and recently lost one of her aging pets that sent her into a state of high grief. She has bloating, poor digestion, hasn't slept normally in weeks because of her grief, tremors in her legs, with spinning bean pulses in her *cùn* 寸 / *guān* 關 positions, and empty *chǐ* 尺 position. Her tongue is swollen, pale with a glassy ice-like coating.

I treated kidney divergent points on the back, *tiān zhù* 天柱 / celestial pillar (Bl 10) and *shèn shū* 腎俞 / kidney shu (Bl 23) with moxa, *yīn gǔ* 陰谷 / yin valley (Kid 10), *shēn mài* 申脈 / extending vessel (Bl 62), *gān shū* 肝俞 / liver shu (Bl 18) and *dà cháng shū* 大腸俞 / large intestine shu (Bl 25) with moxa. I then turned her over and treated her at Kid 3 (*tài xī* 太谿) with *tōng lǐ* 通里 / penetrating the interior (Ht 5) (opposite and unilaterally), *gōng sūn* 公孫 / grandfather grandson (Sp 4) with *nèi guān* 內關 / inner pass (PC 6) to open the *chōng mài* 衝脈, and abdominal points such as *zhāng mén* 章門 / cycle gate (Liv 13) and *guān yuán* 關元 / gate of origin (Ren 4) with moxa. Her main herbal formula is *fù zǐ lǐ zhōng wán* 附子理中丸 / aconite accessory root pill, but since she had recently recovered from pneumonia and bronchitis, during that time I had given her formulas such as *chái hú guì zhī gān jiāng tāng* 柴胡桂枝干姜汤 / bupleurum,

---

[103] See my examples at the end of *"Thoughts on Repairing (Mending) the Broken Vessel (Ring),"* pg. 239-240

cinnamon twig and dried ginger decoction, and *xiǎo chái hú tang* 小 柴胡湯 /
minor bupleurum decoction with *Líng guì zhú gān tāng* 苓桂術甘湯 / poria,
cinnamon twig, white atractylodes and licorice decoction.

Stephen: Well said! Indeed this capacity of releasing potential to heal is one
of the keys to understanding biologic flow dynamics, so important in the
context of circulation. Besides the rice kernel image, the ideogram for *jīng* also
contains the character *qīng* 青, the color blue-green. Green is the color of our
tiny blue-green planet spinning in space. Green to me has the ecological sense
of "going green," honoring the gift of life we find in our smallest connections to
Nature, mother earth providing us with nourishment.

The *Nàn Jīng* authors however state that the kidneys store a second spirit-
consciousness in addition to *jīng*.

Zhì 志 - Which as a spirit-consciousness related to cognition is defined as a
sense of purpose, passion, drive, will-power, perseverance, determination. The
pictogram shows a tiny seedling emerging from the ground, with the heart-
mind beneath it. This captures the spirit of a plant reaching up to the sky. One
can see the close relationship between *jīng* and *Zhì* as they relate to seed and
sprout, to the spirit of manifesting our potential that defines the arousal / vitality
we feel in nature which is so critical to our survival amidst the challenges and
changes of life.

And lastly we have the two spirits *Yì* 意 and *Zhì* 智 that are housed in the
spleen.

Yì 意 - As a spirit-consciousness related to cognition is translated as thought,
intention, idea, meaning. The ideogram contains the heart-mind beneath the
character of a mouth with something in it, meaning a tone or sound. The
heartbeat is the intention of the heart to do something. The heart-mind's
intention is to circulate ideas. Our constant stream of thoughts carries the
intention of thinking things out. The spleen is responsible for processing
information (not just in the form of food), transforming and transporting it to
the various places it belongs.

Zhì 智 - Translated as knowledge, intelligence, comprehension, or "know-
how" is sometimes translated as wisdom. The ideogram is said to show an
arrow on the left and a mouth on the right which by itself means understanding
zhi 知 and when the sun is placed below it, gives a bigger feeling of "Aha! Now
I get it."

The *Nàn Jīng* completes the human circulatory map by pointing out that there
are many different kinds of human knowing. Intuitive knowing of the heart.
Factual knowledge of the lung. Spatial and directional knowing of the liver and

of course inferential and conceptual knowledge of the kidneys. As we see in Zhāng Shìxián's diagram, the spleen-soil sits at the very center of the mandala for a reason!!!

Its job is to contain all these ways of knowing, to connect them all so that they're all related, so that they tell a story. This is the digestion of information and transformation into meaning *zhì yì* 智意. In western psychology it may, in some ways, be akin to what is called "working memory." This is the spleen's ability to hold different ideas in one's mind at the same time.

Z'ev: This is where Antonio Damasio's concept of "distributed mind" (i.e. consciousness) from his book *The Strange Order of Things: Life, Feeling, and the Making of Cultures* comes in (*fig. 2.9*).

Damasio challenges the traditional views by proposing that the "mind" is not solely confined to the brain but instead is distributed across the entire body. This perspective reinforces the concept of a unified relationship between the mind/body, and the dynamic interactions between the brain, body's physiological states, and environment. Consciousness is not "brain-centric" as in neuroscience, it is distributed throughout the body/mind and "stored" in its various aspects in the *zàng* 臟 and extraordinary fu (*qí héng zhī fǔ* 奇恆之腑). When consciousness is distributed throughout the organism, we are no longer "top heavy," relying only on the brain and ignoring the body's role. A prime modern example is the "brain-gut connection," where essential neurotransmitters in the brain are produced and synthesized in the gastrointestinal tract. There is a "feedback system" between the GI tract and the brain, and recent research about the microbiomes indicates that one of the best ways to treat brain/CNS disorders is by cultivating the gut microbiome with "neurobiotics." Early Han dynasty texts state that "the viscera store emotions and qì."[104] Specifically in *Língshū* 6, "*wind and cold harm the form, while grief, fear, rage and anger harm the qi.*"[105]

---

[104] Hsu, *"Pulse Diagnosis in Early Chinese Medicine: The Telling Touch,"* pg. 26: *"the viscera, rather than gaining importance within medicine as proto-anatomical entities may have become medically significant as storage places for feelings and qi."*

[105] ibid., pg. 37.

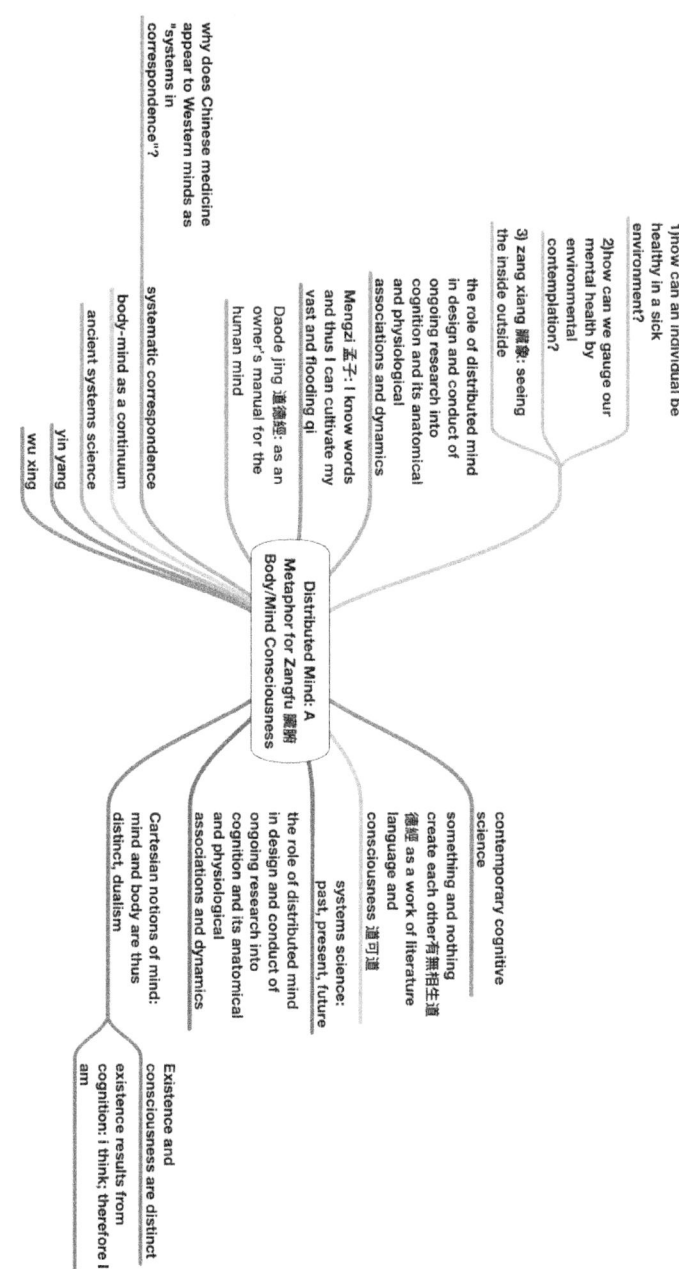

Figure 2.9 - Distributed Mind[106]

---

[106] Original diagram by Ken Rose, updated/revised by Z'ev Rosenberg.

Stephen: In our current digital society, the problem of too much information can all to easily overwhelm us, leading to accumulation disorders emanating from the spleen. This manifests as obsessive overthinking, worry, procrastination and of course phlegm which the spleen then passes on to the lung causing further confusion, fixation, agitation, anxiety and a breakdown of mandala, a sign of our times.

Z'ev: Unfortunately the "false flag" education in TCM is a prime culprit. The material is based on rote memorization rather than synthesis and deep connection and understanding. It leads to spleen accumulation, and counterintuitive lifestyles and study habits that lead to spleen vacuity issues.

In my 23 years teaching at a TCM school, while I had some 'academic freedom' to teach from my source texts, experience and understanding, there was always the pressure to teach to school, state and national exams, which pressed the education into a more didactic, "flatlined" approach based on memorization of separate points, herbs, illnesses and protocols. This completely eliminated the real time observations revealed in the clinical mandalas Stephen describes here. The focus was on *zàngfǔ* 臟腑 diagnosis (called, inaccurately eight principle/*bā gāng* 八綱 diagnosis), which is the basis of TCM herbal practice, where formulas are fitted to specific *zàngfǔ* syndromes in a fixed manner. This works poorly, in my opinion with acupuncture/moxibustion unless one studies more sophisticated physicians such as Qín Bówèi 秦伯末 (1901-1970). One case comes to mind of a regular patient in the school clinic who had a different intern and supervisor every week, and looking over their file in a clinical review class I noted that each week the patient had a different diagnosis, formula and acupuncture treatment based on entirely disconnected *zàngfǔ* diagnoses.

Stephen: The *Lǎozǐ* advises that this condition of overthinking requires purging the clutter, closing the doors (shut down your computer), settle the dust, to ensure healthy mind-body-spirit circulation in navigating our ever-changing relationships, that enables us to maintain a grounded sense of "orderly chaos."

Z'ev: Living the lessons of Tang dynasty mountains and rivers poetry is essential. Hikes in nature, experiencing the sentience of the universe. I like to view herbal medicine as a condensation of environmental *qì* applied to the body/mind. Classical formulas are designed to raise, lower, scatter, and condense *zhèng qì* 正氣/correct *qì*, and expel *xié qì* 邪氣/perverse *qì* from the channel system. A formula such as *dìng zhì wán* 定志丸/settle the will pill, for example, will fortify the kidneys and heart/mind while concurrently *kāiqiào* 開竅/opening the orifices of the mind and heart.[107]

Stephen: Living according to the multidimensional mandalic principles of the map described in *Nàn Jīng* 34, implies that we live as relational beings, always in context with our surroundings, never as isolated absolutes. These relationships define the health of our circulation, give meaning to our life and enable us to continuously transform.

---

[107] For a detailed discussion of *dìng zhì wán* 定志丸/settle the will pill, see *Afterglow: Ministerial Fire and Chinese Ecological Medicine*, pg. 123-127 and "*Meditations on Dìng Zhì Wán* 定志丸 *(Settle the Emotions Pill)*." *Journal of Chinese Medicine*, no. Issue 135 (June 2024): 48–51.

Wǔxíng 五行 **Relationships and Causality in the *Nàn Jīng* 難經**

Stephen Cowan & Z'ev Rosenberg

"Two conditions - gravity and a livable temperature range between freezing and boiling - have given us fluids and flesh. The trees we climb and the ground we walk on have given us five fingers and toes. The "place" (from the root 'plat': broad, spreading, flat) gave us far-seeing eyes, the streams and breezes gave us versatile tongues and whorly ears. The land gave us a stride, and the lake a dive. The amazement gave us our kind of mind. We should be thankful for that and take Nature's stricter lessons with some grace."
- Gary Snyder[108]

Stephen: "Fluids and flesh" as Gary Snyder says, are the essence of our healthy adaptation to life on planet Earth. The *Nàn Jīng* 難經 advances such an understanding of the way we follow the laws (*fǎ* 法) of Nature, as originally put forth in the *Nèijīng* 內經. However the *Nàn Jīng* emphasizes the dynamic flow of fluids through the flesh and organ networks. The *wǔxíng* 五行 / five movements (phases) and the *yīnyáng* 陰陽 dynamics have their origins in the *Yijīng* 易經 / *Classic of Changes* where they were correlated with our internal and external landscapes. The relationship between organ networks communicate through vessels just as rivers and streams run through the valleys between mountain ranges. It's important to remember that the fluids are not independent of the flesh anymore than are the rivers independent of the mountains. The mapping of the *wǔxíng* five movement-phases follow this nature-based logic of relationships, *yīnyáng* being the fundamental relativity of all life.

In *Sùwèn* 素問 5 we find the process of the five phases functioning as resonances (*gǎn* 感), microcosms "humming," as Sabine Wilms says [109], with the imagery / metaphors (*xiàng* 象) of Heavens and Earth. Throughout the *Nàn Jīng* this understanding of how the relational rhythms between the five phases is

---

[108] Snyder and Hass, *"The Practice of the Wild,"* pg. 31.

[109] See Wilms,,*"Humming with Elephants: The Great treatise on the Resonant Manifestations of Yin and Yang: A Translation and Discussion of Chapter Five of the Yellow Emperor's Inner Classic Plain Questions."*

expressed as health or disease under the influence of the natural *kè* 剋 and *shēng* 生 cycles. Just as the paths which streams and rivers take will always depend on the nature and contours of the mountainside, likewise the pathways that our blood vessels, nerves and fascia form will always depend on their five phase relationships. The *Nánjīng* authors recognized that diseases manifest whenever the harmonic flow within these relationships is cut off.

As with any landscape, everything in the classics was mapped in such a way as to help the clinician more effectively navigate the cyclical rhythms of the five phase relationships. *Nánjīng* Difficulty 40 takes the question of these relational correspondences even further. As Unschuld translates:

"The explanation given in the answer has been interpreted by some authors as referring, for the first time in this book, to a relationship among the five phases that is more sophisticated than the sequences of mutual generation (shēng) and destruction (kè) quoted earlier. This third relationship among the Five Phases is known as wǔxíng zhǎng shēng 五行長生 *(literally, five phase long life/birth)."*[110]

It is the inter-relationships *between* the phases explained in *Nàn Jīng* 40 that offer an ecological map of how the four directions/four seasons awaken our senses which in turn affect the liveliness of organ function. For example, *Nàn Jīng* 40 states that lung/sense of smell corresponds to metal phase which comes to life during the earthly branch *sì* 巳 which happens to be the summer season (corresponding to fire). Thus metal is awakened during the fires of summer and this is how the *Nàn Jīng* explains why the heart *controls* the sense of smell.

As mentioned in the earlier chapter on the maps of Zhāng Shìxián 張世賢 the example here offers an extensive perspective of this dynamic third relationship (time) that correlates with our lifespan: the four seasons being a metaphor for raising a child thus demonstrating a revolutionary kind of *"ring without end"* mandala as follows:

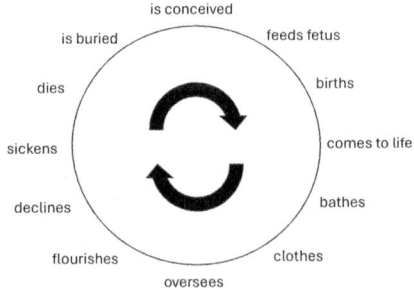

Figure 2.10 - Developmental Sequence Mandala

---

[110] Unschuld (2016), *"Nan Jing: The Classic of Difficult Issues,"* pg. 339.

This developmental sequence (*fig. 2.10*) generates an elaborate map of interrelations based on the 12 earthly branches as follows:

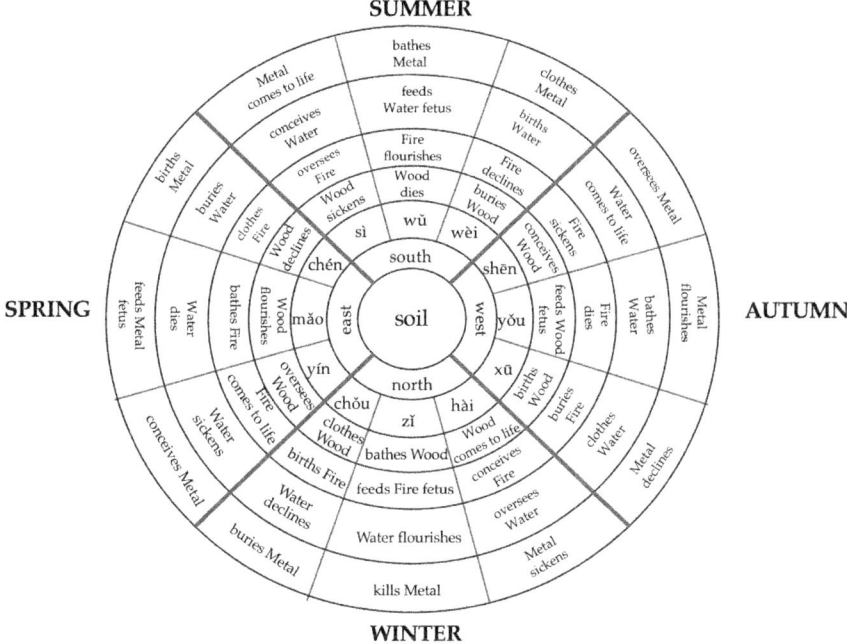

Figure 2.11 - Nàn Jīng 40 Map

Zhāng's map (*fig. 2.11*) enables us to see the multi-dimensionality of inter-relations between the four seasons and the five phases. For example, it describes how Wood (plant life) flourishes in spring, (while simultaneously) Water (ice) dies, Fire is bathed, and the Metal fetus is fed. Following this logic, Metal flourishes in autumn, (while simultaneously) Water is bathed, Fire dies and the Wood is fed. It is this simultaneity that releases us from the linear-logic progression of the five phases so often depicted in modern Chinese medical literature.

Péng Zĭyì 彭子益 (1871-1949) said "*the circular dynamic of the five elements is completely integrated and cannot be separated; the human body is also thus. Diseases of the five elements (phases) are all due to a loss of this circular dynamic, which in turn leads to separation of their individual roles and loss of integration. The role of the middle qi is to maintain the integration of the five elements.*"[111]

---

[111] McMahon, "*Circular Dynamics of Ancient Chinese Medicine I,*" pg. 1.

Zhāng's map clearly emphasizes the central role of earth/soil in maintaining relational integrity. As it was conceived in the ancient *Yìjīng*/*Book of Changes* and *luò shū* 洛書/inscription of the river *luò* and *hé tú* 河圖/yellow river map (*fig. 2.12*). Soil/Earth is the "fifth" movement/phase that sits in the middle of the other four movements.

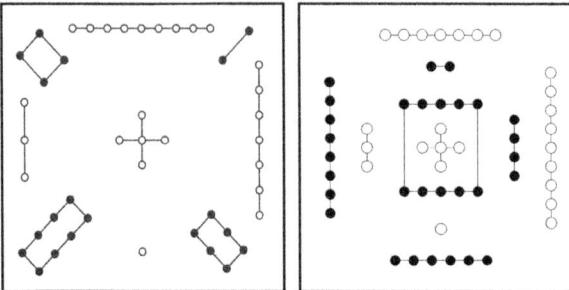

Figure 2.12 - Luò Shū 洛書/Inscription of the River Luo (left) and Hé Tú 河圖/Yellow River Map (right)

This soil-phase is right beneath our feet and represents the very ground we stand on. Like a GPS system, it personalizes our relationship with Nature, telling us where we are at any given moment. It is the center that ensures that the four directions, four seasons, four "other" *xíng* 行 movement-phases always relate to each other! The *Yìjīng* tells us that from the still point center, we can witness the reality that the only constant is change (*biàntōng* 變通) and that all change and transformation is nothing but relationships. In the clinical mandala described in our previous chapter, the central position of the earth/soil spleen corresponds to the spirit-consciousness of *zhī yì* 知意, meaning/understanding which can only come from how we relate to the world around us. Chinese medicine is emphatic that this relational stance is never absolute but always relative to the context of circulating seasons. Indeed this is how the *Yìjīng* generates meaning (*zhī yì*) within the Space-Time that one happens to be in. Lǐ Dōngyuán 李東垣 highlighted this Earth-centric circulation in the *Pí Wèi Lùn* 脾胃论 stating:

> *"the spleen qi spreads essence which gathers in the lungs and frees the flow of water passageways, transporting fluids down to the urinary bladder. Water essence spreads in the four directions and the five channels run side by side in agreement with the four seasons, five viscera, and the measurements of yin/yang. This is how normalcy is kept."*[112]

For me, understanding this dynamic ecological *wǔxíng* 五行 map was a life-changing event that transformed my medical career. 30 years ago, Efrem

---

[112] Li, & Flaws, *"Li Dong-Yuan's Treatise on the Spleen & Stomach: A Translation of the Pi Wei Lun,"* pg. 4.

Korngold taught me how to use the classic *wǔxíng* map (*fig. 2.13*) with each patient in recording their history and symptoms according to their correspondences in order to determine which dynamic dyads and triads are causing disorder to manifest. This is a completely different way of understanding complexity and causality than I had been taught in the linear-logic of Western medicine.

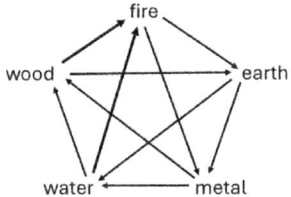

Figure 2.13 - Wǔxíng 五行 Map

Because each of us has a unique constitutional orientation within the five phases, the *wǔxíng* map helps clarify why the same disharmonies may express themselves differently in different individuals, thus making the treatment extremely personalized.

In practice I've adapted this dynamic mapping to explain symptom causality to parents and children. Assessing a child's primary constitutional style, I then explain the relationship with the other four element/movement-phases, calling the *shēng relationships* "the helpers" which promote healthy flow of *xuèqì* 血氣 and allow a person to effectively share their natural gifts with the world. I call the *kè relationships* "the challengers," which help promote resilience in the face of change. We need both helpers and challengers to be in healthy balanced flow in order to grow. Furthermore, in observing the way children grow, I have come to realize that our constitutional orientation is not a fixed archetype, but rather, is constantly being colored by the particular phase of life we find ourselves in. This ensures the complexity of life is constantly alive and changing.

This explains why a person suffering from a liver-spleen disharmony will express a different degree of symptoms depending on their primary constitutional orientation at a particular phase of their life as well. For example someone who has a primary Fire constitution versus someone with a primary Metal constitution in the face of a wood-soil/*kè* imbalance, will manifest different symptoms in accordance with the orientation of the *wǔxíng* map:

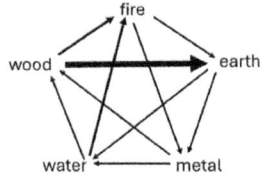

Figure 2.14 - Wood Overacting on Earth

In the first scenario above, Fire depends on its *shēng* helper cycle (wood/earth) for smooth flow of circulation (physically, cognitively and spiritually. When Wood overtakes the Earth/Soil (liver/spleen disharmony) (*fig. 2.14*), exaggerated symptoms of heat and agitation are likely to be the presenting symptoms.

In the second scenario, Metal depends on its helper Earth/Soil for nourishment but when Wood is challenging Earth/soil, it causes Metal to be prone to symptoms of accumulation of damp phlegm produced by spleen and respiratory symptoms ensue due to further invasion of wind (wood) (*fig. 2.15*).

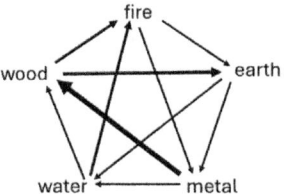

Figure 2.15 - Metal Overacting on Wood

The *wŭxíng* map, as elaborated in the *Nàn Jīng*, is yet another example of Chinese Medicine's effective way of navigating complexity, by seeing the ecological causes and conditions of disease patterns. This ensures that our perceptions remain fresh and open to changing relationships each time we meet a patient, selecting acupoint combinations and prescribing herbal medicines appropriate to that particular moment in time, always with the intent on promoting healthy flowing circulation. As a famous Chinese medicine quote by Lǐ Zhōngzǐ 李中梓 stated in the *Nèijīng Zhī Yào* 内经知要, "*tōngzé bù tòng bù tōngzé tòng* 通则不痛 不通则痛 "*when there is healthy flow there is no suffering. When there is suffering, there is no healthy flow.*"

Z'ev: This concept of *tōng* 通 represents the natural flow and movement within the body, mirroring the circular dynamic of the five elements. This dynamic is completely integrated and cannot be separated; the human body is also thus. When this *tōng* is balanced, energy, blood, and vital substances circulate smoothly, ensuring harmony and health. Diseases of the five elements arise when this circular dynamic is disrupted, leading to stagnation (no-flow) or excessive movement (too much flow). Both conditions disrupt the unity of the five elements, which in turn leads to a separation of their individual roles and loss of integration.

Zang-Energy	No Flow (Deficient) (Too Little)	Excessive Flow (Too Much)
Liver Wood Rising	*Too Little Fire Qì Stored in Water* • No sweat • No urine • No bowel movement • Abdominal pain • Intercostal pain • Delayed menstruation	*Too Little Metal Qì* • Spontaneous sweating • Excessive urination • Nocturnal emission • Fever • Dizziness • Tinnitus • Leucorrhea and shortened menstruation in women
Lung Metal Gathering	*Too Much (Excessive) Rising of Wood Qì* • Excessive sweating • Dizziness • Fever • Cough • Wheezing • Nocturnal emission • Excessive urination • Diseases of atrophy	*Too Little Expansive Fire Qì* • Aversion to cold • Constipation • Epigastric stuffiness • Absent Sweating
Heart Fire Opening/Expanding	*Too Little Fire in Wood, No Rising* • Blood obstruction • Spiritual lassitude • Lack of flavor in the mouth • Blood cold	*Too Little Middle Qì Thus Too Little Metal Qì Descending* • Pain in the tongue • Pain in the throat • Palpitations • Frustration

Kidney Water Storing	*Too Little Gathering Metal Qì* • Floating yang • Dizziness • Fever • Edema of the feet	*No Symptoms of Too Much* Storing Kidney-Water Yang
Spleen Earth Transport	*Too Little Attachment* • Abdominal fullness • Food stasis • Vomiting • Diarrhea • Heaviness of the four limbs • Lassitude of the entire body	*Too Much Attachment* • Earth Qì Stagnation (Too much solid) • Too Little Transformation & Transportation
Minister Igniting/Warming	*Too Little Yuán Qì Storage* • Cold in the lower half of the body, • The kidneys will be cold, Spleen Stomach function will be poor, • With difficulty controlling both urination and bowel movements.	*No Too Much!* *(No Too Much Yuán Qì)* • But failure of Minister fire to descend = • Burning heat in the exterior • The greater the burning heat is without, the more deficient the minister fire is within

Thoughts on *Shēntǐ Tú* 身体圖/Body Maps:
Channels, Terrains and Clinical Gaze

Z'ev Rosenberg & Stephen Cowan

Z'ev: The crux of the problem in understanding Chinese medicine and its foundational theories is how modern biomedicine and Westernized cultures view nature and the human organism. This misunderstanding is specifically seen with channel theory. Whereas modern Western anatomy views the "stuff" and contents of internal organs, vessels and structures, Chinese medicine's main interest was to map the terrain at the exterior of the organism based on the *Nèijīng* 內經 principle of *zàng xiàng* 臟象/visceral manifestation, imaging the interior by location and timing in locations that resonate with the interior structures. This view of the human organism as a landscape, has been a defining template of Chinese medicine since formative years in the Han dynasty. Without adapting, studying and embodying this specific "clinical gaze," as Foucault defined the doctor's view of the human organism[113], we will find it impossible both to understand and practice Chinese medicine effectively beyond protocols and point/herb prescriptions. We may use needles and herbs as our tools and without this clear understanding we will not have a solid foundation. It is not the technology of medicine that defines the system, but the underlying principles and theories that are practiced.

Viewing the various representations of acupuncture channels and *xué* 穴/holes, we see that there is little attempt to accurately display what the human body looks like either inside or outside. These are diagrammatic representations of movements, transformations, and locations in time and space. Just as topographical maps of landscapes are not what the landscape actually looks like, but rather serve to effectively navigate the terrain which we are choosing to explore, the *Nàn Jīng* 難經, *Sùwèn* 素問, and *Língshū* 靈樞 are precision maps based on time, location, transformation and movements in the human organism, never losing sight of how these resonate with earthly landscapes, which breathe, expand, contract, transform according to and in relation with the laws of *yīnyáng*, season, phase, and direction.

---

[113] Michel Foucault's *The Birth of the Clinic (Routledge, 2003)*, and the discussion regrading this in my previous books, *Returning to the Source* (Singing Dragon, 2018) Chapter 4 and *Ripples in the Flow* (Singing Dragon, 2019) Chapter 2.

As Paul Unschuld points out in his book *What is Medicine: Western and Eastern Approaches to Healing,* the body does not speak with its own language outright. Modern (Western) anatomy is no more "real" than a representational grid. Symptoms, signs, colors, structures, must always be interpreted by the human mind. Western anatomy is just another, more "materialistic" interpretation of the "stuff" that makes up the human being, broken into smaller and smaller parts. Valuable, yet limited.

The value of Chinese medicine today, is to provide an alternative perspective of human life and health, a philosophy that is both ecological and curative to humanity, sentient beings and the earth itself. To heal oneself is to heal the earth, to heal the earth is to heal oneself. Polluted streams resonate with veins and arteries clogged by cholesterol and plaque, toxic landfills with guts accumulated with toxins.

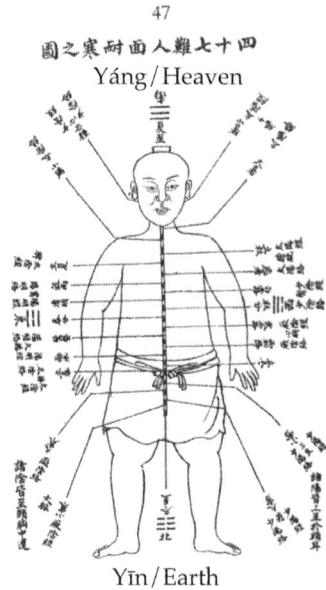

Figure 2.16 - Nàn Jīng 47 Map[114]

Stephen: Zhāng's anatomic map of *Nàn Jīng* Difficulty 47 (*fig. 2.16*) is a good example of the Chinese clinical gaze. The question asked is: *"Only man's face can stand cold. Why is that so?"*[115] To illustrate the answer to this question by mapping the dynamic terrain of "movements, transformations, and locations in time and space," as Z'ev says, we can see Zhāng's mapping of Qíbó's response:

---

[114] Unschuld (1986), *"Nan-ching: The Classic of Difficult Issues,"* pg. 707 - Zhāng Shìxián 張世賢's map entitled *"Nàn Jīng 難經 47: The Human Face is Resistant to the Cold.*

[115] Unschuld (2016), *"Nan Jing: The Classic of Difficult Issues,"* pg. 376.

"*The human head is the meeting place of all the yang [vessels]. All the yin vessels reach into the neck and chest from which they return. Only all the Yang vessels reach upward into the head. Hence they let the face endure the cold.*"[116]

Z'ev: *Nàn Jīng* 47 is largely based on *Língshū* 靈樞 38, which is a sublime expression of the role of the physician plays as architect and artisan, based on the laws of heaven/human/earth and the mapping of the acupuncture channels:

匠人不能釋尺寸而意短長，廢繩墨而起平水也，工人不能置規而為圓，去矩而
為方。知用此者，固自然之物，易用之教，逆順之常也。

"*An artisan must not neglect foot and inch, and estimate lengths. [He must not] disregard measure tape and ink, and attempt to create a plane surface. A worker must not discard the compass when he draws a circle, and must not lay aside the ruler when he generates a square. To know how to use these [tools], is a matter of course. These are instructions that are easy to use, and they entail the regularity of movements contrary to and in accordance with the norms.*"
-*Língshū* 靈樞 38[117]

Here Qíbó is clearly stating the importance of basing clinical practice on the foundations based on these laws. When applied to conundrums as described in *Nàn Jīng* 47 "*Only Man's Face Can Withstand Cold*," these foundations allow one to apply the logic that all of the *yáng* channels rise to the head to nourish the sense organs with *yáng qì*, blood and essence. The warmth generated by this movement keeps the face warmer than the extremities, which are not as critical to human life as a hierarchy.

Continuing in *Língshū* 38, here is a concrete metaphor demonstrating how we can view the channel flows and work to restore their potency and health:

臨深決水、不用功力、而水可竭也。循掘決沖，而經可通也。此言氣之滑澀、
血水清 濁，行之逆順也。

"*If one is faced with a deep [pond] from which the water is to be drained without the use of force, the water can be drained entirely nevertheless. This is done by digging a hole to open a runoff, and the stream can pass through it. That is meant by "whether the [flow of the] qi is smooth or rough, and whether the blood is clear or turbid, this is where a movement contrary to or in accordance with the norms is realized.*"[118]

---

[116] ibid., pg. 376.

[117] Unschuld, "*Huang Di Nei Jing Ling Shu: The Ancient Classic on Needle Therapy*," pg. 394.

[118] ibid., pg. 394.

The Chinese physician views the body as a landscape, and acts to open up streams and ponds, secure the flow of *qìxuè* and fluids, following the laws of *shùn* 順 and *nì* 逆. While this is a completely different "mind set" from modern biomedicine, there is nothing difficult or contrived in adapting this view of life and practicum. It is no accident that the Chinese medical classics were largely influenced by philosophical works and the lives of its authors, including the *Yìjīng* 易經, *Lǎozǐ* 老子 and *Zhuāngzǐ* 莊子, along with the great "Mountains and Rivers" poets.

The Space-Time Map of *Xuèqì* 血氣: *A Radical Rethinking of Blood-Qì*

Stephen Cowan & Z'ev Rosenberg

"In the world described by quantum mechanics there is no reality except in the relations between physical systems. It isn't things that enter into relations but, rather, relations that ground the notion of 'thing.'"
- Carlo Rovelli[119]

Stephen: *Nàn Jīng* 難經 Difficulty 32 is a further development of the space-time map of life put forth in *Nàn Jīng* 30 which introduces the *Ring Without End* principle of *yíngwèi* 營衛 circulation.[120]

While *Nàn Jīng* 31 traces the source of *yíngwèi* to the *sānjiāo* 三焦 (triple warmer), *Nàn Jīng* 32 examines the correlation between special anatomic locations of the heart and lung above the diaphragm (in the upper burner) as a metaphor for the intimate relationship of *xuèqì* 血氣/blood-*qì* that defines the source of vitality in life. It poses an interesting question: why are the heart and lungs located in a specially-dedicated space in the chest, anatomically separated from the other organs in the body? In this profound question, we see the sage-physicians clearly attempting to correlate metaphoric meaning to anatomical location.

Z'ev: We should, of course, address the diaphragm as separation of above and below in the body, and the role of the fascia.

Stephen: Yes indeed. The whole idea of membranes is an important topic when discussing the *sānjiāo*/Triple Burner function which the classics say is the master of the waterways (aka. fluid dynamics). In *Nàn Jīng* 38, Lǐ Jiōng 李駉's commentary states that *"the Triple Burner is nothing but membranes attached to the upper, central and lower openings of the stomach (digestive system). The triple burner has a name but no form"*[121] This idea of membranes as a special place of activity,

---

[119] See Rovelli, and Segre, *"Reality is Not What it Seems: The Journey to Quantum Gravity."*

[120] See MindNode in *Appendix II: Blueprints and Charts from Z'ev's Notebook* pg. 291.

[121] Unschuld (2016), *"Nan Jing: The Classic of Difficult Issues,"* pg. 332.

functioning as a meeting place for exchange is a radical reimagining of anatomic structure. From this perspective, we can see the *sānjiāo* functions as part of the Earth phase, related to digestion but also as a process of exchange anywhere in the body, particularly as it relates to blood perfusion in the lung where oxygen and carbon dioxide are exchanged. Again, this highlights the concept of membranes as part of the communication system within the body.

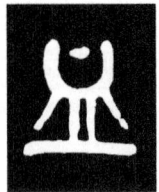

Figure 2.17 - Xuè 血

Dating back into shamanic neolithic times there was a human conception of blood as a sacred substance. The oracle bone ideogram (*fig. 2.17*) shows a sacrificial chalice with a drop of blood thought to represent a sacred ritual that honors what makes us alive. Paleontologists find evidence of ritual sacrifices of blood around the world.

The concept of blood as a living substance comes closer to "*xuèqì*," as a coupled relationship reflecting *yīn-yáng* inter-being. Blood without *qì* is like stagnant water sometimes referred to as "dead water." In *Nàn Jīng* Difficulty 32, there is a clear emphasis on the importance of circulation as the key to life. The idea of Blood/Qì circulation being fundamental for living relates to the statement in *Sùwèn* 素問 5 "*that yīnyáng is the basis and beginning of life.*" I think *Nàn Jīng* 32 is providing this statement from the *Nèijīng* 內經 with a clear anatomic correlation.

Z'ev: I also appreciate the various locations in *Língshū* 靈樞 and *Sùwèn* where blood oaths are taken!!

Stephen: By this logic we can see an important sequence in *Nàn Jīng* 32:

血爲榮, 氣爲衛

Xuè wèi róng, qì wèi wèi

The *wèi* 爲 here has multiple (simultaneous) connotations: to function as, to make, to become, to *represent* as the passage states:

"Blood represents (or functions as) nourishment for the body (yíng 營)" "Qi-breath represents (functions as) immune protection for the body (wèi 衛)"

相隨上下,謂之榮衛

"They accompany each other, moving up and down (in the organism) and are called yíng 營/wèi 衛."[122]

This idea of blood/*qì* traveling together, *xiāng suí* 相隨, literally going hand-in-hand or accompanying each other in the form of *yíng* 營/*wèi* 衛, drives home the point of why the heart and lung are such a fundamental couple for circulation and why the Chinese anatomists understood their special location above the diaphragm in the upper burner. Indeed we see this special positioning reflected in the *cùn* 寸 pulse position of heart and lung.

Z'ev: Beautiful! Teeming with metaphor and poetry! This section also reveals the hierarchical approach of Chinese philosophy in the Han dynasty…emperor, minister, etc.

Stephen: In modern western physiology, there is a concept of Heart Rate Variability (HRV) which explains the special relationship between respiration and heartbeat as a fundamental key to health. When the heartbeat is in synch with respiration, speeding up with inhalation and slowing down with exhalation, there is a healthy autonomic balance between sympathetic and parasympathetic nervous systems. HRV is an *emergent property* of interdependent regulatory systems which operate on different time scales to help us adapt to environmental and psychological challenges. HRV has been shown to be useful in predicting morbidities from common mental (e.g., stress, depression, anxiety, PTSD) and physical disorders (e.g., inflammation, chronic pain, diabetes, concussion, asthma, insomnia, fatigue), all of which increase sympathetic output and create a self-perpetuating cycle that produces autonomic imbalance and greater allostatic load. Thus, autonomic nervous system (ANS) dysfunction is a systemic common denominator of poor health and associated with acute and chronic illness and a risk factor for such serious health issues as cancer survivorship, cardiovascular disease and myocardial infarction, stroke, and overall mortality.[123]

Z'ev: I've observed my own HRV variability using an app on the Apple Watch for sometime now. It is interesting how overexposure to heat, exhaustion/poor sleep, and emotional strain affect the HRV levels! It is interesting to me that a rigidly regular heartbeat ratio indicates issues with heart function, whereas a certain amount of variability, i.e. chaos is necessary as an indicator of human health. From my thinking, this means that the heart needs to be flexible and responsive to both external/environmental changes, internal emotional/function variables, and circadian rhythms. When the

---

[122] *Nàn Jīng* 32 translation/interpretation S. Cowan.

[123] See Shaffer and Ginsberg, *"An Overview of Heart Rate Variability Metrics and Norms."*

communication between *xīn* 心 / the emperor and the other officials, functions channels and substances is compromised, this is when perverse *qì* can take hold in the areas that are not in touch with *shén* 神. *Shén* here means body / mind self awareness, the aspect of the heart that is in absolute communication with every cell, tissue, function nook and cranny of the organism.

Stephen: "Allostatic load" is a modern concept that I think relates here to the special location and relationship of the heart and lung. It refers to the cumulative burden of chronic stress and life events. It involves the interaction of different physiological systems at varying degrees of activity. *"When environmental challenges exceed the individual ability to cope, then allostatic overload ensues."*[124] I am thinking here about all the stressed out teenagers I treat who are complaining of shortness of breath, hyperventilation and sleep disorders. When I first examine them, I notice that they breath with their chest rather than their belly (the way babies do.) The second thing I notice is that their pulse has no relation to their respiratory rate. This is an objective sign of their being in a disembodied state. I explain to them that when their heart is not listening to their lungs, all kinds of chaos is generated. Blood and *qì* aren't coupled so of course they have a sense of life-threatening dread. The first thing I do even before needling, is have them practice releasing the diaphragm in order to help reduce the tension in their chest and give space / time for the heart to reconnect to the lung rhythms. This simple exercise enhances the treatment.

Nàn Jīng 32 further advances the conception of a "space-time map" of the living organism that has practical applications in assessing and treating illness. This map takes the principle presented in *Sùwèn* 5, that *yīn-yáng* relationships are the basis of life and death, expanding it to conceptualize an anatomic basis of how breath (oxygenation?) and circulation of blood together provide the vital nutrients and motive force for healthy living. The unified coherent circulation of *xuèqì* through the vessels allows the various organs to stay in communication and relationship with each other and with the environment. The qualities of these relationships can be assessed through the pulses.

Z'ev: The *Nàn Jīng* is too often ignored for what it is, a refinement of the great *Nèijīng* treatises. It is written as haiku, it's meaning condensed into precise text, and the mandalic charts accompanying the difficulties translated here are a tool for illuminating the text. I also like what you've said about how the original texts (*Nèijīng / Nàn Jīng*) are meant to be digested and interpreted in order to allow new expressions of our medicine in each era.

Stephen: Our development from infancy recapitulates our development as a species. As we've seen in earlier chapters, from a developmental perspective,

---

[124] Guidi, Lucente, Sonino, and Fava. *"Allostatic Load and Its Impact on Health: A Systematic Review."* pg. 11.

we humans have naturally evolved a capacity to map space and time as we grow. Initially as a young child learns to move their body and navigate their surroundings, they begin to recognize familiar landmarks, mapping relationships between objects as a way of orienting themselves to place. These are known as "spatial cognitive maps." As language emerges in labeling objects, children go on to create "time maps" which eventually enables them to formulate "relationship maps." It is these relational maps that were so important in the Chinese medicine classics understanding of meaning that enabled them to navigate change in space over time. From these relationships they could begin to understand causality of disease processes just as a child of 4 or 5 years old begins asking "why" and develops "causal maps." Child development research has shown that children by 5 years old develop an innate sense of life force (*qì* 氣), and are able to differentiate what is "alive" and what is "dead." They can understand that their stuffed animal is not really alive, it's just a representation of a living thing. This is one of the many ways that children have taught me about the heart of Chinese medicine.

Z'ev: Rudolf Steiner, in his conception of Waldorf Education, touches on this. Waldorf Education was designed to respect the development of the various capabilities and expressions of a child's developing consciousness, emotionally, cognitively and socially. Teaching a mind conceptual material before it is ready is damaging to spleen *qì* and its expression as *yì* 意 and potentially the *shén* 神 itself.

Stephen: I think this concept of our human capacity to construct space-time maps of our life diverged somewhat in the evolution of Eastern and Western thinking. Kuriyama says *"the history of the body is ultimately a history of ways of inhabiting the world."*[125] The Greeks (and later Descartes) developed a discrete separation between mind and body, wherein the mind-thought lives "outside" of nature, Ideas such as Truth and Perfection, having a kind of eternal "out-of-body" quality. Whereas the Chinese never conceptualized a split between mind and body, or for that matter, body and landscape, constructing their space-time maps more in line with modern quantum physics, that is, as microcosmic resonances.

Z'ev: Lest we forget that despite the dichotomies between Greek and Chinese conceptions of the universe, along the Silk Road one thousand years ago medical traditions were being transported between Tibetan, Chinese, Indian, Greek, Persian and Middle Eastern civilizations. It is interesting to note where integration largely occurred (in Tibetan medicine, for example, which has elements of Ayurvedic, Greco / Arabic (Galenic) and Chinese medicine, but less so in China and India. In other words, we can see, for example that both Tibetan

---

[125] Kuriyama, *"The Expressiveness of the Body and Divergence of Greek and Chinese Medicine,"* pg. 237.

and Chinese medicine have adapted the three position *cùn* 寸, *guān* 關, and *chi* 尺, diagnostic method of vessel diagnosis[126], whereas channel theory never permeated any system outside of Chinese medicine. Rather, a predominantly "humoral theory" was the governing paradigm.

---

[126] See Hsu, "*A Hybrid Body Technique: Does the Pulse Diagnostic Cun Guan Chi Method Have Chinese-Tibetan Origins?*"

Thoughts on Yùn Tiěqiáo 惲鉄樵: *Maps and Reality, Metaphor and Structure*

Z'ev Rosenberg & Stephen Cowan

"The study of Chinese medicine is the study of the microcosm of the human body.… The original study of the human body as a microcosmic reflection was abandoned because the way of understanding the universe was lost, and with it, the way of understanding Chinese medicine. … The only remedy for this deviation is to rediscover the true method of researching Chinese medicine. The result of such a method is to immediately grasp the macrocosm. If one grasps the macrocosm, naturally they will also grasp Chinese medicine."[127]
- Péng Ziyì 彭子益 (1871-1949)

Z'ev: Whenever one looks at the human being through the lens of physics (process, *qì* transformation, cosmology) or biology (forms, structures, tissues and layers), one is simply mirroring complimentary perspectives of each other. In reference to the need for Chinese medicine to find its proper place in the modern world, one must, as Volker Scheid says *"re-emphasize that Chinese medicine has access to the body of flesh and blood without needing to take a detour through biomedicine as an important first step in this process."*[128] How this will be done is a matter of much conjecture and essential creativity. This creativity, we propose, needs to be based within the long tradition of Chinese medicine; which has its foundations in the culture and linguistics of the Han dynasty medical canon. Chinese medicine is as much a way of viewing the world, requiring the practitioner to train one's "clinical gaze," as applied to diagnostics and treatment. Without contextual understanding and textual study, a uniquely adaptable "Chinese medicine" is impossible to manifest, specifically in a modern world whose world view is dominated by biomedicine.

Stephen: Chinese medicine, like the ideographic language it is rooted in, is concerned with the ongoing unfolding of relationships in time-space. Just as any ideogram functions as both verb and noun and will depend on the context

---

[127] McMahon, *"Circular Dynamics of Ancient Chinese Medicine I."*

[128] Volker, and Yun. *"Yun Tieqiao and the Disappearance of the Body from Chinese Medicine."*

it finds itself in for meaning, so too, is the body perceived as simultaneously verb and noun intimately dependent on the contextual time-and-space process it exists in. This dynamic view is the foundation of the systematic correspondences inherent in Chinese medical thinking. That the cosmos speaks *through* us, resonating (*gǎnyìng* 感應) with the patterns of the stars, moon, sun, wind, seasons, plants and animal life around us, represents what noted psychologist Carol Dweck calls "*Growth Mind*" thinking in contrast to "*Fixed Mind*" thinking that is so common in Western analytic sciences.[129] Fixed mind thinking is a highly compartmentalized perspective driven by rigid labels that limit the possibilities of change. Western medicine is ruled by fixed mind diagnoses founded on so called *objective* measurement as the rule for diagnostics. If you can't measure it, it doesn't exist. Growth mind thinking, on the other hand, is process-driven and Dr. Dweck has shown in elegant research that it is this kind of thinking that is the key to success in life. Chinese medicine is inherently driven by "growth mind" thinking. The Sage doctor sees a world of constantly transforming events that she may consciously choose to temporarily freeze into a pattern of discrimination but she recognizes that life exists as flowing beyond such distinctions. Thus the clinical gaze, pulse, and environmental influences carry much more weight in making decisions on treatment than laboratory tests which are mere snap-shots of a moment in time that has already passed.

Stephen: As we have been saying throughout this book, Chinese medicine is rooted in the Daoist-Confucian concern with relationships. Rather than isolating events, our relationship to the world around us (Daoist) and to each other (Confucianist) rely on metaphor to describe these connections and treatment options. This stands in stark contrast to the reductive perspective of Western medicine that emerged from Cartesian mind-body split. Freud, and even more so, Jung, opened a "new" dimension to medicine that approached the mind through metaphor. For centuries, Chinese medicine viewed the body in much the same metaphoric way.

In Western medicine, unfortunately, metaphoric language is all too often disregarded as unscientific. What is of central concern in diagnosis is objective measurements. Take vessel (pulse) diagnosis for example. what matters in Western diagnostics is the beat count and beat to beat rhythm that reflects Newtonian physics of linear mechanics. Whereas in Chinese medicine, in vessel diagnosis, not only are there six different positions and three (or more) depths to be examined (utterly missed by Western trained physicians) but there is a whole metaphoric language used to describe what the clinician encounters. Qualities of roughness or smoothness, floating or sinking, wiry, or soggy all serve as metaphors for disease processes. These "*ripples in the flow,*" as Z'ev calls them, though subjective, define in highly specific terms, the context of a

---

[129] See Dweck,"*Mindset: The New Psychology of Success.*"

patient's condition and its pattern of change over time. The location of time (pulse) in space (body), *qì* and blood (*qìxuè* 氣血) is what quantum physics and philosophers like Heidegger call the time-space continuum.

Z'ev: With the advent of modern twentieth century Western medical treatments, (e.g. antibiotics, pain medications, steroids, surgical techniques, radiography) suddenly acute life-threatening emergencies were dramatically and effectively controlled. In the wake of political upheaval and modernization in China, Yùn Tiěqiáo's attempt to preserve Chinese Medicine's place in this new world required him to make statements such as:

> "*Heart disease in the Inner Canon is not the heart disease of Western medicine. Skilled Western medicine doctors can cure serious diseases; Chinese medicine practitioners who have grasped the essence of the Inner Canon can also cure serious diseases. The same goal is reached by different routes.*"[130]

Texts such as the *Nàn Jīng* 難經 have been deeply studied as to their underlying principles, applied to the issues at hand in each generation. Just as the seasons change and transform, each generation of physicians has found new inspiration and interpretations of this work for their patients, writing commentaries in order to make these writings relevant.

Stephen: In a sense, Yùn Tiěqiáo seems to be saying; ok, sure, if you're having a heart attack or an acute life-threatening infection, go to the ER but remember, there's more to life than acute emergencies and Chinese medicine has an important place in treating (and preventing) these. In fact, acute life-threatening emergencies account for a small percentage of overall health problems in the USA. This was for me, as a physician, an eye-opening realization. I was trained in some of the best hospitals in New York but when I went out into practice I found that all my training left me with little to do to address the vast number of modern epidemics of our time, the chronic and recurrent inflammatory processes that are not classified as "medical emergencies".

> "*The six warps are recordings of symptoms in the human body ordered through bounded definitions. Hence, one can say that after one gets ill the six warps come into being, but when one is not ill these entities do not exist.* "
> -Yùn Tiěqiáo (1878-1935)[131]

Z'ev: The *liù jīng* 六經 / six warps as developed in the *Shānghán Lùn* 傷寒論 can be reinterpreted, adapted to any medical era or disease process due to its innate flexibility, and it is no accident that there are multiple schools of thought

---

[130] Volker, and Yun, "*Yun Tieqiao and the Disappearance of the Body from Chinese Medicine.*"
[131] ibid.

on this text and branch philosophies that have produced their own medical schools (*wēn bìng* 温病, *sānjiāo* 三焦). As Volker Scheid has pointed out in his work, great physicians such as Yè Tiānshì 葉天士 (1667–1747) and Wú Jūtōng 吳鞠通 (1757-1841) sought not to "reinvent the wheel," but to adapt the *Shānghán Lùn* 傷寒論 to the warm epidemics they observed during the Qing dynasty.

We now find ourselves in a new era, post-industrial, post-modern, a time of great instability, chaos and human over-reach in the natural world. This proto-Anthropocene era requires new strategies and interpretations to treat the coming era of novel viruses, epidemics and pathogens released and mutated as forests burn and polar ice caps melt. As we observed the recent novel virus pandemic, new strategies and interpretations have emerged. What we are proposing in this book is a return to the classics as a basis for applying the ancient wisdom of metaphoric medicine that sees body function as mirroring what's happening ecologically and in the socio/economic realms in our world.

Stephen: There's a trend these days in the USA to "westernize" Chinese medicine in order to make it more acceptable to the general public and to the conventional Western medical establishment. I see the so-called functional medicine movement with its test-based decision-making as no more than another version of western medicine and yet, I'm seeing it becoming a draw for many American acupuncturists today. There are many factors underlying this trend. Economics certainly plays an important role. An acupuncturist coming out of training these days has huge loans to pay back somewhat comparable to USA medical students.

Additionally, I think there may be an urge to appear more "scientific" (by using more objective lab tests) with their patients who are concurrently being treated by western medical practitioners. Furthermore, by and large, American acupuncturists are not often trained as apprentices, a tradition that has a long history in China before the Mao era and so once they graduate, they are left without sagely guidance and must rely on protocols they memorized in school. Without the serious study of the classics, particularly the cultivation of metaphor in medicine, it is understandable that there would be lack of confidence and trust in the medicine that might underlie their attraction to functional medicine as a compromise between Chinese and Western medical approaches. While functional medicine tests have their place as an alternative to conventional Western lab testing, in examining possible metabolic causes for chronic conditions related to diseases of modern life, it is our hopes that we can with this book re-inspire an appreciation for the collected empirical wisdom contained in the classics so that it will bring greater trust in, and application of, classical Chinese medicine's metaphoric approaches to meeting the needs of our patients today.

Softness, Relaxation, Rooting and Flow as Principles of Chinese Medicine

Stephen Cowan & Z'ev Rosenberg

"Comparing the musculature portrayed in Vesalius' anatomy and the total absence of muscle in the acupuncture man, we see almost irresistibly a puzzle about blindness, about how observant Chinese doctors overlooked, strangely, one of the most prominent features of the human body."
- Shigehisa Kuriyama[132]

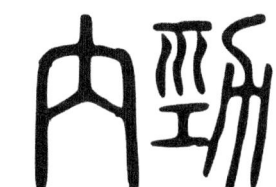

Figure 2.18 - Nèi Jìn 內勁[133]

Stephen: Contrary to Kuriyama's idea that the Chinese were blind to muscle as an anatomic component, there is a long history in China of differentiating "inner strength" (*nèi jìn* 內勁) (*fig. 2.18*) from "outer muscular force (*lì* 力). Comparing the two forms of body maps, West and East, that developed through the ages, I am again struck by a fundamental difference in context between Western Medicine and Eastern medicine. During my early years of training in Western medicine, having studied stiff corpses to map human anatomy, by the time I entered the hospitals for residency, I became keenly

---

[132] Kuriyama, *"The Expressiveness of the Body and the Divergence of Greek and Chinese Medicine,"* pg. 111.

[133] *Nèi jìn* 內勁 / inner strength or tenacity. The character *jìn* 勁 shows the underground waterway, the very same character which we see in describing the channels (*jīng* 巠) and the medical classics. In *jìn*, next to this image of the waterway, there is an image of the muscles of the shoulder (*lì* 力 meaning force). The waterway radical gives the sense soft, relaxed, rooted, flow that transforms the meaning of muscular force.

aware of the level of pervasive fear that had unwittingly been generated by this corpse-based map of life.

Simultaneously, I had begun my study of *tàijí quán* 太極拳 which emphasized the use of softness, relaxation, rooting and flow as a means of generating health and self-defense. In *tàijí*, one speaks of "tenacious strength" as distinguished from muscular force, the former having root and flexibility, the latter being more rigid. When employed, tenacity is likened to a strong vine which is pliable while muscular force is said to be like a stiff dead stick.

This observation of softness as strength dates back to the *Yìjīng* 易經 and is reiterated by *Lǎozǐ* 老子:

> *"Nothing in the world is softer and weaker than water*
> *But for attacking the hard and strong, there is nothing like it!*
> *For nothing can take its place.*
> *That the weak overcomes the strong*
> *And the soft overcomes the hard*
> *This is something known by all*
> *But practiced by none."*
> -*Lǎozǐ* 78[134]

Professor Cheng Man-ching 郑曼青 (1902-1975) said that *"tenacity is alive, force is dead"* and *"tenacity is the resilience or tone of living muscle however relaxed it may be."* [135] I think back to those stiff corpses I studied in my early medical education and find this idea of tenacity highlights a fundamental difference between what I've experienced as Western and Eastern medical approaches to healing. Perhaps this is why the Chinese anatomic drawings preferred to emphasize the power of the internal landscape over the outer muscular form. The medical maps that Western medicine tend to employ create a rigid system of force to attack disease. This force requires a certain tension to maintain control in order to strike hard and oppose an enemy; the overuse of steroids and antibiotics is an example of such strong force. The tension required to maintain that force is generated by and in turn perpetuates fear: the fear of the unknown, fear of loss of control, fear of making a mistake. I've experienced that stress-based tension in my own body while working within the fear-based New York City hospitals back in the 80s when violence, AIDS and crack wars were wreaking havoc on families. The rigid protocol-driven maps we learned were certainly effective in acute life-threatening emergencies but generated enormous adverse effects that were considered acceptable collateral damage in

---

[134] Wu, *"Tao Teh Ching,"* pg. 159.

[135] Cheng,*"Tai Chi Chuan, A Simplified Method of Calisthenics for Health and Self-Defense,"* pg. 47.

light of the battle-field mentality at that time. What's more, this heavy handed approach was utterly ineffective in promoting long term health.

My first job after training was medical director of the Asthmatic Children's Foundation, a rehab hospital for children suffering from chronic medical conditions who had been repeatedly hospitalized and could not get off their medication. Coming from the inner city, these children were stuck in an acute care system that kept them rebounding over and over again, being discharged and readmitted, crises after crises. They came to my center located up in the country, with little hope of getting off their steroids and bronchodilators which had taken a terrible toll on their bodies. The fear in their eyes, and the eyes of their parents was palpable. Because these children were admitted for prolonged stay to stabilize their condition, I had the opportunity to develop a holistic program that provided proper nutrition and exercise. Recognizing that the system I was trained in was not actually improving their health, forced me to "think outside the box." This was a *pivotal* moment in my career. Having privately studied meditation, Daoism and *tàijí* for some time, I took the bold move of applying those principles to my patients. The radical idea that soft and gentle overcomes hard and forceful became a motto of my approach.

The first program I introduced was to have all kids (and staff practice gentle qigong breathing exercises each morning. This alone had a remarkable effect on the kids stamina, reducing their anxiety (and the anxiety of the staff). As the kids got a little stronger, I then began taking them on hikes in the woods around the property, a natural "rooting" experience most of these children had never had. I cannot overstate the importance of the "green' power, that time in Nature has on physical and mental health, though this was not never mentioned to us in our training in the hospitals of NYC back then. The exposure to the natural shapes of trees and rocks had the effect of softening their perceptions, shifting from a more rigid black & white mindset towards a process (*Dào* 道) growth mindset. With each hike, measurements of lung function improved, sleep improved and medication use reduced. Furthermore, I brought in organic food, which most of these children had never seen nor eaten before, having been raised in the relative "food deserts" of the inner city. To my utter surprise, within a few weeks, a number of these kids were for the first time able to miraculously be weaned off *all* their medication! When I went back to the hospital centers that had referred them to tell them of this miracle, the specialists simply refused to believe me, calling it *coincidence*. They could not see beyond what they believe. For me this would be impetus to go deeper into the study of Chinese medicine that would change my life and career.

We witnessed that same paralyzing fear generated by the Western medical system again during the recent COVID pandemic. Western medicine cannot see the role that diet and environment play in our responses to infection, not to mention the fear-producing tension transmitted by the medical establishment to the body, which amplifies symptoms and wreaks havoc on the immune resilience. These so-called "soft sciences" of healthy eating, breath-work and exposure to Nature are simply not on their radar. Persistent emergency thinking begets persistent emergency response. From a physiological perspective, having persistently tense muscles will cut off blood flow, causing stiffness and pain as we harden our stance in the world and brace ourselves to fight an enemy. This survival mode is unsustainable and ultimately uproots our sense of well-being, diminishing our ability to effectively care for ourselves or others. What's more, we saw how the medical staff living within this fear-based environment suffered themselves. Perhaps this is why there is such a high burnout rate among Western-trained doctors today.[136] According to the AMA, physician burnout rates spiked to 63% in 2021. The research concluded that "findings of this study suggest that this burnout pattern is a potential threat to the ability of the US health care system to care for patients and thus needs immediate solutions."

In contrast, I think one of the primary reasons that Chinese medicine has had the *tenacity* to last thousands of years is because its maps are rooted in the principle of flow rather than force (*lì* 力). The *tàijí* principle of "inner strength" (*nèi jìn* 內勁) implies softness, relaxation, root and flow in order to promote healing through the circulation of *xuèqì* 血氣. This is the very nature of applying *tuīná* 推拿, acumoxa and herbs. Maybe this difference is the reason why when I try to explain the concept of "*qì*" to Western physicians, they look at me dumbfounded and struggle to accept it. They simply have no map or context in which to see it.

Z'ev: This is a beautiful summation of your discovery of tenacity versus sheer force in the practice of medicine. Chinese medicine has always had embedded military metaphors, such as the relationship of *wèi qì* 衛氣 and *yíng qì* 營氣 constructive or 'camp' *qì*. As it says in *Língshū* 靈樞 71:

> "The guard qi (wèi qì 衛氣) appear as the wild and fast ones among the aggressive qi. At first they move into the regions of the partings of the flesh (còu lǐ 腠理) and the skin in the four limbs. They never rest. During the day they move in the yang realm. During the night they move in the yin realm."[137]

We also discuss the *jīn jīng* 筋經/sinew channels, innovative grouping of ropy tissues that we call tendons, muscles and ligaments. It is essential that we emphasize in training new practitioners in the Chinese medical arts that we make these distinctions clear, as most educational programs in the West do not. We must base training on the original, authentic medical manuals, the Han

---

[136] Ortega, et.al. "*Patterns in Physician Burnout in a Stable-Linked Cohort.*"

[137] Unschuld, "*Huang Di Nei Jing Ling Shu: The Ancient Classic on Needle Therapy,*" pg. 632.

dynasty medical classics. Without original principles, clear terminology and practical applications, it is all too easy to become confused about how to actually apply Chinese medicine in the real time clinical situations that confront us in the 21ˢᵗ century. I was also on the "frontlines" of 1980's health care crises, working with HIV, cancer and asthmatic patients, among other serious conditions. In those days (in Denver/Boulder, Colorado) it was much easier for a practitioner of Chinese medicine to work with patients in hospital and doctors' office setting, and I did both alongside my independent practice. I assisted in V-back births, treated cancer patients in oncology wards, and conducted research on HIV and Chinese Medicine.

Getting back to the conundrum of understanding and applying classical Chinese medicine and it's texts (*Nèijīng* 內經/*Nàn Jīng* 難經,/*Shānghán Lùn* 傷寒論), as you also point out, musculature is real, physical anatomy is real. We do not need to "replace" it with a solely "energetic" approach, we simply need to reframe the physical anatomy in the more dynamic, cosmic perspective of Chinese medicine which sees the physiology of humans as an expression of the interactions of heaven, earth, celestial and movements in time. Our profession is presently having a crisis, wondering if a harsh, physical approach to acupuncture (ignoring herbal medicine, and probably moxibustion as well) is "better" when focused on structures rather than the traditional channel system. This is simply the result of not understanding the clarity and practicality of the channel systems described in the classical acupuncture literature, and being seduced by such methods as "dry needling" which are clearly inferior to the more intensive methods described in such sections as the "Nine Needles" in *Língshū* 靈樞 1 and other chapters as well. Like homeopathy, Chinese acupuncture medicine has a variety of approaches to needling from gentle/subtle to surgical, and needles that correspond to the intensity of the disorder. The main factors to consider in this regard are:

1) Gauge and length of needles
2) Insertion technique (including depth and stimulation)
3) Frequency of treatment
4) Number of needles
5) Timing (chronobiology, consideration of time of day, season, stem and branch, lunar and seasonal cycles).

Stephen: Ultimately, soft does not mean passive or ineffective. And there is nothing wishy-washy about being relaxed and rooted. Learning needling techniques, herbs (and how to relate to your patients, for that matter) must start with self-cultivation in order to counter the rather muscular Western fixed mind belief that strength means hard, rigid power. Otherwise, one cannot promote the flow of life. As *Lǎozǐ* 老子 76 says: *"Things that are hard and rigid are the companions of death. Things that are soft and supple are companions of life."*[138]

---

[138] Ames and Hall, "*Dao De Jing: Making This Life Significant: A Philosophical Translation*," pg. 195.

Circadian Maps 難經晝夜節律圖: *The Secret of Time in Chinese Medicine*[139]

Z'ev Rosenberg & Stephen Cowan

Z'ev: We now will explore perhaps the most complex and imbedded maps within classical Chinese medicine, and in our opinion the most important aspect of diagnosis and treatment. As I pointed out in *Afterglow: Ministerial Fire and Chinese Ecological Medicine*, the center point of stillness and potentiality in the human being is *yuán qì* 原氣 / source *qì*. "*What is unfathomable in yin /yang are the changes/biàn huà* 變化 *of origin yuán qì*" and "*allowing the original qi of the body to heal without action.*"[140] *Yuán qì* always lies at the source of human life, and from this center of tranquility arise the movements and changes of *yīnyáng* 陰陽 through the patterns that underlie human life and health. The core circulation is described by Péng Ziyì 彭子益 (1871-1949)'s as the *Circular Dynamics of Chinese Medicine*, the *qì huà* 氣化 / *qì* transformations beginning at heaven's root at winter's solstice arrival, when the first yang line appears in the hexagram 24 ䷗, *Fù* 复 / Return. The other node is the yin starting point of *qì* transformation, "moon cavity," at summer's solstice arrival, when the first broken line of *yīn* appears. This creates the circular motion, with earth at the center, *yáng* rising, and *yīn* descending. This is the central "wheel" of flow, movement and transformation of human life. This same circadian dynamic of the seasonal hexagrams through the body is illustrated by Zhāng Shìxián 張世賢 map (*tú* 圖) for *Nàn Jīng* 難經 23 (*fig. 2.19*).

---

[139] See MindNode in *Appendix II: Blueprints and Charts from Z'ev's Notebook* pg. 288.

[140] Farquhar, "*A Way of Life: Things, Thought, and Action in Chinese Medicine*," pg. 133-5.

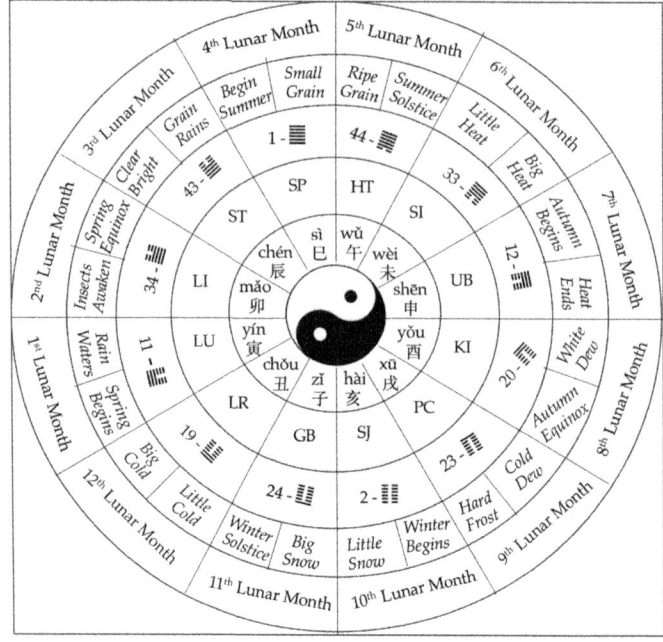

Figure 2.19 - *Nàn Jīng* 23 Map[141]

Stephen: Zhāng Shìxián's map reveals some interesting relationships that *Nàn Jīng* 23 discusses. The question asked is whether we can measure the three *yīn* and three *yáng* vessels of the hands and feet. The answer given is quite remarkably detailed for all conduits and even includes the *qiāo* 脈 - foot walker vessels (giving the impression that the extraordinary vessels are not independent of the 12 conduit circulation.

人兩足蹻脈，從足至目，長七尺五寸，二七一丈四尺，二五一尺，合一丈五尺

"Man has in both feet the walker vessels, they extend from the feet to the eyes. they are seven feet five inches long."[142]

After describing the precise measurements of the vessels, *Nàn Jīng* 23 makes a remarkable statement:

---

[141] Translation of diagram 23 created by Zhàng Shìxián (1510) of the circulation and maintenance of warmth throughout the body.

[142] Unschuld (2016), *"Nan Jing: The Classic of Difficult Issues,"* pg. 241.

皆因其原，如環無端，轉相灌溉

[The movement through] all of them returns [again and again] to its origin, as a ring without end, with [the qi and blood] pouring from one [conduit] into the next, thus revolving [through the entire organism].[143]

This is a reiteration of *Língshū* 靈樞 15 and is the first time in the *Nàn Jīng* 難經 where we see the term *rú huán wúduān* 如環無端, *"like a ring without end."* What I find interesting in Zhāng Shìxián's map is his emphasis on the correlation of time of day / season with the organ networks as well as the tidal hexagrams. It raises a question for me as to whether the Han doctors were making those precise measurements of the conduits based solely on physical dissection or were more likely making metaphoric measurements based on the space-timing of the seasonal cycles! This perhaps addresses the debate over how often dissection guided their understanding of *qì* function.

Z'ev: The *Sùwèn* 素問, *Língshū* 靈樞, *Nàn Jīng* 難經, and *Shānghán Lùn* 傷寒論, all have several chapters that discuss these celestial movements and transformations through time, which we will discuss below. The most effective therapy in Chinese medicine works with these circadian maps to establish normal flow and recover normative function and transformation / metabolism.

These maps are embedded in the Han dynasty medical canon. A full nine chapters, reportedly added by Wáng Bīng 王冰, compiler of the *Sùwèn*, deal with *wǔ yùn liù qì* 五運六氣 / five movements six *qì* theory, the most elaborate calendrical maps that apply to predicting health in illness in yearly, seasonal and monthly cycles. However, there are embedded theories throughout the texts, and we will describe several of these maps below.

I. *Sùwèn* 26 (*Bā Zhèng Shénmíng Lùn* 八正神明論)

"All laws of piercing require an observation of the qi of sun, moon and stars, and the eight cardinal [turning points] of the four seasons..... When heaven is warm and sun is bright, then blood in man is rich in fluid. and guard qi is at the surface... When heaven is cold and sun hidden, blood in man congeals, so that [its flow] is impeded, and guard

---

[143] ibid., pg. 242

is in the depth."[144] The position of the *qì* is determined in view (of the luminaries of heaven) moving the position of their light.

Zhāng Zhìcōng 張志聰 comments:"*one conforms with the cold and summer heat of heaven, with the cold and warmth of the sun, with the fullness and depletion of the moon, and with the movement of the stars.*"[145] Just as the heavens and earth follow specific patterns and movements, so does the human entity. We are influenced by tides, seasons, movement of constellations, and the angle of the sun. Recent research on autoimmune disorders such as multiple sclerosis indicate that these illnesses are more common in far northern latitudes where sunlight is generally very indirect. Rowan Jacobsen in his article *Against Sunscreen Absolutism* writes that scientists observed a global pattern called the "latitude effect" over a century ago. After accounting for factors like income, exercise, and smoking, they found that people living at higher latitudes experience higher rates of various diseases, particularly autoimmune disorders like multiple sclerosis, compared to those in lower or middle latitudes.[146]

Observations of the movements of heavenly *qì*, constellations, sun and moon and seasonal *qì* are essential in choosing acupuncture treatment. Continuing in the text:

> "*at the time of beginning crescent moon, blood and qi originate as essence, and the guard qi begins to move. When the disk of the moon is full, blood and qi are replete; the muscles and the flesh are firm.When the disk of the moon is empty, the muscles and the flesh wane, the conduits and the network [vessels] are depleted and the guard qi leaves.The physical appearance exists all by itself.It is therefore that one follows the seasons of heaven in regulating blood and qi.*"[147]

The text goes on to describe how a master practitioner can read the relationship of the human *qì* to heaven and earth, sun and moon, constellations and seasons, even when there are no observable symptoms. In other words, diagnosis must include a mapping of the relationship of a human being in time and space to these conditional factors, and specifically by vessel diagnosis and

---

[144] Unschuld, Tessenow, and Zheng, "*Huang Di Nei Jing Su Wen: An Annotated Translation of Huang Di's Inner Classic - Basic Questions, 2 Volumes,*" pg. 433-435.

[145] ibid., pg. 433.

[146] See Jacobsen, "*Against Sunscreen Absolutism.*"

[147] Unschuld, Tessenow, and Zheng, "*Huang Di Nei Jing Su Wen: An Annotated Translation of Huang Di's Inner Classic - Basic Questions, 2 Volumes,*" pg. 434-435.

palpation, observation, sound, scent and complexion can read the medical history of the patient and predict outcomes and tendencies to illness.

II. *Sùwèn* 素問 27 (*Líhé Zhēn Xié* 離合真邪)

"All these shifts towards imbalance of the camp and guard [qi] are generated by depletion and repletion, not because an evil qi has entered the conduits from the outside."[148]

In this chapter, *xié qì* 邪氣 is seen as a disruptive force, such as a sudden wind rising violently, causing the main waters to gush up in breakers and rise like ridges in the fields. Or as Wáng Bīng 王冰 notes, *"when wind enters the conduit vessels, they react in the same way."*[149]

The *Nàn Jīng* 難經 and *Língshū* 靈樞 teach us that the interface of *xié qì* and *zhèng qì* 正氣 is the key to diagnosing illness through vessel diagnosis. When the *xié qì* is strong, and overwhelms a person with normal *zhèng qì*, we drain the *xié qì*. When the patient is weak, we strengthen the *zhèng qì* to overcome *xié qì*. When illness is in the *yáng* aspect (exterior), we can attack *xié qì* directly. If it reaches the yin aspect (interior) however, we must strengthen the *zhèng qì*. This is how we develop long term treatment strategies when dealing with chronic illnesses.

III. *Nàn Jīng* 難經 30

This chapter in the *Nàn Jīng* 難經 reiterates and expands on *Língshū* 18, on the *wèi qì* and *yíng qì* following each other. Zhāng Shìxián 張世賢 draws upon the times of day, the *wǔ* 午 hour (11 AM to 1 PM) being the time when *qīngqì* 清氣/clear *qì*, transforms to *yíng qì*. The *zhuóqì* 濁氣/turbid *qì* transforms to *wèi qì* after the gong hour (text says *zǐ* 子 hour), from 11 PM to 1 AM. In the morning, at the *yín* 寅 hour (3 AM to 5 AM, there is a great meeting in the vessels at *cùn kǒu* 寸口, where the vessels at the inch mouth are palpated.[150] A clear description of *"a ring without end."*

---

[148] ibid., pg. 447-448.

[149] ibid., pg. 448-449.

[150] See Zhāng Shìxián 張世賢 's comments Unschuld (2016), *"Nan Jing: The Classic of Difficult Issues,"* pg. 288.

IV. A *Shānghán Lùn* 傷寒論 View of Interior and Exterior Disorders

At this point, we need to discuss the relationship of the internal, denser, more physiological nature of the *zàngfǔ* 臟腑 / viscera / bowels and associated sense organs and tissues, such as the liver with the *jīn* 筋 / sinews, and eyes. All of these, including *yíng qì*, are relatively yin in nature, whereas *wèi qì* and the main channel circulation is more *yáng* and external in nature. Therefore, the channel system is swifter and quicker to respond to environmental changes. Also *wèi qì* flows at the surface of the body (outside the channels), constantly shifting and responding to stimuli from both inside and outside. Stephen has noted that the metal phase (lung-gut-skin) represents our interface with the external environment. In addition, the internal viscera / bowels, being more dense, are slower to pick up signals of disharmony or change, and are less flexible. It is for this reason that in the *Shānghán Lùn*, there is a hierarchical relationship of transference of pathogenic *qì* from exterior to interior. Illness in the channels, such as *tàiyáng* 太陽 disease can easily be expelled by venting the exterior, or harmonizing *yíng qì* and *wèi qì* as described in *guì zhī tāng* 桂枝湯 / cinnamon twig decoction. Next are *yáng* bowel channels and bowels, which require more effort to expel pathogenic *qì*. All of the *yáng* bowels have "exit routes" to the exterior, so in herbal medicine we can use purging / precipitation, vomiting, or urination to release these pathogens. In the yin stages of illness, the internal yin viscera are affected, and being solid, slow, dense and filled with blood hold on to pathogenic *qì*, often without the body's immune function or eliminative capacities being alerted. This is potentially a very dangerous state of affairs, as organic illnesses and degeneration of function can occur without the patient being aware until there is a full blow disease process underway, an "enemy within." This process is at the root of many autoimmune disorders, cancers, kidney failure, heart disease and many other life threatening illnesses.

V. *Língshū* 靈樞 18 and *Nàn Jīng* 難經 49 & 50

老者之氣血衰，其肌肉枯，氣道澀，五藏之氣相搏，其營氣衰少而衛氣內伐，故晝不精，夜不瞑。

"In old [persons] the qi and the blood (xuèqì 血氣) are weak. Their muscles and their flesh wither and the paths of their qi are rough. The qi of the five long-term depots (wǔzàng 五臟) strike at each other. The camp qi (yíng qì) are weak and diminished, and the guard qi (wèi qì) attack their own interior."[151]

---

[151] Unschuld, *"Huang Di Nei Jing Ling Shu: The Ancient Classic on Needle Therapy,"* pg. 262.

In visceral manipulation, the internal organs in the abdominal region are seen as analogous to a solar system, where each organ has a specific space, gravity and rhythm. As I've discussed in previous writings, the internal organs have a *yīnyáng* 陰陽 rhythm of "breathing," in other words expansion and contraction, and can be said to be healthy when this process is uninhibited. However, when there are lesions, scars, damage to the diaphragm by surgery, erosion of structure and function (by poor diet, alcohol, obesity, lack of exercise), the organs become crowded, inhibited and lose their equilibrium with the "organ community" that requires full cooperation with all of the *zàngfǔ* 臟腑 to establish human health. The *Nàn Jīng* and *Língshū* brilliantly emphasize this as interior evils, where the five phases and their associated *zàngfǔ* overact on each other, or compensate for weakened function. This can express itself emotionally or in specific symptoms discussed in such chapters as *Nàn Jīng* 49 and 50, which traces the five evils (depletion evils, repletion evils, robber evils, weakness evils and *zhèng* 正/regular evils. The *Nàn Jīng* further developed (based on the *Língshū*) an acupuncture treatment system based on the *wǔ shū xué* 五俞穴/five transporting points. Dr. Yoshio Manaka describes this phenomenon as "isopathy," or resonance between channel locations/points to restore equilibrium to both the channels and their associated viscera and bowels.[152]

Stephen: It's interesting to note that emerging Western research has demonstrated just how critical circadian rhythms are for healthy neuroimmune function as well as autonomic control of blood flow. Recent research indicates that "there appears to be a balance of circadian factors, inflammatory molecules, neurotransmitters, and physiological mechanisms governing vaso-hemodynamics that govern sleep regulation."[153] Indeed we now know that every cell in the body has an internal clock that is *"listening to (and responsive to) environmental circadian rhythms thus shaping who we are."*[154] What's more, *"the vagus nerve is considered to play a key role in the circadian rhythm."*[155] There is growing research that highlights the critical functions of the vagus nerve, the

---

[152] Additional chapters that discuss the relationship of *wèi qì* 衛氣 and *yíng qì* 營氣 in the *Língshū* 靈樞 include: Chapters 76 (Movements of Guard Qi), 52 (Guard Qi), and 41 (Yin/Yang, Sun/Moon), 16 (Camp Qi).

[153] Zielinski, and Gibbons, *"Neuroinflammation, Sleep, and Circadian Rhythms."*

[154] Van Drunen, and Eckel-Mahan. *"Circadian Rhythms as Modulators of Brain Health During Development and Throughout Aging."*

[155] See Smets, et. al, *"Chronic Recording of the Vagus Nerve to Analyze Modulations by the Light–Dark Cycle."*

main component of the parasympathetic nervous system, involved in the regulation of immune response, wound healing, digestion, heart rate, and control of mood. Healthy vagal tone can detect microbiota metabolites through its afferent branches, transferring this gut information to the central nervous system. Thus the vagus nerve has direct two-way communication with microbiome/macro-biome continuum. Stephen Porges has done revolutionary work defining the many functions of the ventral vagus nerve in order to resolve chronic illness and trauma thereby promoting what he calls "the social-engagement network. It is interesting to note that both sympathetic and parasympathetic functions are directly influenced by the so-called endogenous circadian rhythms. *"Results during wakefulness indicate that the circadian pacemaker may control both the sympathetic and vagal limbs of the autonomic nervous system. Vagal tone was maximal during the circadian phase corresponding to the usual sleep episode (although these measurements were made in the absence of sleep) with an acrophase at 4 am to 5 am.*[156] *Sympatho-vagal balance was minimal between 9 am and 1 pm.*[157] *[Unbalances in these] endogenous circadian rhythms in ANS function may contribute to mortality from cardiovascular disease and nocturnal asthma."*[158]

Here we can see current western medical research attempting to catch up to what the ancient sages of Chinese medicine already knew, that our cosmic connection to the moon and sun cycles is, as *Nèijīng* 內經 and *Nàn Jīng* texts repeatedly emphasize, critical to living a healthy, balanced life of longevity.

VI. *Língshū* 靈樞 41: Commentary on "Yīnyáng Jì Rì Yuè 陰陽繫日月 "The Ties Between Yīn and Yáng, Sun and Moon"

Z'ev: In this chapter, the human form is delineated as to correspondences with heaven and earth. *"[The region] from the lower back upward is heaven. [The region] from the lower back downward is the earth."*[159] This chapter then establishes that "the twelve conduit vessels of the feet correspond to the twelve months. *"The moon emerges from the water.*[160] *Hence what is below is yin. The ten fingers correspond to the ten sun [orbits]."*[161] Continuing the correspondences of the

---

[156] This corresponds to the Lung phase according to chrono-acupuncture maps.

[157] This corresponds to the period of maximum *yáng qì* flow.

[158] Hilton, et.al, *"Endogenous Circadian Control of the Human Autonomic Nervous System."*

[159] Unschuld, *"Huang Di Nei Jing Ling Shu: The Ancient Classic on Needle Therapy,"* pg. 409.

[160] i.e. yin essence, according to Zhāng Jǐngyuè 張景岳.

[161] Over a ten day period…Unschuld, *"Huang Di Nei Jing Ling Shu: The Ancient Classic on Needle Therapy,"* pg. 409-410.

twelve earthly branches and their associated lunar months control the *yáng* and *yīn* foot channels. The hand *yáng* and *yīn* channels are controlled by the ten celestial stems. Between the 12 earthly branches and 10 heavenly stems, we have the basis of *wǔ yùn liù qì* 五運六氣 / five movements six *qì* theory. The text goes on to categorize the channels and viscera in terms of *yáng* within *yīn*, and *yīn* within *yáng*.

足之陽者，陰中之少陽也；
足之陰者，陰中之太陰也。
手之陽者，陽中之太陽也；
手之陰者，陽中之少陰也。

The yang [conduit] of the feet are the minor yang in yin.
The yin [conduits] of the feet are the major yin in yin.
The yang [conduits] of the hands are the major yang in yang.
The yin [conduits] of the hands are the minor yin in yang.

其於五藏也，
心為陽中之太陽，
肺為陽中之少陰，
肝為陰中之少陽，
脾為陰中之至陰，
腎為陰中之太陰。

As for the five long-term depots:
The heart is the major yang in yang.
The lung is the minor yin in yang.
The liver is the minor yang in yin.
The spleen is the extreme yin in yin.
The kidneys are the major yin in yin. [162]

Finally, the "human *qì*" or *zhèng qì* 正氣 circulate through the months in such a manner that needling is not recommended at a time when this *qì* are said to be located in these channels. A more elaborate system of channel/point prohibitions can be found in such texts as the *Yellow Emperor's Toad Classic / Huángdì Hámá Jīng* 黃帝蝦蟆經.

---

[162] ibid., pg. 412-3.

VII. Chronobiology in Biomedicine, and the Importance of Acupuncture in Regulating Circadian Rhythms

Z'ev: As long as the central biologic clock is communicating with a peripheral clock during the day, processes including DNA repair, mitochondrial activity (energy management), metabolism, and the natural cell cycle can be kept on track. If these mechanisms can be explored in more detail and controlled to some extent, then it could be a significant step towards keeping parts of the body in better health for longer as we get older. *"Our study reveals that minimal interaction between only two tissue clocks, one central and the other peripheral, is needed to maintain optimal functioning of tissues like muscles and skin and to avoid their deterioration and aging,"* says biologist Pura Muñoz-Cánoves, from the Pompeu Fabra University in Spain at the time of the research."[163]

These central (yin aspect of the body, associated with *yíng qì*) and peripheral (*yáng* aspects of the body, associated with *wèi qì*) of circadian clocks that need to be "communicating" and "controlled" beg the question: how is this to be done? More pharmaceutical interventions, which tend to be very one-sided and local interventions with potential side effects? Or is there a way to treat our patients systematically so that the body/mind's self correcting mechanisms are activated?

Clearly, Chinese medicine has been aware of these circadian clocks for centuries, and sought to regulate them through lifestyle, living with the seasonal changes (sleep, clothing, cooking, activity and rest) and focusing the mind on specific seasonal aspects (planning in winter, active participation in summer). Therapeutically, the dynamic maps of acupuncture and moxibustion, needles and fire therapy recorded in the *Língshū* and *Nàn Jīng* specifically work with time and timing. This includes five phase acupuncture involving the five transporting points, the eight extraordinary vessels, harmonizing *yíng qì* and *wèi qì*, five movements/six *qì*, solar and lunar phases, and seasonal rhythms. Herbal internal/medicine strategies were also formulated in this manner, and different formulas were designed to harmonize with seasonal *qì*, time of day, and the circulation of *qìxuè* 氣血 in the channels

---

[163] Nield, *"Keeping the Body's Multiple Clocks in Sync Could Be the Secret to Slowing Aging."*

The Celestial Dance: *Integrating Time and Astronomy in Chinese Medicine*

Anne Shelton Crute

Chinese medicine, at its core, operates on the principle that the human body is a microcosm mirroring the macrocosm of the earth and heavens. As such, understanding the relationship between the human being and the landscape becomes crucial for understanding and treating health. The channel system and its functions are analogous to streams and rivers, influenced by location and weather. However, to fully grasp the interconnectedness of life, we must consider the celestial dimension, integrating time, astronomy, and astrology into our understanding of health and disease. This chapter will explore the historical precedents, philosophical underpinnings, and practical applications of this integration, emphasizing the importance of aligning with the rhythms of the cosmos.

Historical Precedent: Humans as Part of a Wider Sense of Nature

The concept of the human being as intrinsically linked to both the earth and the heavens is deeply rooted in Han dynasty Chinese thought and continues throughout Chinese history. Classic texts, such as the *Nèijīng* 內經, provide ample evidence of this interconnectedness.

> *"The traditional Chinese belief in the harmony of nature was based on the close relationship between heaven (tiān天), earth (dì 地), and man (rén 人), the so-called 'three powers' (sāncái 三才). This worldview conceived of the harmonious cooperation of all matters within the universe, arising from the fact that they are all parts of a hierarchy of wholes forming a cosmic, organic pattern, and obeying the internal laws of their own natures."*[164]

This highlights the holistic worldview of Chinese medicine, emphasizing the interdependence of all things within a cosmic framework. The human being is not separate from nature, but an integral part of it.

---

[164] Yoke,"*Chinese Mathematical Astrology: Reaching Out to the Stars,*" pg. 12.

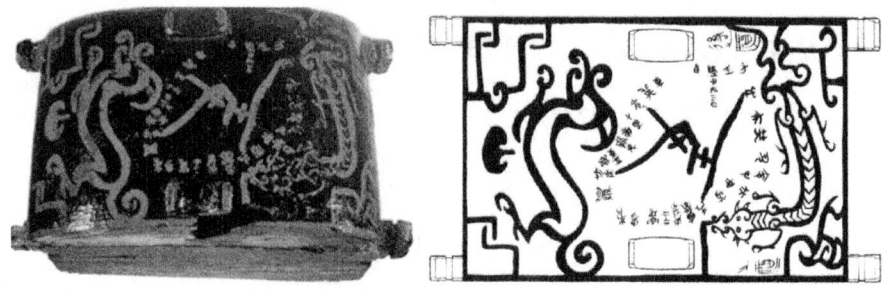

Figure 2.20 - Dragon and Tiger Constellations flanking the Dipper and Twenty-Eight Lunar Mansions from the Tomb of Marquis Yǐ 乙 of Zēng 曾[165]

In Chinese thought, celestial phenomena exert profound influence on human affairs, and classic texts of our tradition suggest that our destinies are intertwined with the rhythms of the cosmos. The Han dynasty classic *Huáinánzi* 淮南子 emphasizes the point, "*Men's lives are reflected in the movements of Heaven.*"[166] Even older sources recognize the movement of *Běidǒu* 北斗, the Northern Ladle and its related star, Polaris, aka the North Star, the Polestar, or Alpha Ursae Minoris. (*fig.2.20*) Several hexagrams in the *Yìjīng* 易經 reference various constellations and celestial events such as the solstices, including 1 ䷀ *qián* 乾 / Heaven; 26 ䷙ *dà xù* 大畜 / Great Store; 29 ䷜ *kǎn* 坎 / Pit; and 30 ䷝ *lí* 離 / Oriole. In the *Yìjīng*, Polaris and the the Northern Ladle are seen as a crucial point of orientation, guiding us to understand the nature of change and patterns, just as it guides us in navigating the night sky.[167] We see this described in the following quote:

> *"The Dipper is the [Supernal] Lord's carriage. Revolving in the center, it oversees and controls the four directions, separates yin from yang, establishes the four seasons, equalizes the five elemental phases, shifts the seasonal nodes and angular measures, and fixes the various cycles—all are tied to the Dipper."*[168]

Records of Chinese astronomy go so far back that we know pre-Han Chinese cultures recognized stars other than Alpha Ursae Minoris in the position and function of the Polestar.[169] The Chinese tradition of observing the sky is so

---

[165] Adapted from Shi, *"The Astronomical Meaning of Some Jade Artifacts Unearthed at the Lingjiatan Site. 2: The Jade Pigs,"* pg. 509 referencing MHP (The Museum of Hubei Province), 1989. *Tomb of Marquis Yi of State Zeng*. Beijing, Cultural Relics Publishing House.湖北省博物馆.曾侯乙墓[M].北京:文物出版社，1989 (in Chinese.).

[166] Walters, *"The Complete Guide to Chinese Astrology,"* pg. 177.

[167] Schipper, *"The Taoist Body,"* pg. 108.

[168] Pankenier, *"Astrology and Cosmology in Early China: Conforming Earth to Heaven,"* pg. 243.

[169] Yoke,*"Chinese Mathematical Astrology: Reaching Out to the Stars,"* pg. 140.

longstanding that some constellations used are no longer visible to us, yet their effect is still included as useful in calculations for human wellbeing.

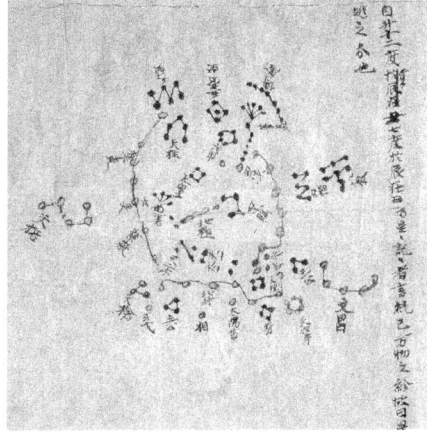

Figure 2.21 - Dūnhuáng 敦煌 Cave Star Chart[170]

Many maps and records of the skies show as many as 2000 years of unbroken astronomical data collection (*fig. 2.21*). The interconnection of our *qì* and the stars emphasizes the value of our conduct in the resonance between ourselves, the land, and cosmos. Kwok Man-Ho writes:

"In Chinese thought, there is a triad…[consisting of] Heaven, Earth and Humanity. The interaction of Heaven and Earth is made through us. We can put the universe out of harmony by disturbing the balance of yin and yang…or we can restore the balance through right actions and thoughts. In the end, Chinese astrology presents us with a picture of our current relationship to the great cosmic forces which shape all life and give measure to all lives. But, it presents us with the challenging possibility of change, because we are also part of the cosmic force which molds and gives meaning to life."[171]

The sky was considered to reflect the virtue of the Imperial leadership. *Figure 2.22* shows an image of harmony in the sky, *"said to appear when the ruler is enlightened, ministers are worthy, and the whole realm is in accord."*[172] When things were going awry in the nation, it was attributed to personal misconduct on the part of the Emperor. Such problems were said to be foretold by astronomical events such as comets and eclipses. In this way, we can see a theory of resonance between cosmological order, societal events, and personal conduct.

---

[170] ibid., pg. 141.

[171] Kwok, *"Complete Chinese Horoscopes,"* pg. 20.

[172] Dunhuang Star Chart showing the North Polar region (British Library Or.8210/ S.3326).

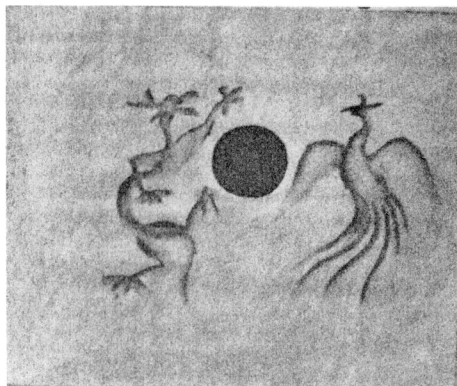

Figure 2.22 - Sun Flanked by a Dragon and Phoenix[173]

Astronomical and astrological knowledge were one and the same science, and were so highly valued that they were functionally classified. Additionally, at this time *"there was virtually no distinction between the historian and the astrologer."*[174]

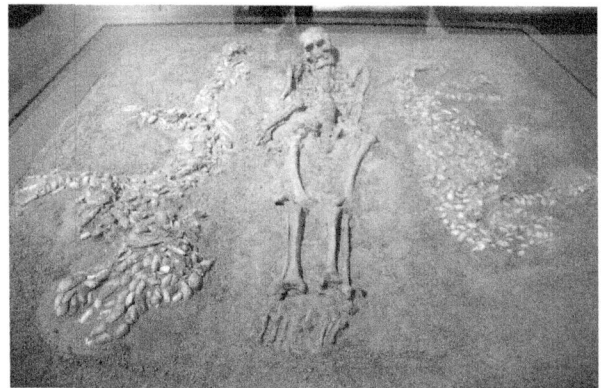

Figure 2.23 - Neolithic Burial at Xīshuǐpō Site in Púyáng濮陽[175]

The intricacies of the sky were indeed a sort of secret code hiding in plain sight with use since at least Neolithic times (*fig. 2.23*). This wisdom, over time, seamlessly integrated into Chinese culture and philosophy, impacting many

---

[173] Pankenier, *"Astrology and Cosmology in Early China: Conforming Earth to Heaven,"* pg. 490.

[174] Nakayama, *"Academic and Scientific Traditions in China, Japan, and the West,"* pg. 4.

[175] Human burial and shell mosaics in the shape of the dragon and tiger constellations from *Xīshuǐpō* 西水坡, *Hénán. Yǎngsháo* 仰韶 culture. National Museum Beijing. Ref. : Li Liu and Xingcan Chen : *The Archaeology of China*, 2012, pg. 197.

aspects of Chinese life ranging from governmental function to ritual practice, from mythology to medicine.

We can see by the time of the Song dynasty *qí mén dùnjiǎ* 奇門遁甲 text on military strategy *Huángdì Yīnfú Jīng* 黃帝陰符經/*Yellow Emperor's Secret Military Warrant Manual*[176] a telling example of the refinement of scientific and cultural integration evidenced by the following quote:

> *"The mystery of how Yin and Yang move in the ascending or the descending order is difficult to comprehend. The two solstices indicate the way back to the numbers one and nine in the Nine Palaces (jiǔgōng 九宮). When one comes to understand the 'pattern' (lǐ 理) of Yin and Yang, Heaven and Earth will all come within one's grasp."*[177]

This concept of *lǐ* 理, or "pattern," as described in the *Huángdì Yīnfú Jīng*, would also be a cornerstone of Neo-Confucian thought, and would later be refined by thinkers such as Zhūxī 朱熹 (1130–1200). The Neo-Confucianists saw *lǐ* as an inherent natural law, as well as a guiding principle for self-cultivation and moral clarity. By reflecting on earlier Daoist and Confucian ideas and integrating cosmology with moral philosophy, the Neo-Confucianists reinforced the belief that understanding cosmic patterns is essential to achieving harmony in both personal and governmental conduct. It's applicability to human life, as the next section will demonstrate, is far reaching.

Neo-Confucian Concepts: *Lǐ* 理, *Qì* 氣, and *Shù* 數

To appreciate the philosophical depth of the integration of Heaven, Earth, and Man, we must understand the Neo-Confucian concepts of *lǐ* 理 (cosmic organic pattern), *qì* 氣 (material-energetic substrata within time), and *shù* 數 (predestination/ mathematics/ calculation). *Lǐ* represents the inherent order and structure of the universe, the underlying principles that govern all things. *Qì* is the vital force that animates and manifests this order. *Shù*, often associated with mathematics and divination, helps us to decipher these patterns and understand our place within them.[178] The neo-Confucianist Kaibara Ekken 貝原益軒 (or Ekiken) (1630 - 1714) writes:

---

[176] The *Huángdì Yīnfú Jīng* 黃帝陰符經 described here is completely different in nature and context from the sixth century CE Daoist *Huángdì Yīnfú Jīng* 黃帝陰符經/ *Yellow Emperor's Scripture on the Hidden Talisman* text which contains the same name and is a central text in early internal alchemy (*nèidān* 內丹) traditions and in the early *Quánzhēn* 全真/Complete Perfection movement.

[177] Yoke,"*Chinese Mathematical Astrology: Reaching Out to the Stars*," pg. 87.

[178] ibid., pg. 12-13.

"As for principle, it is inherent in material force; principle and material force should not be divided into two things. There is no temporal connection of before and after between them. There is no spatial relationship of separation or combination"[179]

These concepts provide a framework for understanding the interconnectedness of all things. Our bodies are not separate entities, but are expressions of *qì* shaped by *lǐ*. By understanding *shù*, we can gain insight into our inherent patterns and tendencies, allowing us to navigate our lives with greater awareness.

With or without knowing it, this is what we treat in clinic. When we recognize patterns in the pulse and tongue, we are keying into wider patters of *lǐ*, or cosmic order, that extend quite literally through all of manifestation, right down to the level of the individual. When we intervene and support our patient's physical harmony with acupuncture, we are adjusting *qì*. When we apply an awareness of our timing, whether by use of seasonal awareness, *qì* nodes, *tōng shū* 通书, or other means like Chinese astrology, we are refining that adjustment by considering *shù*, the mathematical rhythm.

The 60-Year Cycle: Mathematics Beyond Materiality

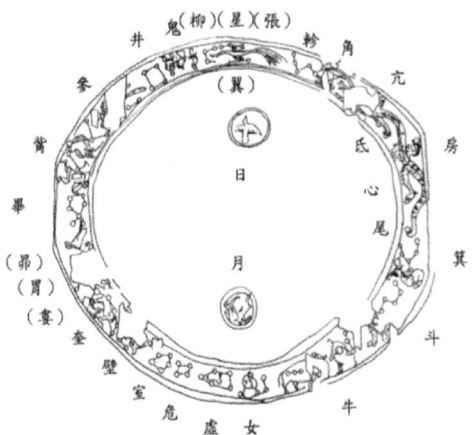

Figure 2.24 - Progression of the Lunar Lodges from the Ceiling of a Han Dynasty Tomb at Xī'ān Jiāotōng 西安交通 University[180]

A cornerstone of the Chinese understanding of time is the 60-year cycle. This system, born from the creation of a lunisolar calendar and the observations of

---

[179] Kaibara, and Tucker *"The Philosophy of Qi: The Record of Great Doubts,"* pg. 88-89.

[180] 莊, "得 "意" 忘 "形"-漢墓壁畫中天象圖的轉變過程研究, "pg. 7.

Jupiter's movements, reflects a sophisticated grasp of cosmic rhythms. Throughout history, we have used the positions of the moon and sun to coordinate human activities with time, ascribing various names and mythology to each lunar and solar position (*fig. 2.24*). What these have in common is an Earth-based model of wisdom that loosely lines up across cultures, directly connected to planting and harvesting cycles, and extending into all arenas of human life from the utilitarian to the sacred.

Many cultures have used Jupiterian cycles as a scale to understand larger time-scapes than the lunar months and solar year, however the Chinese took this observation a step further: into the math.

The true movement of Jupiter, which orbits the sun approximately every 12 years, deviates slightly from a perfect 12-year cycle. By multiplying this cycle by five and synchronizing it with the movements of the moon and the sun, the Chinese arrived at a 60-year cycle. This larger cycle is made up of smaller sub-cycles designated by stems and branches, thus abstracting from the purely observational to a mathematical understanding of time and space.

In the West, we often perceive mathematics as an intellectual overlay onto physical reality, a view rooted in material absolutism. However, the Chinese ancients recognized that abstract numbers possess a truth that transcends physical manifestation. This insight, which modern Western science has only recently begun to grasp through quantum mechanics and advanced physics in the last century, reveals that the underlying mathematical structures are perhaps more fundamental—possibly even more true—than the reality they describe.

The Chinese system extrapolates into larger movements and patterns with great accuracy. It is a system which takes observations from nature and utilizes its rhythms. Per the *Huáinánzi,* these rhythms are then understood within an even larger framework of *hùn dùn* 混沌, or primal chaos, in which pattern naturally arises, continues for some time, and later dissolves.

Chinese theories of time—of which the 60-year cycle is but one—are perfect examples of these rhythmic patterns of nature. When properly understood and applied, they are no longer viewed as a hokey relic of unpolished folk medicine. With study, we can embrace these elegant theories and apply them to modern medical practice.

The Problematic Gregorian Calendar and the Wisdom of the Chinese Almanac

The Gregorian calendar, while widely adopted for its practical utility, presents a subtle yet significant challenge to our understanding of natural temporal rhythms. The misalignment between our standardized timekeeping and the actual progression of seasonal changes can have far-reaching implications for our perception of time, health, and societal functioning.

There is a discrepancy between the Gregorian demarcation of the seasons and their observable, natural transitions. For instance, the calendar's designation of the vernal equinox as the first day of spring contradicts the gradual onset of spring-like light conditions that can be observed weeks earlier, especially in northern latitudes. We experience the days growing warmer and longer, blossoms blooming on the trees, while the calendar tells us that we are still in the midst of winter. Similarly, the summer solstice—the longest day of the year—is inexplicably marked as the beginning of summer, rather than its obvious peak. Even without weather changes to match our cultural ideas about the seasons, what theChinese calendar is showing us is the portion of light and dark, of available yin and *yáng qì*. Our human conduct can and should match this seasonal movement for optimal health and wellbeing.

The fundamental misrepresentation of natural time cycles on the Gregorian Calendar can have profound effects on our clinical practice and broader societal perspectives. The Gregorian calendar subtly discourages alignment with natural patterns. This impacts our ability to recognize and respond to emerging trends. It distorts our capacity to make timely adjustments in personal and professional life. It robs us of the appropriate orientation to synchronize our physiological rhythms with natural cycles.

The repercussions of this temporal disconnect extend beyond individual health and psychology to societal functioning. It can impair our collective ability to identify and address emerging issues, such as in the case of climate change. When we have not learned to acknowledge the early stages of basic phenomena, it makes it more challenging for us to recognize and respond to changing conditions. This is why we come into crisis in societal and economic issues. This is also why our patients often arrive in clinic with full-blown disease.

Chinese Medicine practitioners work to correct this misalignment for our patients. We educate our patients on traditional worldview of natural systems. We attenuate our patients to the rhythms of nature using therapeutic treatments such as acupuncture and herbal medicines. Our medicine fosters a culture that values proactive engagement with change rather than reactive fear.

Traditional systems like the Chinese almanac offer a more nuanced approach to timekeeping. Rooted in careful observations of celestial and terrestrial phenomena, such systems provide a framework for understanding the cyclical nature of *qì*. As Kristofer Schipper notes, "*The cycle of days and seasons, of centuries and ages, of the cosmic rhythm, is the working of the Dao. Hence the sacred nature of the calendar.*"[181]

The misalignment between our standardized calendar and natural time cycles is more than a mere inconvenience. It reflects a deeper disconnection from the rhythms of nature, potentially impacting our health, decision-making processes, and societal resilience. Recognizing and addressing this disconnect may be crucial for fostering a more harmonious relationship with our natural environment and improving our collective ability to navigate change.

Practical Application: Aligning with Time Through Chinese Almanac and Astrology

The integration of Chinese almanac and astrology into acupuncture practice aligns with the holistic principles of Chinese medicine. We view our patients as unique expressions of time and space. This approach profoundly enriches our clinical experience with individual patients. It is supported by both ancient texts and contemporary scholarship.

The *Sùwèn* 素問 emphasizes the intrinsic connection between time, space, and the human body. *Sùwèn* 66 reminds us that all things manifest as part of a progression, when it is their time. It states, "*Heaven has the five agents; they control the five positions.*"[182] These five positions correspond to the cardinal directions on the compass and center. The *Sùwèn* highlights that our experiences are intimately linked to electromagnetic fields of the earth and sky, with celestial influences varying based on their directional relationship to us.

This holistic view necessitates a treatment approach that goes beyond targeting the physical body alone. Roger Ames articulates this perspective in his work on Confucian ethics:

"*In classical correlative cosmology, the term 'body,' like any predication of qi, must of course be used advisedly; everything is a continuous field of qi manifesting itself at once as 'lived body' and as 'environs,' as 'physical' and as 'spiritual,' as 'forming' (ti) and as 'functioning' (yong), as 'temporal' (shi) and as 'spatial' (jie), as 'persistent' (tong) and as 'flux' (bian).*"[183]

The understanding of the body as a multidimensional expression of *qi* supports the integration of astrological and almanac-based considerations in clinical practice. Stated simply, it matters not only how we treat our patients,

---

[181] Schipper, *"The Taoist Body,"* pg. 23.

[182] Unschuld, Tessenow, and Zheng, *"Huang Di Nei Jing Su Wen: An Annotated Translation of Huang Di's Inner Classic - Basic Questions, 2 Volumes"* pg. 173.

[183] Ames, *"Confucian Role Ethics: A Vocabulary,"* pg. 57.

but when and where. Historically, such an interdisciplinary approach is not without precedent. Kristofer Schipper notes that Daoist priests collaborated with "Confucianist specialists," including acupuncturists, astrologers, and geomancers, in ritual healing practices.[184]

In modern acupuncture practice, integrating almanac and Chinese astrology, aka *zǐwēi dòushù* 紫微斗数, aka Polestar astrology, provides a framework for a more comprehensive understanding of patients. Practitioners can consider a patient's birth data alongside other diagnostic information such as lab work, tailoring treatments to harmonize cosmic, ancestral, and earthly rhythms with constitutional tendencies. When the wide view of Chinese philosophy is properly applied, ancient and modern tools can be integrated easily and utilized for that which they are best suited.

Powerful tools such a *zǐwēi dòushù* allow for more personalized and holistic treatment strategies that address not only physical symptoms, but also the patient's position within a broader order. *Zǐwēi dòushù* evaluates an individual's expression of the time in which they are born in comparison with the arrangement of their free will and fate patterns. Although contemporary Western culture tends to consider free will and fated predispositions as mutually exclusive, the traditional East Asian view considers both to be true and relevant. Furthermore, fate and free will exist on a continuum with one another. These values are what can be assessed using traditional *zǐwēi dòushù*.

If skeptics are wary of terminology like "fate" and "free will," we can remind them that these principles are a matter of common sense. Despite Western New Age spiritual culture sensationalizing terms such as these, the traditional philosophical interpretation is entirely pragmatic and grounded. For instance, if one is born into an English-speaking culture and family, one may certainly apply free will to learn another language, but there would also be a strong fated tendency to speaking English. These concepts of fate and free will are not so foreign to Western medical thought. Consider the modern field of epigenetics. One may be born with a more fated predisposition for alcoholism, yet one may apply free will to avoid drinking.

When we bring traditional Chinese astrological tools into clinic, we can understand prognosis on a larger framework. Does our patient present with an illness that time itself may clear? Is our role as doctor one to educate the patient about longterm management or can we see a clear path to complete healing? Is the illness medical and therefore responsive to standard application of treatment? Or, is fate playing out through the body, requiring a re-examination of the life path? When we use calculations to help our patients understand

---

[184] Schipper, *"The Taoist Body,"* pg. 74.

auspices and coordinate with the dance of time, their health and general wellbeing improves.

Ultimately, there are many tools available to consider a patient's case in a multidisciplinary way. Availing tools which employ time, such as the astrological chart and the daily guidance of the almanac, practitioners can select acupuncture points, herbal formulas, and make lifestyle recommendations that align with both the individual's constitution and disease process, as well as the larger *qì* nodes, open points, and expressions of time in the environment.

The Importance of Context: Countering Reductionism

The efficacy of Chinese medicine has been well-demonstrated through both scientific studies and patient experiences. Yet, there is a growing trend toward reductionism that threatens to weaken its foundational strengths. Increasingly, practitioners are adopting a modern, professionalized approaches that emphasize specialization—refining their offerings to niche populations or specific diseases.

While this may appear to enhance expertise, it risks undermining the broader, integrative understanding that is central to the philosophy of Chinese medicine. The true strength of this system lies in its ability to approach health and disease holistically, guided by deep theoretical knowledge and cosmological principles. When practitioners cultivate this broader understanding, they develop exceptional diagnostic skills and the capacity to treat a wide range of patients effectively. Conversely, when one's practice is limited to treating only fertility or oncology, for example, it may reflect a reliance on a collection of techniques rather than a comprehensive grasp of the root causes of disease.

This reductionist trend is further exacerbated by the push to distance Chinese medicine from its contextual roots in time, astrology, and philosophy. The argument often made is that these elements are unnecessary now that Chinese medicine's efficacy has been validated through modern scientific frameworks.

However, to abandon these contextual aspects is to strip the medicine of its essence. We end up with medicine based on protocols, applied without due consideration of the individual in time-space. In truth, our point selections and formulas are only as good as our diagnoses. Our diagnoses are only as sophisticated as our cosmological understanding of the manifestation of disease within the larger, organic picture.

When practitioners integrate the essence of Chinese medicine philosophy, they think in a broad and associative manner, cultivating reasoning skills that are grounded in deep study and self-cultivation. This holistic training fosters not only intellectual understanding, but also emotional and spiritual growth, enabling practitioners to approach their work with compassionate, heart-centered focus.

This integrative approach is not new; it is deeply rooted in Chinese thought. For example, during the Song dynasty, Confucian training emphasized the importance of a well-rounded education that included government, history, calligraphy, music, and even oracle. Such breadth was seen as essential for developing leadership capable of solving complex problems for the populace. Similarly, in Chinese medicine, proficiency arises from cultivating oneself in diverse areas of knowledge and practice.

As Xúnzǐ 荀子 (310-238 BCE) wrote in the third century BCE:

"Heaven has its seasons, Earth has its resources, and man has his government. For this reason, it is said that they may form a triad. If one abandons that which allows him to form a triad, yet longs for the triad, he is deluded."[185]

This triadic relationship underscores the interconnectedness between humanity and the natural world—a principle at the heart of Chinese medicine's diagnostic and therapeutic methods. Maintaining a broad perspective allows practitioners to treat patients with greater depth and nuance while safeguarding the integrity of this ancient healing tradition.

Harmonizing with Heaven: Benefits in Clinic and Beyond

The traditional view of Chinese medicine offers an opportunity to opt into a more connected experience of reality, allowing us to align with natural order. It brings us closer to a state of flowing harmony, which is the ultimate goal of this work for all of us: doctor and patient alike.

The complexity and urgency of our modern conditions so often lead us to a state of distraction and disconnection. Chinese medicine provides a path to genuine satisfaction by helping us embrace reality as it is, rather than as we wish it to be. The gap between those two only reflects the healing work we have to do, both individually and as a society.

This work shows us that we can experience ourselves connected to and expressing as the landscape, the waterways, the stars. Kristofer Schipper's observes,

"The body appears as one and many at the same time. The head, thorax, and abdomen are described as distinct sections, and on each level one finds the sun, moon, and Pole

---

[185] Kaibara, and Tucker, *"The Philosophy of Qi: The Record of Great Doubts,"* pg. 62.

Star (as well as the Dipper constellation with which it is associated). At the same time, each section retains its own essence and together the three form a complete landscape."[186]

This microcosmic view of the body reflects the macrocosmic order, the medicine alchemizing a direct experience of our bodies as nature.

By cultivating this traditional view, we gain access to a deeper understanding of our place within the natural world. The celestial maps embedded within our bodies serve as guides, illuminating the reciprocal relationship we experience with and as nature. This perspective not only enhances clinical practice, but also extends its benefits beyond the realm of medicine. It offers a framework for harmonious living in all aspects of life.

Integrating time, astronomy, and astrology into Chinese medicine is not an expansion but a recognition of what has always been an essential part of its foundation—understanding the human being as an integral part of the cosmos. These ancient methods have been integral to Chinese medical practice. Thus enriching the practice rather than contradicting modern clinical methods. By embracing the wisdom of the Chinese almanac, exploring the insights of astrology, and aligning ourselves with the rhythms of time, we can bring greater awareness to these fundamental aspects of healing and transformation, both for ourselves and our patients.

---

[186] Schipper, *"The Taoist Body,"* pg. 74.

Charting the Inner Ecosystem Through Chinese Medical and Daoist Alchemical Body Maps

Daniel Schrier

In the Chinese medical and Daoist traditions, the human body is visualized and mapped as a living landscape (*jìng* 境). Both share similar views of the body as a country (*guó* 國), shaped by the natural contours of the surrounding environment. As outlined in *Sùwèn* 素問 8, Chinese medicine sees each of the *zàngfǔ* 臟腑 organs as a governmental official with specific roles. Daoism, paints the body as a vast realm full of forests, gardens, rivers, terraces, mountains, caverns, temples, monasteries, towers and palaces, habited by various celestial and terrestrial animals, gods, and spirits reflecting the interdependence of the human and the environment.[187]

Three ways in which these two traditions viewed/mapped the body was via the

1) External views of the body's surface
2) Internal anatomical views
3) Symbolic/alchemical imagery

Each of these mapping systems serve distinct purposes and reflects a unique understanding of the body, knowledge systems, and spiritual practices.

External Views of the Body's Surface

Many of these maps have a focus on the body's surface anatomy, highlighting the channels and acupuncture points visually through drawings and text. During the Song dynasty, the Bronze Man (*zhēn jiǔ tóng rén* 针灸铜人) statues allowed these maps to be a key tool for medical education and training (*fig. 2.25*). These visual aids would further assist the viewer in understanding *qì* flow and locating the various points to heal the body.

---

[187] Schipper, *"The Taoist Body,"* pg. 100.

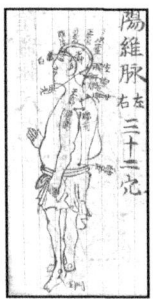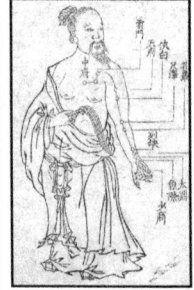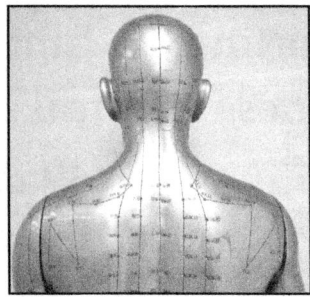

Figure 2.25 - Acupuncture Channel Maps[188]

In addition to channel mapping, Chinese medicine also utilizes a variety of diagnostic maps such as the tongue, the pulse positions, the eyes, ears face and hand/palm to aid in diagnosis (*fig 2.26*). Each of these serves as microcosmic reflections of the body's internal state, forming a complete and interconnected method for understanding changes/imbalances within the body.

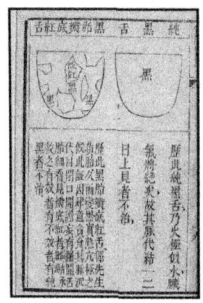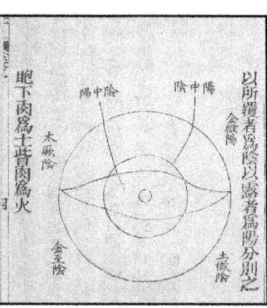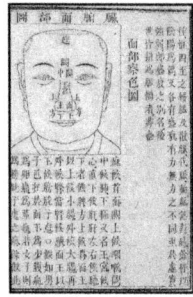

Figure 2.26 - Tongue, Eye, and Physiognomy Maps [189]

Chinese medicine texts, such as the *Zhēnjiǔ Jiǎyǐ Jīng* 針灸甲乙經 and *Língshū* 10 & 74, describe hand/palm maps. While palm diagnosis (*zhǎng zhěn* 掌診) is no longer a primary diagnostic tool in modern Chinese Medicine, it was one of the main diagnostic method used by Master Tung. Hand maps additionally play an important role in Daoist practice; where they are integrated into incantations, meditation, healing rituals, and other divination practices. Certain positions on the hand are linked to specific energetic or cosmological forces such as the *bāguà* 八卦, five phases (*wǔxíng* 五行), Twelve Earthy Branches (*shí'èr dìzhī* 十二地支) (*fig. 2.27*), Ten Heavenly Stems (*tiāngān* 天干) and the

---

[188] Picture taken by D.Schrier of handwritten manuscript given as gift in 2013 (left); *Lung channel of hand taiyin with point names, Chinese woodcut*. Wellcome Collection. Source: <u>Wellcome Collection</u>.(center); Picture taken by D.Schrier of bronze man replica, (right).

[189] *Tongue morphology: Heitai biandi hongshe, Chinese woodcut*. Wellcome Collection. Source: <u>Wellcome Collection</u>. (left). *C19 Chinese eye diagnosis chart showing Yin and Yang division*. Wellcome Collection. Source: <u>Wellcome Collection</u>.(middle) *Physiognomy diagnosis chart, Chinese woodcut, 1817*. Wellcome Collection. Source: <u>Wellcome Collection</u>.(right)

Twenty-Eight Star Constellations (*èrshíbā xiù* 二十八宿). These hand positions play a role in both daily greetings among Daoists, as well as within more formal ritual performance. One example is the *tàijí shǒuyìn* 太極手印 mudra, also known as the *zǐwǔjué* 子午訣. This mudra is formed by placing the left thumb on the *zǐ* 子 point on the right hand, with the right thumb touching the *wǔ* 午 point on the right hand, thus creating a *tàijí* 太極 symbol with one's hand. This, mudra also establishes a connection between fire and water. This is one of the fundamental alchemical mudras and commonly used in meditation practice.

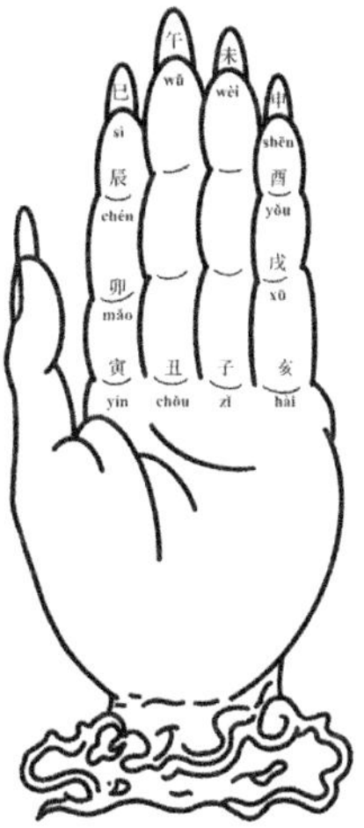

Earthly Branch	Lunar Month	Time	Organ	Outer Energy	Inner Energy
zǐ 子	11th	11pm-1am *Midnight*	GB	Wood	Water
chǒu 丑	12th	1am-3am	LR	Wood	Earth
yín 寅	1st	3am-5am	LU	Metal	Wood
mǎo 卯	2nd	5am-7am *Sunrise*	LI	Metal	Wood
chén 辰	3rd	7am-9am	ST	Earth	Earth
sì 巳	4th	9am-11am	SP	Earth	Fire
wǔ 午	5th	11am-1pm *Noon*	HT	Fire	Fire
wèi 未	6th	1pm-3pm	SI	Fire	Earth
shēn 申	7th	3pm-5pm	BL	Water	Metal
yǒu 酉	8th	5pm-7pm *Sunset*	KI	Water	Metal
xū 戌	9th	7pm-9pm	PC	Fire	Earth
hài 亥	10th	9pm-11pm	SJ	Fire	Water

Figure 2.27 - Twelve Earthly Branches Hand Pattern & Correspondences[190]

Other maps include the *dǎoyǐn* 導引[191] maps/charts, which display static and dynamic postures aimed at instructing on methods for promoting health and longevity. However, these maps often require accompanying textual explanations and personal/oral instruction (*kǒujué* 口訣) for proper practice. These practices tend to be static, focusing on specific postures or "movements" for particular purposes rather than continuous full-body motion. By integrating breathing control, stretching and twisting the arms and legs, and mental focus, these movements helps to direct the flow of *qì*, creating a harmonious balance between *qì* and blood in the body. This, in turn, aids in preventing illness, as well as improving one's overall health and vitality.

---

[190] Image adapted from *Dùrén Shàngjīng Dàfǎ* 度人上經大法/*Great Rites of the Book of Universal Salvation.*

[191] Guided stretching or stretching and breath work - *Dǎo* 導 - to guide *qì*, the internal vital energy of the body, so as to create an internal balance, & *yǐn* 引 - to stretch the body so as to gain strength & flexibility. *Dǎoyǐn* is sometimes referred to as "Daoist Yoga" which is a mistaken translation and category.

161

One of the earliest and famous examples of this type of map/chart is the *Dǎoyǐn Tú* 導引圖/*Diagram of Internal Pathways*[192] (*fig. 2.28*), uncovered in the *Mǎwángduī* 馬王堆 manuscript (168 BCE), which illustrates 44 health exercises. One could view this as a fully integrated movement sequence, however, it is much more likely that each movement shown was for a particular condition. The *Dǎoyǐn Tú* depicts many movements that are performed while standing; while others being done kneeling or sitting. The *Dǎoyǐn Tú* illustrates *qì* development training to help aid in alleviating illness. Its imagery helps viewers remember the 44 movements and to help choose which movement would be most appropriate for the presenting condition.

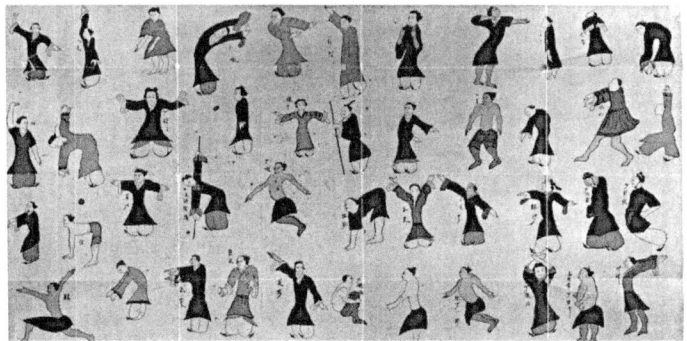

Figure 2.28 - Reconstructed Dǎoyǐn Tú 導引圖 Diagram[193]

We can also see similar *Dǎoyǐn Tú* charts such as Chén Tuán 陳摶's[194] (d. 989) *Chén Xīyí Xiānshēng Èrshísì Qì Zuògōng Dǎoyǐn Zhìbìng Tú* 陳希夷先生二十四氣坐功導引治病圖/*Master Chénxīyí's Twenty-Four Nodes Seated Exercises of Guided Stretching for Curing Ailments*. This text outlines a series of twenty four exercise techniques, corresponding to the twenty-four solar terms (*èrshísì jiéqì* 二十四節氣) to help prevent diseases, and maintain health during the seasonal changes throughout the year. These twenty-four movements detail the energetic mapping of the body's inner seasons, allowing one to embody and attune themselves with seasonal vibrations.

---

[192] This is not a Daoist map/chart and was not originally called the "*Dǎoyǐn Tú*." This name was given by archaeologists and interpreters.

[193] *Dǎoyǐn Tú* 導引圖/*Guiding and Pulling Chart, Mǎwángduī, tomb 3 (closed 168 BCE)*. The original is in the Hunan Provincial Museum, Changsha, China. © Wellcome Library, London, L0036007.

[194] A mountain hermit, immortal, & the patron saint of *Huàshān* 華山. He is known for his sleep exercises (*shuìgōng* 睡功), 24 seasonal *dǎoyǐn* exercises mentioned above, physiognomy, *Yìjīng* studies (*yìxué* 易學) and creating the *Wújí Tú* 無極圖 diagram which would become famous in Neo-Confucian circles and provide the basis for the Zhōu Dūnyí 周敦頤's *Tàijí Tú* 太極圖.

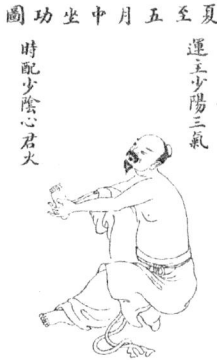

Figure 2.29 - Summer Solstice (Xiàzhì 夏至) Exercise Chart [195]

For instance, the movement associated with the summer solstice/*xiàzhì* 夏至 (*fig. 2.29*) which occurs during the fifth lunar month,[196] is practiced during the *yín* 寅 (3-5 AM) and *mǎo* 卯 hour (5-7 AM).[197] This practice involves one kneeling in a seated posture, stretching their hands out with fingers interlocked under one's foot, and then stretching the foot outwards. The movement is repeated 35 times (5×7), alternating between the left and right foot. The practice concludes with the clicking of the teeth, inhaling the clear (*qīng* 清) and exhaling the turbid (*zhuó* 濁), then swallowing the salvia which was produced in the mouth.[198] This particular movement is beneficial for conditions regarding stagnations due to wind damp (rheumatism); as well as wrist, knee, ankle and arm pain. It also alleviates discomfort from hot palms, pain in the kidney region, pain in the waist and spine and a general feeling of heaviness of the body.[199]

Internal Anatomical Views

While internal organ anatomical study might have had a less prominent role in Chinese tradition as compared to Western medicine, anatomical observations

---

[195] Komjathy, *"Electronic Supplement to Traces of a Daoist Immortal."*

[196] This period of time marks the peak of Summer, with the longest day and the shortest night of the year. The Sun's longitude at 90° and falls roughly around June 21st-22nd of the Gregorian calendar and lasts for 15 days.

[197] Note: There is no mention however if these movements should be done on the exact day of the solar node or during this 15 day period.

[198] Adapted from Komjathy, *"Traces of a Daoist Immortal: Chén Tuán* 陳摶 *of the Western Marchmount,"* pg. 391.

[199] Adapted from Komjathy, *"Traces of a Daoist Immortal: Chén Tuán* 陳摶 *of the Western Marchmount,"* pg. 391.

and measurements were documented in classical literature such as *Língshū* 靈樞 12 and *Nàn Jīng* 難經 41 and 42. During the late Five Dynasties (902-979 CE) and Song periods (960-1279 CE), there was an emergence of illustrations depicting only the torso and internal organs without outlining the body's external contours, some including detailed depictions of individual viscera. There is also a series of texts with representations of the trunk and the organs *(fig. 2.30)* dating from the late Jin dynasty (936–947) preserved in the Song-Yuan Dynasty text, *Xiūzhēn Shíshū* 修真十書/*Ten Books on the Cultivation of Perfection* (1250), as well as illustrations from Yuan Dynasty in the *Huá Tuó Xuánmén Nèizhào Tú* 華陀玄門內照圖/*Hua Tuo's Images for Internal Visualization According to the Mystery School (1273).*

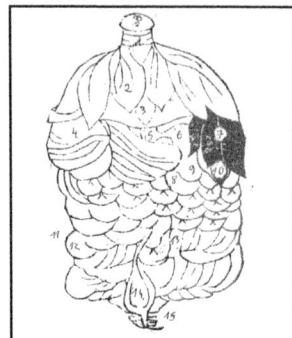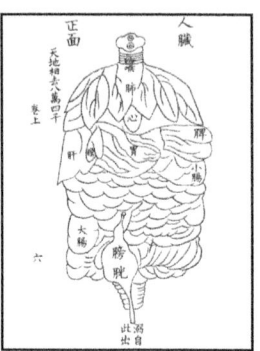

Figure 2.30 - Xiūzhēn Shíshū 修真十書 (left) & Huá Tuó Xuánmén Nèizhào Tú 華陀玄門內照圖 (right)[200]

As Stephen mentioned in *Stream Waters (Jīng Shuǐ 經水)*[201], the Han dynasty physicians went beyond merely calculating size and form; they understood the profound interconnection between the flow of blood in the human body and the movement of streams and aquifers in nature. They recognized that this dynamic circulation served as a form of irrigation, vital for maintaining the health and balance of the human landscape.

Symbolic/Alchemical Views

The symbolic/alchemical body is central to Daoist practices, since it represents the body as a microcosm of the cosmos/universe (*yǔzhòu* 宇宙) and is the site of and for spiritual transformation. Daoist texts depict the body as a sacred space, such as a mountain, which is inhabited by various body gods and spirits. These representations serve both ritualistic and meditative purposes,

---

[200] Lo, and Barrett, "*Imagining Chinese Medicine*," pg. 58-59.

[201] See "*Stream Waters (Jīng Shuǐ 經水)*," pg. 59-666

guiding one through *cúnxiǎng* 存想 / visualized practice and *nèiguān* 內觀 / inner observation[202] to achieve immortality / spiritual enlightenment.[203]

While the Daoist view of the body as a landscape inco ikerporates elements forests, gardens, rivers, terraces, mountains, caverns, temples, pagodas, monasteries, palaces, gods, and spirits, all which highlight various access points and landmarks which engage the subtle body. We often see a strong emphasis on mountains in many of these maps. The significance of this extends beyond physical mountains and the practice of mountain seclusion. Mountains serve as powerful metaphor for meditative practices. In this context, we can look at the Daoist phrase "*rù shān* 入山" which translates as "entering the mountains," as a reference to ascending the altar to perform Daoist rituals, as well as engaging in meditation practices.[204] The "mountain" represents a sense of stillness inside of us. This concept is reflected in the mountain trigram ☶ (*gèn* 艮), which also appears doubled in hexagram 52 ䷳, and shares the same name (*gèn* 艮). Because the mountains are the closest place to where heaven and earth meet, and they offer a sense of *yīnyáng* stability and balance. This connection of mountains to meditation is also reinforced by Xuē Tàilái 薛泰來 (1923–2001)[205] who in a conversation with Bill Porter said "*If you want to find a place to practice, you have to go into the mountains.*"[206] While Xuē Tàilái suggests physically going to the mountains to find this stillness in order to practice, one can also look to the inner mountains within one's body to find this stillness.

Examples of charts that depict the body as a mountain can be found in the *Tǐxiàng Yīnyáng Shēngjiàng Tú* 體象陰陽升降圖 / *Diagram of the Ascent and Descent of Yīn Yáng in the Body* (*fig. 2.31*) This map depicts the human body viewed from the front (left) and back (right), illuminating the flow of the lesser celestial circuit (*xiǎo zhōu tiān* 小周天). In this diagram, the governing (*dū mài* 督脈) and conception (*rèn mài* 任脈) vessels, trace parallels watercourses, encircling a landscape of which encompasses a mountain. This imagery reflects the body's hidden topography, where energies rise and fall like mist over these sacred peaks.

---

[202] These are two of the five major types of Daoist meditation which include 1) Apophatic or Quietistic Meditation (including *jìngzuò* 靜坐 / *xīnzhāi* 心齋 / *zuòwàng* 坐忘) 2) Visualization (*cúnxiǎng* 存想) 3) Ingestion (*fúqì* 服氣) 4) Inner Observation (*nèiguān* 內觀) & 5) Internal Alchemy (*nèidān* 內丹).

[203] Komjathy, "*The Daoist Tradition,*" pg. 135-137 & Schipper, "*The Taoist Body,*"pg. 100.

[204] Komjathy, "The *Daoist Tradition,*" pg. 135-137.

[205] A 24th generation Huàshān 華山 lineage Daoist.

[206] Porter, "*Road to Heaven: Encounters with Chinese Hermits,*"pg. 80.

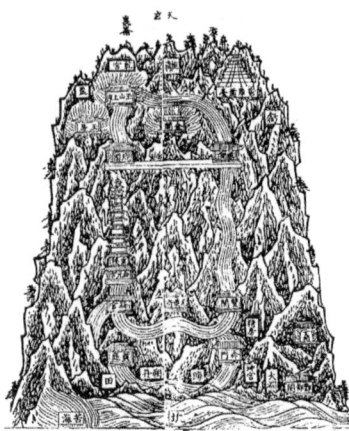

Figure 2.31 - Tǐxiàng Yīnyáng Shēngjiàng Tú 體象陰陽升降圖/Diagram of the Ascent and Descent of *Yīnyáng* in the Body[207]

As Stephen mentioned in his introduction *The Art & Science of Seal Form Characters*,[208] one could look at *huán* 環/ring; loop; to encircle, as a metaphor for the microcosmic orbit, also referred to as the lesser celestial circuit (*xiǎo zhōu tiān* 小周天) and the waterwheel (*héchē* 河車). The *Nèijīng Tú* 內經圖/*Map of the Inner Landscape* (*fig. 2.32*) also displays this celestial circulation. The microcosmic orbit, is a *nèidān* 內丹/inner alchemy technique, which involves the circulation of transformed vital essence up the governing vessel and down the conception vessel, allowing the body to become an integrated whole, or *huán* 環/ring. This movement of energy aids in awakening the subtle body. When combined with the cultivation of stillness, it fosters deep integration and transformation within the body. This image in *Figure 2.31* reminds us that we are the mountain, as we embody it's energy within us.

There are many body maps (*shēntú* 身圖) which play a significant role in charting alchemical transformation, such as Lǐ Jiǒng 李炯's *Nèijīng Tú* 內經圖/*Map of the Inner Landscape*, the *Huǒhòu Tú* 火候圖/*Firing Processing Map*, Chén Tuán 陳摶's *Wújí Tú* 無極圖/*Diagram of Non-Differentiation* and Zhōu Dūnyí 周敦頤's *Tàijí Tú* 太極圖/*Diagram of the Great Ultimate*. Two maps/charts of particular importance are the *Nèijīng Tú* 內經圖/*Map of the Inner Landscape* and the *Xiūzhēn Tú* 修真圖/*Map for Cultivation of Reality*, which incorporate numerous visual metaphors representing the human body and illustrating specific processes of alchemical transformation. The following section will explore some of the key symbols and images found within these two maps.

---

[207] Huang,"*Picturing the True Form: Daoist Visual Culture in Traditional China*,"pg. 79.

[208] See Stephen's introduction "*The Art & Science of Seal Form Characters*," pg. 25-29.

Nèijīng Tú 內經圖/ Map of the Inner Landscape

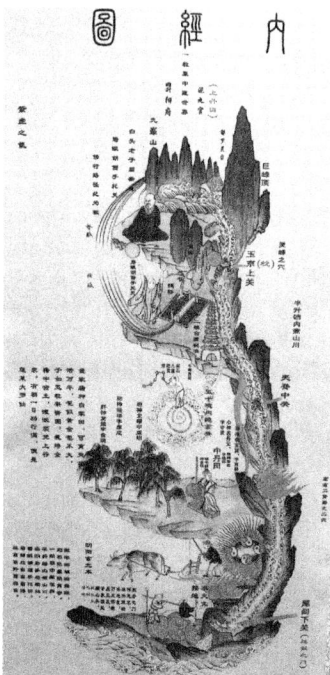

Figure 2.32 - *Nèijīng Tú* 內經圖/ Map of the Inner Landscape[209]

The *Nèijīng Tú* 內經圖 (*fig. 2.32*) is a one of the most famous Daoist body maps *(shēntú)*, which serves as a visual representation of internal alchemy practices, *nèigōng* 內功, and the microcosmic orbit, aimed at cultivating health, spiritual enlightenment, and harmony with the *Dào* 道. Created during the Qing dynasty, and carved into a courtyard wall of the *Báiyún Guàn* 白雲觀/White Cloud Monastery in Beijing,[210] the diagram combines physiological, energetic, and cosmological elements to illustrate the Daoist body as a cohesive map and guide for self-cultivation, with the aim of achieving harmony within the body and unity with the *Dào* 道. The integration of metaphors of nature throughout the map reflects the Daoist understanding of the human body as a sacred microcosm of the universe. This map depicts a person from the side, with the bottom representing the base of the torso and the top representing the head.

---

[209] Picture by D.Schrier from personal scroll, all images of the *Nèijīng Tú* 內經圖 shared in this text are from this source.

[210] *Báiyún Guàn* 白雲觀/White Cloud Monastery is the seat of contemporary Quánzhēn 全眞 Daoism, and the headquarters of the Chinese Daoist Association (*Zhōngguó Dàojiào Xiéhuì* 中國道教協會).

This map is full of natural and cosmic imagery, depicting the body as a sacred landscape, that includes rivers, mountains, and celestial bodies such as the sun and moon. These images convey the body's dynamic energy flow and spiritual potential and point to how the practitioner engages in the actualization and refinement of these internal landscapes. The intention is to reinforce the Daoist belief that the body mirrors the cosmos, with its internal geography reflecting the external world.

Rivers and streams symbolize the flow of energy throughout the body. These streams connect various elements, illustrating the interconnectedness of the body's energy pathways.The spine is depicted as a flowing path resembling a mountain range with water flowing, and symbolizing the central channel of energy of this map the *dū mài* 督脈/governing vessel. Mountains represent the spiritual ascent and the heights of enlightenment. The head as a series of mountain peaks, symbolizing the ultimate goal of reaching enlightenment. Temples and pagodas represent spiritual centers or gateways where transformation occurs. For instance, the temples within the spine align with the Three Passes (*sān guān* 三關) and mark key points for meditative focus. The celestial symbols such as the sun and moon reflect the balance of *yīnyáng* forces. These celestial symbols are often located in the head region, with the left eye depicted as the sun (*yáng*) and the right eye as the moon (*yīn*). This duality highlights the need for balance in Daoist cultivation, as practitioners harmonize opposing forces within their bodies to achieve spiritual equilibrium.

The *Nèijīng Tú* features the three passes or energetic gates (*sān guān* 三關), which are critical spiritual/energetic gateways located along the spinal column, as a path connecting the lower abdomen to the cranial region (*fig. 2.33*). Each pass represent stages in the practitioner's meditative ascent toward internal alchemical transformation. This path mirrors the flow of *qì* in meditation practices, particularly the lesser celestial circuit (*xiǎo zhōu tiān* 小周天), where energy circulates through the governing (*dū mài* 督脈) and conception (*rèn mài* 任脈) vessels. The three passes are depicted and discussed below:

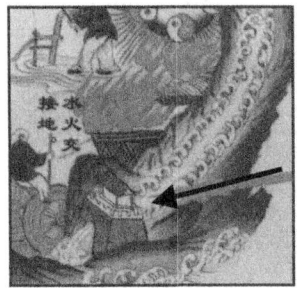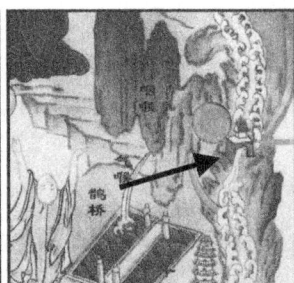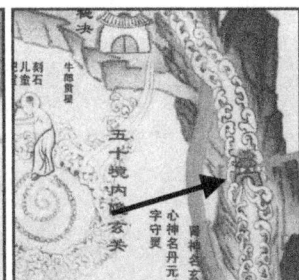

Figure 2.33 - Nèijīng Tú 內經圖 (Three Passes)

Lower Pass - Wěi Lú 尾閭/***Tailbone Gate*** (*fig. 2.33 left*) - Is located at the base of the spine (tailbone) and represents the starting point for circulating *qì* energy. This pass corresponds with the acupuncture point *cháng qiáng* 長強 (Du 1).

Middle Pass - Jiā Jǐ 夾脊/***Narrow Ridge*** (*fig. 2.33 middle*) - Is situated in the mid-spine, and serves as a checkpoint for refining energy and aligning internal processes. This pass corresponds with the acupuncture point *fēng fǔ* 風府/palace of wind (Du 16).

Upper Pass - Yù Zhěn 玉枕/***Jade Pillow*** (*fig. 2.33 right*) - Is positioned at the base of the skull, and symbolizes spiritual ascent and enlightenment. This pass corresponds with the acupuncture point *nǎo hù* 腦戶/brain's door (Du 17)

The diagram highlights the three energy centers (three elixir fields (*sān dāntián* 三丹田). These energetic centers store and transform vital essence (*jīng* 精), energy (*qì* 氣), and spirit (*shén* 神) and are essential for transforming physical vitality into spiritual essence. The *dāntián* act as reservoirs of life energy and are integral to achieving immortality in Daoist alchemical practices. The symbolic imagery reflects the Daoist emphasis on harmony between both the physical and spiritual realms. The three energy centers and their associated imagery are as follows:

The Lower Dāntián (Jīng 精*)* (*fig. 2.34*) is associated with the base of the torso and is represented by a lake, symbolizing *jīng* 精 essence. This essence resides first at the kidneys and then descends to the *huìyīn* 會陰/meeting of yin (the perineum and associated with acupuncture point Ren 1). This region is important for initiating the *nèidān* process. Through the use of intent and sealing this region, the practitioner reverses the flow of *jīng* where it then becomes conserved, stored, recirculated and transformed. Regarding this reversion, we can look at this energy "bubbling up" as in the acupuncture point *yǒng quán* 湧泉/bubbling spring (Ki 1). This is the first point on the kidney meridian, and connects to *kǎn* 坎 ☵ (water/kidneys), the storehouse of the vital essences.

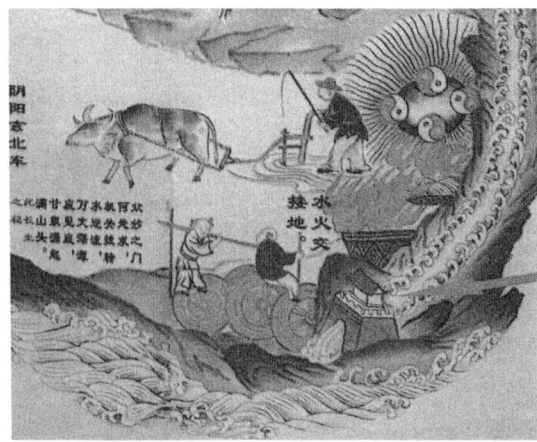

Figure 2.34 - Nèijīng Tú 內經圖 (Lower Dāntián)

The *Nèijīng Tú* 內經圖 depicts various agricultural representations/ metaphors for cultivation. In the lower region of the map, we see two people which represent the *yīnyáng* 陰陽 energies, operating a waterwheel (*hé chē* 河車). This symbolizes the initial stages of using breath and intention to rotate the body's *qì* within the lower abdomen. This rotation raises the *jīng* to the lower *dāntián*, which is the center for the body's foundational energy. We see a *lú* 爐/ "furnace" symbolized by flames representing the expansion of *qì* around the *huìyīn*, further supporting the *dāntián's* energetic role in *nèidān* practice. Above this "furnace" the *dāntián* is depicted with four rotating *tàijí* 太極 symbols emitting heat, reflecting its proper function in Daoist alchemy. It symbolizes the harmonization of the *wǔxíng* 五行/ five phases through attentiveness on the lower elixir field, and the smooth rotation of energy circulation. As well as the transforming power of the five phases within the four cardinal directions.

The image of the plough boy and his ox suggests the practitioner's focused attention on the process of alchemical transformation, especially on the conservation, transformation and circulation of *jīng* and *qì*. In alchemical practices, the ploughing ox serves as a metaphor for the kidney water and the process of energy rising upwards along the backbone.

Through this practice, the practitioner must also focus their intent on various locations in the body, especially on *wěi lú* 尾閭/tailbone gate (the coccyx)[211], which is also identified as *cháng qiáng* 長強 /long strong (Du 1), the first point on the governing vessel. The other locations where one would focus their intent includes *qì hǎi* 氣海/sea of *qì* (the abdomen), and *mìng mén* 命門/ gate of life (between the kidneys) to help increase this fire and circulate the *qì*.

---

[211] Which is also one of the *sān guān* 三關 (*fig. 2.33 left*).

The Middle Dāntián (qì 氣) (*fig. 2.35*) is associated with the body above the diaphragm; in particular, the heart region within the chest cavity where emotional energy is refined and spirit is housed.

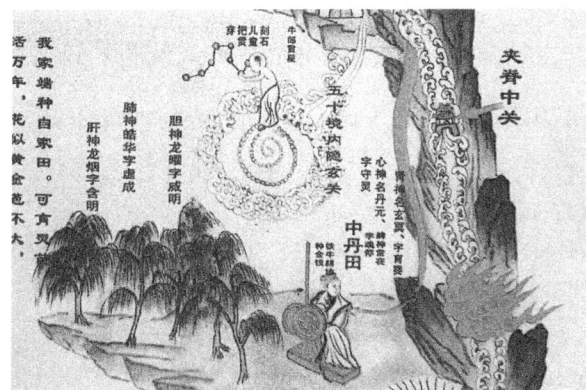

Figure 2.35 - Nèijīng Tú 內經圖 (Middle Dāntián)

The middle *dāntián* is represented by a set of five trees known as the "mulberry grove" (*sāng lín* 桑林) associated with the Liver's spirit and the five phases, the Cowherd Boy (Niú Láng 牛郎), associated with the Heart's spirit and *yáng* aspect along with the Weaving Girl (Zhīnǚ 織女), associated with the Kidney's spirit and *yīn* aspect. The Western star Altair in Aquila corresponds to the Cowherd Boy, who is depicted holding the Northern Dipper (Ursa Major). The Weaving Girl, corresponding to the Western star of Vega in the Lyra constellation. These two figures symbolize the balancing of Water/*kǎn* 坎 ☵ (Kidneys) and Fire/*lí* 離 ☲ (Heart) which is essential for spiritual progression. The Weaving Girl embodies the intuitive Earthly wisdom, while the Cowherd Boy represents spiritual elevation. Their reunion[212] is facilitated by a bridge of magpies, which mirrors this alchemical mixing of Kidney & Heart essences.

The Cowherd Boy (Niú Láng 牛郎) sits on the middle *dāntián*, depicted by a swirl, which symbolizes the movement of *tàijí* within one's core. This could represent the "mixing" of Fire and Water to take place, as well as represent the Sea of Qì and Blood. He interacts with the Big Dipper (*běidǒu* 北斗), the seven-star constellation central to Daoist cosmology, symbolizing the balance of *yīnyáng* and the connection to higher consciousness. Through the stilling of one's Heart's this enables the stability/balance needed for spiritual transformation and facilitating transcendence.

---

[212] On the 7th day of the 7th lunar month of the Chinese calendar, a myriad of magpies are said to fly up to the Milky Way, creating a "magpie bridge" to reunite Zhīnǚ 織女 and Niú Láng 牛郎 as lovers again for a single day.

Since the middle *dāntián* is associated with the heart region. Because Chinese medicine views the tongue as the sense organ associated with fire and the heart, we could see that anatomically, what the Cowherd Boy is standing on is a "tongue." This "tongue" is surrounded by fluid, representing the "jade fluid" (*yù yè* 玉液)[213] or "sweet dew" (*gānlù* 甘露) which is the saliva produced when the "magpie bridge" is formed in the body when the tongue touches the roof of the mouth. This tongue posture connects the governing (*dū mài*) and conception (*rèn mài*) vessels; which is also depicted in the upper *dāntián*.

The flames we see next to the Weaving Girl and below the middle pass (*jiā jǐ* 夾脊)(*fig. 2.33 middle & 2.35*) represents *mìng mén* 命門 / gate of life. This location is the starting point for the *jīng's* transformational process into *qì* and the region corresponds to the acupuncture point *mìng mén* 命門 / gate of life (Du 4).[214]

The Upper Dāntián (Shén 神) (*fig. 2.36*) - This area depicts the head and symbolizes the advanced stages of practice and the seat of spiritual enlightenment and mental clarity. Key images in this section are mountains, Lǎozǐ 老子, a "blue eyed foreign monk (Bìyǎn Hú Sēng 碧眼胡僧),[215] a pagoda, a pool with a bridge, and two orbs (the sun and the moon).

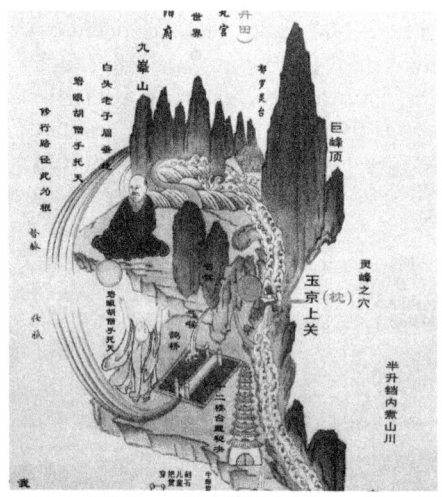

Figure 2.36 - Nèijīng Tú 內經圖 (Upper Dāntián)

---

[213] Also known as Jade Nectar (*yù jiāng* 玉漿).

[214] This point has the function of tonifying the kidneys, regulating the governing vessel, and supporting the spine.

[215] The "blue-eyes monk" is often associated with Bodhidharma, a semi-legendary Buddhist monk who lived during the 5th or 6th century CE. He is said to have traveled from India to the Shaolin temple and is credited as the transmitter of Chán 禪 Buddhism to China (a merging of Daoist and Buddhist cultivation practices).

As we visually move along this pathway, we see a twelve tiered pagoda.[216] This can represent the rings of the trachea, emphasizing proper neck alignment during meditation. These tiers could also represent the two-hour earthly branch (*dìzhī* 地支) time periods. Beyond the pagoda, there is a square pool with a bridge extending across it and followed by two rainbows, one emerging from the bridge and one descending from the mountains. What is symbolized here is is the placement of the tongue to the roof of the mouth, and the connection of the governing (*dū mài*) and conception (*rèn mài*) vessels. This bridge creates the connection of the microcosmic orbit/lesser celestial circuit (*xiǎo zhōu tiān* 小周天). The bridge is liked to the magpie bridge, the pool to the jade fluid (*yù yè* 玉液),[217] the lower rainbow, the conception vessel (*rèn mài*) and the upper rainbow represents the governing vessel (*dū mài* 督脈). Within in these two rainbows are five separate beams, which represent the five elements and the five stages of development.

The depiction of Lǎozǐ in meditation represents the physical body in practice, the *yīn* aspect. The "blue eyed foreign monk" (Bìyǎn Hú Sēng 碧眼胡僧) with arms outstretched holding the heavens represents Bodhidharma, who represents the mind, and the *yáng* aspect. The two of them appearing together symbolizes the coming together of Daoism and Buddhism in an important cross-cultural cultivation practice, as well as representing the dual cultivation of *mìng* 命/life destiny and *xìng* 性/innate nature. The placement of Lǎozǐ (*yīn*) over the blue-eyed monk (*yáng*) can suggest the idea of *yīn* blending within *yáng*, and *yáng* blending within *yīn*.[218] In late medieval *nèidān* lineages, these two individuals represent alchemical ingredients: Lǎozǐ symbolizes lead (*qiān* 鉛) and is associated with *yuán shén* 元神/original spirit, dragon, fire, perfect *yáng* and *xìng* 性/innate nature. While the blue-eyed monk symbolizes mercury (*gǒng* 汞) and is associated with *yuán qì* 原氣/source *qì*, tiger, water, and perfect *yīn* and life destiny (*mìng* 命).

The two "orbs" in the upper portion of the *Nèijīng Tú* 內經圖 represent the sun (celestial *yáng*/left eye) and the moon (celestial *yīn*/right eye) and are anatomically associated with the practitioner's eyes. Lǎozǐ is placed between them, representing our own consciousness and the need to look inward to help illuminate one's internal landscape, via inner observation (*nèiguān* 內觀) meditation techniques.

---

[216] Pagodas have been used symbolically to represent the harmony between Heaven and Earth. Traditionally pagodas have square bases, rooting it to the "Earth" and have circular or octagonal tiers to represent the union of Heavens.

[217] Saliva produced during Daoist practice and is a component of forming the elixir of immortality.

[218] This blending could also represent Hexagram 11 *Tài* 泰 ䷊/Peace the perfect balance between heaven and earth, both moving in their appropriate directions.

The mountains representing *Kūnlún* 崑崙 at the top of the map depict the Nine Peaks (*jiǔfēng* 九峰).[219] These peaks are associated with the Daoist subtle body and are used in Daoist meditation methods. The second most elevated peak, represents *bǎi huì* 百會 / one hundred meeting (Du 20), this directs the Heavenly *Qì* into the Níwán Palace (*níwán gōng* 泥丸宮). Right above the middle peak, there is a small orb, which represents the extraordinary acupuncture point, *yìntáng* 印堂 / hall of impressions (M-HN-3).

Xiūzhēn Tú 修真圖/Map for Cultivation of Reality

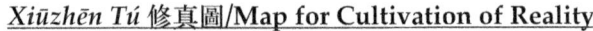

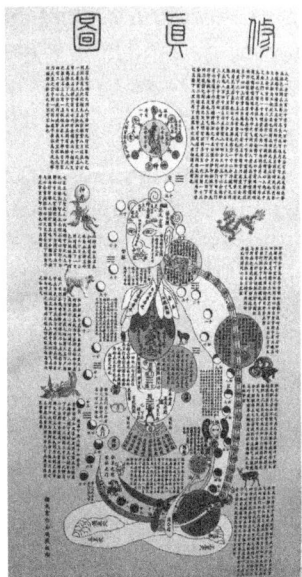

Figure 2.37 - *Xiūzhēn Tú* 修真圖/ Map for Cultivation of Reality[220]

The *Xiūzhēn Tú* 修真圖 / *Map for Cultivation of Reality* (*fig. 2.37*) is often paired with the *Nèijīng Tú* and shows many of the theories and views associated with the viscera and their functions. The *Xiūzhēn Tú* is more intricate than the *Nèijīng Tú*, as it introduces and emphasizing cosmological elements, Chinese medicine, and alchemical principles, reflecting the body as a microcosm of the universe.

---

[219] Also referred to as the Nine Palaces (*jiǔgōng* 九宮) which relate to nine "mystical cranial locations" which include the Hall of Light (*míngtáng* 明堂), Grotto Chamber (*dòngfáng* 洞房), Elixir Field (*dāntián* 丹田), Flowing Pearl (*liúzhū* 流珠), Jade Emperor (*yùdì* 玉帝), Celestial Court (*tiāntíng* 天庭), Secret Perfection (*jīzhēn* 機真), Mysterious Elixir (*xuándān* 玄丹), Great Sovereign (*tàihuáng* 太皇).

[220] Picture by D.Schrier from personal scroll, all images of *Xiūzhēn Tú* 修真圖 discussed in this text are from this source.

Similarly, this map serves as both a guide and a symbolic representation of the body's internal pathways, illustrating its transformative potential to harmonize the body, mind, and spirit with the cosmos. Its symbolism highlights the significance of environmental awareness and the refinement and cultivation of internal energies.

The anatomic map depicts a human figure in frontal view, divided into three sections—lower, middle, and upper—each corresponding to specific energetic, physiological, and spiritual aspects of the body. Surrounding the image, we see thirty alternating black and white circles symbolizing the lunar cycle, as well as the animal spirits of six internal organs.[221]

Surrounding the figure is a depiction of the seasonal and lunar cycles, illustrating their effects on the body's energetic flow. The thirty alternating black and white circles represent the lunar cycle. The lunar phases impact both the lesser celestial circuit (*xiǎo zhōu tiān* 小周天) and the waterwheel (*héchē* 河車). The energy movement depicted starts from the new moon, located at the perineum, and rises along the back of the body along the governing vessel (*dū mài*) to the full moon above the head. This represents the 15 day waxing phase, during which the moon transitions from *yīn* to *yáng*. The waning phase, illustrates the moon's shift from *yáng* to *yīn*, moving from the full moon back to the new moon. This phase connects to the front of the body and corresponds with the conception vessel (*rèn mài*).

The twenty-four circles[222] represent the vertebrae of the "spine"correspond with the twenty-four seasonal solar nodes (*èrshísì jiéqì* 二十四節氣) of the Chinese calendar, thus making visible the relationship between environmental *qì* and human spirit/vitality, which we saw in Chén Tuán 陳摶's *Chénxīyí Xiānshēng Èrshísì Qì Zuògōng Dǎoyǐn Zhìbìng Tú* 陳希夷先生二十四氣坐功導引治病圖 / *Master Chénxīyí's Twenty Four Nodes Seated Exercises of Guided Stretching for Curing Ailments*.

Similar to what we saw in the *Nèijīng Tú*, this aspect of the map depicts three critical gateways or passes, located along the spinal column representing a path connecting the lower abdomen to the cranial region (*fig. 2.36*). This mirrors the flow of *qì* in the lesser celestial circuit (*xiǎo zhōu tiān* 小周天), where energy circulates through the governing (*dū mài*) and conception (*rèn mài*) vessels. Along these passes, we have three animal carts which act as hydraulic vehicles

---

[221] Dragon (Liver); Vermillion Bird (Heart); Phoenix (Spleen); Tiger (Lung); Two-headed Deer (Kidneys); Turtle & Snake (Gallbladder). These are the same as outlined in the *Huángtíng Jīng* 黃庭經 / *Yellow Court Scripture*.

[222] This also has a relation to the trachea & the 12 tiered pagoda as seen in the *Nèijīng Tú* 內經圖.

which work with the waterwheel (*héchē* 河車) to assist the upward movement of energy along the body, and represent specific breathing methods to draw energy upwards through the spine. The three passes and animal carts are:

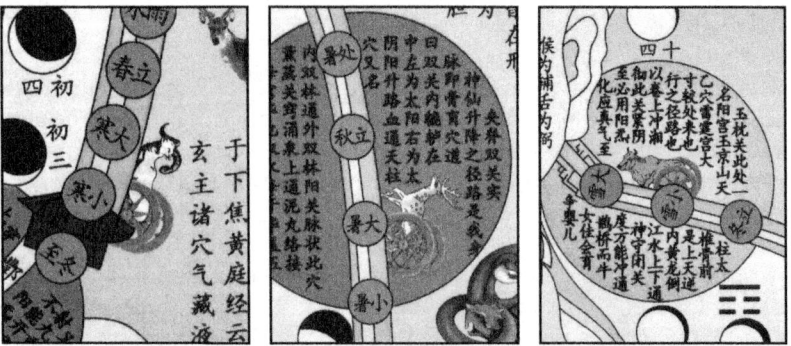

Figure 2.38 - *Xiūzhēn Tú* 修真圖 (Three Passes & Animal Carts)

The Lower Pass (*Wěi Lú Guān* 尾閭關/*Tailbone Gate*) & Goat Cart/*Yáng Chē* 羊車 (*fig. 2.38 left*) focuses on the lumbar region and involves short, sniff like inhalation with little power, this helps to create a bubbling sensation and move energy up the spine.

The Middle Pass (*Spinal Handle/Jiā Jǐ Guān* 夾脊關) & Deer Cart/*Lù Chē* 鹿 車 (*fig. 2.38 middle*) focuses on the thoracic region and involves longer, smooth and gentle breath. This will create a clear and tangible sensation of warmth and bubbling sensation moving upward to the base of the neck.

The Upper Pass (*Jade Pillow/Yù Zhěn Guān* 玉枕關) & Ox Cart/*Niúchē* 牛車 (*fig. 2.38 right*) focuses on moving the warm, bubbling fluid from the neck, through the cervical spine, into the skull, and over the top of the head[223] using powerful deep breath with a little strength.

The Lower Section of the map (*fig. 2.38*) represents the lower *dāntián* and the kidneys. Here we see an individual sitting cross-legged in lotus position, indicating postural guidance. What is interesting is we see inscribed on the soles of the feet *yǒng quán* 湧泉/bubbling spring (Ki 1) and below the knee *zú sān lǐ* 足三里/leg three miles (St 36), showing regions of the body/points that will be of importance for this practice.

---

[223] Before attempting this stage, one must ensure the lesser celestial circuit (*xiǎo zhōu tiān* 小周天) is fully open to avoid pressure buildup in the head, which can cause prolonged discomfort.

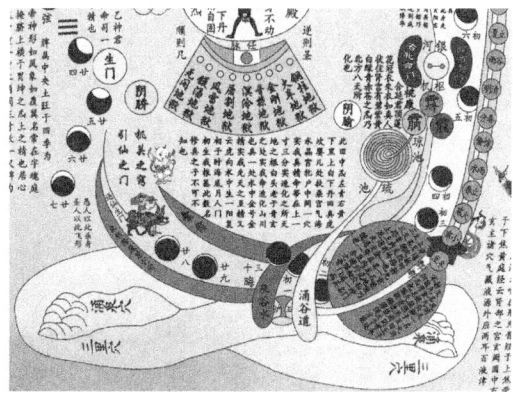

Figure 2.39 - *Xiūzhēn Tú* 修真圖 (Lower Section)

The kidneys shown here are labeled as "mystery"(*zuǒ xuán shèn mén* 左玄腎門) on the right and"female" (*yòu pìn mìng mén* 右牝命門) on the left. These are two terms which represent the transition from the congenital to the acquired realm of existence known as the *"mysterious female" (xuán pìn* 玄牝).[224] Between the kidneys lies the *mìng mén,* which facilitates the flow of energy and water, guided by the *mìng mén huǒ* 命門 火 / life-gate fire.

The Middle Section (*fig. 2.40)* represents the middle *dāntián* and is the location in which *kǎn* 坎 ☵ (water / lower *dāntián*) and *lí* 離 ☲ (fire / upper *dāntián*) mix. The trigram *qián* 乾 ☰ (heaven) at the center symbolizes the elixir and the middle cinnabar field (*dāntián* 丹田). The body's internal organs shown here (heart, lung, liver) are not merely anatomical structures, but vessels imbued with spiritual and alchemical significance. Revealing that the physical body serves as an anchor for the energetic and spiritual dimensions of being, thus aligning the microcosm of the self with the macrocosm of existence.

---

[224] *Xuán pìn* 玄牝/mysterious female is a Daoist technical term that first appears in Lǎozǐ 6. *Xuán* 玄 / mysterious, is a designation for not clinging, signifying a state of non-attachment. *Pìn* 牝 / female, means feminine and gentleness. In some Daoist contexts, it frequently designates original spirit (*yuánshén* 元神) housed in the *zǔqiào* 祖竅 / ancestral cavity, the center of the head. For more on the Mysterious Female, see discussion in chapter *"The Secret Circulation,"* pg. 249-256.

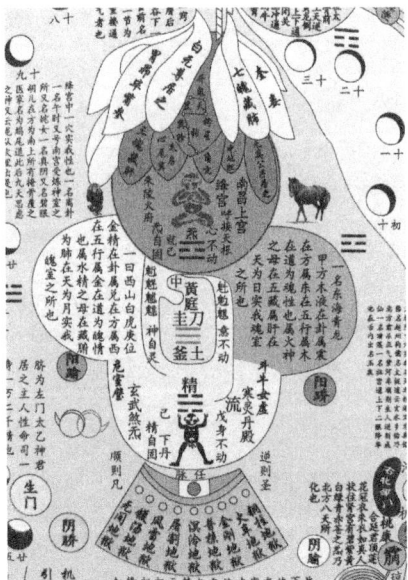

Figure 2.40 - *Xiūzhēn Tú* 修真圖 (Middle Section)

The organs (heart, lung, liver/gall badder) are represented as several petals, similar to that of an inverted flower. At the top, we have the lung drawn as a series of petals with inscriptions for the deity of the lung and the seven *pò* spirits (*qī pò shén* 七魄神). In the center is the heart, which looks like an upturned lotus bud, and in the center is the seven stars of the Northern Dipper (*běidǒu qīxīng* 北斗七星), which opens the path to heaven in both meditation and in ritual. Below the heart is the liver. Like the lung, the liver is depicted petals inscribed with the liver deity and the three *hún* spirits (*sān hún shén* 三魂神).

At the level of the heart, there is a picture of a horse and monkey. These two animals symbolize the two states of the human mind. The monkey mind (*yuánxīn* 猿心) is restless, erratic, and unfocused, jumping from branches to branches (thought to thought) in the tree, which is a common characteristic of the beginner whose thoughts scatter wildly during meditation. The untrained horse mind (*mǎyì* 馬意), is similar in uncontrolled thought processes jumping and galloping from one thought to another.

The symbolism of these two animals connects the horse to the heart/fire and the monkey with the bladder/water. The horse has a direct relationship to *shén* 神/spirit, as the heart is the storehouse of *shén*, which relates to our consciousness. We then can say that the untrained "horse mind" is characterized by spiritual confusion and disorientation. As we tame the mind, we also tame the heart. As this "wild horse" gradually begins to be reined in, and settles down, it cultivates internal harmony, fostering constant stillness and clarity (*qīng jìng* 清靜). A trained horse mind[225] is one which is calm, steady, and disciplined, indicating mastery over one's thought(s) and breath.

At the lower left of this section, around the level of the umbilicus, are two interlocking rings. With no accompanying inscription, their symbolism is open to interpretation. One perspective could view them as the "mysterious pass" (*xuán guān* 玄關), a gateway to higher spiritual realization and the union of original *yīn* and *yáng*, the sacred merging of opposites that which opens the portal to the formation of reality itself. Through sustained practice, practitioners then can transcend mere technique, entering a realm of profound transformation where body, spirit, and cosmos merge into a seamless flow.

The Upper Section (*fig. 2.41*) represents the upper *dāntián* and is the location of the head. The head is the heavenly part of the body and the celestial origin of the individual. It includes layers of celestial realms and the processes required to transcend physical existence. The forehead and nose feature the names of deities, celestial locations, and internal energetic locations such as the muddy pellet (*ní wán* 泥丸) and the celestial eye (*tiān mù* 天目) between the eyes.

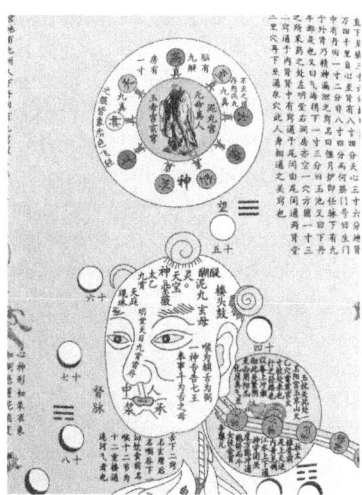

Figure 2.41 - *Xiūzhēn Tú* 修真圖 (Upper Section)

The Muddy Pellet (*ní wán* 泥丸) corresponds to the physical root of the pineal gland and has nine cavities which corresponds to the Nine Heavenly Palaces

---

[225] See *The Daoist Horse Taming Pictures* by Gāo Dàokuān 高道寬 (1195-1277) was created to serve as map for cultivation development and was likely adapted and/or inspired by the Chán (Zen) text Pǔ Míng 普明's *Shí Niú Tú* 十牛圖 /Ox Taming Pictures. Translations of these two text are Louis Komjathy, *Taming the Wild Horse: An Annotated Translation and Study of the Daoist Horse Taming Pictures* (Columbia University Press, 2019) & Red Pine *P'u Ming's Oxherding Pictures & Verses* (Empty Bowl, 2015).

(*jiǔxiāo* 九霄),[226] representing stages toward spiritual immortality through the alignment of one's *yuánshén* 元神 / original spirit.

Sitting above the head is a disc with nine encircled characters, each forming a pair with the character *zhēn* 真 / perfected. Written below it are the names of the Nine Perfected (*jiǔzhēn* 九真).[227] Here, we can see the process of becoming a *zhēnrén* 真人, a true or perfected person. This is one who has attained and mastered the *Dào* 道, and in *Sùwèn 1* we have Huáng Dì 黃帝 describing the characteristics of this individual.

> *I have heard, in high antiquity there were true men (zhēnrén 真人). They upheld [the patterns of] heaven and earth and they grasped [the regularity of] yin and yang. They exhaled and inhaled essence qi. They stood for themselves and guarded their spirit.*
> *Muscles and flesh were like one. Hence, they were able to achieve longevity, in correspondence with heaven and earth. There was no point in time when [their life could have] come to an end. Such was their life in the Way[228]*

The *Nèijīng Tú* 內經圖 / *Map of the Inner Landscape* and the *Xiūzhēn Tú* 修真圖 / *Map for Cultivation of Reality* discussed above illustrate how Daoist mapping of spiritual cultivation depicted a coherent circulation that reflect the ecological forces of Nature, which had a strong influence on the development of Chinese anatomic thinking. These body maps (*shēntú* 身圖) present the body as an extension of the natural world, emphasizing balance, harmony, and the interdependence of internal and external forces. By aligning the body's internal energy flow with natural cycles, such as the movement of celestial bodies, seasonal changes, and the interplay between the five phases, they not only guided practitioners in their spiritual refinement but also reinforced a holistic understanding of human physiology.

---

[226] This refers to the heavenly regions inhabited by Daoist immortals and to the position of the emperor. The Nine Heavens are 1) *Shénxiāo* 神霄 / Divine Heaven, 2) *Lángxiāo* 琅霄 / Pure White Heaven, 3) *Zǐxiāo* 紫霄 / Purple Heaven, 4) *Tàixiāo* 太霄 / Great Heaven, 5) *Qīngxiāo* 青霄 / Azure Heaven, 6) *Bìxiāo* 碧霄 / Emerald Heaven, 7) *Dānxiāo* 丹霄 / Vermillion Heaven, 8) *Jǐngxiāo* 景霄 / Luminous Heaven, 9) *Yùxiāo* 玉霄 / Jade Heaven.

[227] The Nine Perfected are 1) Gāozhēn 高真 / High Perfected, 2) Zhìzhēn 至真 / Realized Perfected, 3) Tàizhēn 太真 / Supreme Perfected, 4) Xūzhēn 虛真 / Void Perfected, 5) Xiānzhēn 仙真 / Immortal Perfected, 6) Xuánzhēn 玄真 / Mysterious Perfected, 7) Shàngzhēn 上真 / Superior Perfected, 8) Shénzhēn 神真 / Divine Perfected, 9) Tiānzhēn 天真 / Heavenly Perfected.

[228] Unschuld, Tessenow, and Zheng, "*Huang Di Nei Jing Su Wen: An Annotated Translation of Huang Di's Inner Classic - Basic Questions, 2 Volumes,*" pg. 42.

Part III:

Circulation &
Channels

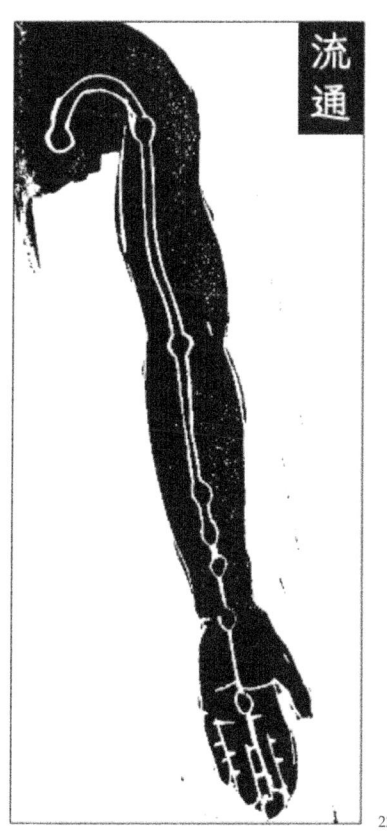

流通

229

Setting the Stage: *Língshū* 靈樞 1

Z'ev Rosenberg & Stephen Cowan

Z'ev: The very first chapter of the *Língshū* 靈樞 reflects on two ways of utilizing the "map" of the body, contrasting points (*xué* 穴 / holes) as *guān* 關/ versus *jī* 機 / pivot, opportunity, motive force, mechanism), finding the essence of practicing acupuncture. All the consecutive chapters that follow in the *Língshū* are difficult to comprehend without the core principles revealed in this chapter. As Qíbó 岐伯; states:

麤守形、上守神。神乎神、客在門。麤守關、上守機，機之動，不離其空。空中之機，清靜而微。

"Unrefined practitioners guard the physical appearance. Outstanding (practitioners) guard the spirit. The unrefined practitioners guard the gate or pass/guān 關. Outstanding practitioners guard the jī 機 motive/pivot"[230]

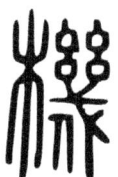

Figure 3.1 - Jī 機

Stephen: *Jī* 機 is a fascinating character. *Jī* is variously translated as "opportunity" (as in *wéijī* 危機 - crisis or "dangerous opportunity"), pivot, mechanism, machine or crucial point. The ideogram (*see fig. 3.1*) is composed of tree / wood radical on the left giving a quality of organic growth to the meaning. On the right is *jī* 幾 that shows two silk threads, a person and a tool

---

[230] I have edited the original translation. I think there may have been some confusion about the sequence the way Unschuld translated *guān* and *jī*: 麤守關，上守機.

that may relate to a loom or weapon. According to the *Shuōwén Jiězì* 說文解字,[231] *jī* 幾 represents guards at the frontier who are attentive to the least movement. One interpretation is that the image of a weapon with two threads of silk implies awareness of the subtle thread-like movement. I find this meaning pertinent to the *Língshū* text here. The superior practitioner is attentive to the slightest movement at the access point (*xué* 穴 / hole) where the spirit (*shén* 神) is felt. The unrefined practitioner is simply needling the points, (*guān* 關 the outer gate) on the physical form based on acupuncture maps and locations.

Z'ev: Here Qíbó emphasizes the importance of differentiating *guān* 關 - the physical gate and *jī*, the subtle presence of motive force, in order to recognize *shùn* 順, to "go with the flow," and *nì* 逆 / counterflow. Much ink has been spilled over the centuries in understanding this subtle differentiation. My understanding is that one senses the immaterial *shénqì* 神氣 enclosed within the physical structures and symptom complex when one visualizes *jī* . The outstanding practitioner does not just mechanically stick needles in the body at point locations. While locations certainly matter, they sense the *jī* within the *guān* 關/gate as the stimulus that occurs in inserting the needle that "sparks" the channel system and awakens the body / mind intelligence. The correct composure, focus, insertion and correct needle and technique awakens the resonance of the system, however this by itself is not sufficient. The superior physician must use this "opportunity" (*jī*) to dive deep, to sense the motive force (*jī*), promoted by the formless source, the *yuán qì* 原氣 / source (original) *qì*, in order to have a complete cure. *Língshū* 1 goes on to say:

機之動，不離其空。空中之機，清靜而微。

"The motion of jī never leaves the enclosed empty space. The jī in the enclosed empty space is clear, calm and subtle."

The ability to perceive the clear, calm and subtle movements within a given acupuncture point takes the utmost refinement in practice. As I discussed in *Afterglow: Ministerial Fire and Chinese Ecological Medicine*[232], the true cure is when the source *qì* heals through non-action (*wúwéi* 無為). *"The root of treating illness*

---

[231] *Shuōwén Jiězì* 說文解字 / Chinese etymological dictionary originally compiled by Xǔshèn 許慎 c. 100 CE, during the Eastern Han dynasty (25–206 CE).

[232] Rosenberg, *"Afterglow: Ministerial Fire and Chinese Ecological Medicine,"* pg. 55-61.

should allow the yuán qì 元原氣/original (source) qi of the body to heal without action."[233] This is the essence of promoting circulation within the body.

The remainder of the chapter discusses techniques of supplementation and drainage, expelling *xié qì* 邪氣 / perverse *qì*, and the tools of the trade (the nine needles). Each needle, entry point and channel must be used precisely in order to gain clinical success, and the dangers of wrong treatment are clearly delineated.

往者為逆、來者為順、
明知逆順、正行無問。

"Those going away, they move contrary to the norms; those coming, they move in accordance with the norms.To clearly know movement contrary to and in accordance with the norms results in a correct conduct leaving no room for questions.."[234]
- Língshū 1

Shùn 順, or to "go with the flow," and *nì* 逆, or counterflow (contrary to the norm) in a short paragraph explain that normalizing the flow of *qì* in the channel system, restoring what is depleted, draining repletions and blockages is the entire key to promoting healthy circulation in acupuncture practice. Without *gǎnyìng* 感應 / resonance, this is impossible. One must first see the entire map, the entire channel system in order to know how to proceed.

疾雖久、猶可畢也。
言不可治者、未得其術也。

"Now, those who are experts in the use of the needles, when they remove an illness, that is as if they pulled out a thorn, as if they cleansed a stain, as if they untied a knot, as if they opened a closure."
- Língshū 1

The practice of acupuncture / moxibustion requires proper self-cultivation: breathing, posture, focus and intention, in order to facilitate the exchange of *qì* between the practitioner and patient, by using the needles or mugwort cones. Then, the practitioner needs to read the maps of the body / mind, and its various depths, locations and flow of *qì*. Season, time of day, receptivity of the patient

---

[233] Farquhar, *"A Way of Life: Things, Thought, and Action in Chinese Medicine,"* pg. 133.

[234] Unschuld, *"Huang Di Nei Jing Ling Shu: The Ancient Classic on Needle Therapy,"* pg. 51.

all come into play. As David White describes it, one needs to guard both *shén* 神 and *jī* 機.[235] One visualizes the channel system, seeing its normal flows, blockages, dark hidden spaces where perverse *qì* resides. *Língshū* 1 describes disease as a thorn that needs to be removed, and reassures us that if we are able to remove the thorn, that even a chronic illness can be completely alleviated.

A few days ago, in early January, a young woman seventeen years old came in with a stubborn head cold and wanted to feel better before she left on a school trip to Poland. I treated her *yángmíng* 陽明 and *shàoyáng* 少陽 channels, plus ST 2.5 on the face directly below *sì bái* 四白 / four whites (ST 2), and the symptoms immediately resolved. Her youth and sensitivity, combined with the appropriate point selection immediately resolved the condition.

I had a similar experience some 35 years ago, when I had traveled to the Bay Area, also in January, to visit a processing facility for Chinese herbal liquid extracts. As soon as I stepped off the plane, I immediately experienced bronchitis with yellow / green phlegm and coughing. The next morning, I went to Efrem Korngold's clinic, and after the acupuncture treatment and a dose of *jīng fáng bài dú sàn* 荊防敗毒散 with *huáng lián wēn dǎn tāng* 黃連溫膽湯, the condition was completely better by the afternoon!

Stephen: The fact that *Língshū* begins with this discussion of *guān* and *jī* seems crucial in cautioning practitioners about treating the territory rather than just the map of points. This reiterates the points we made earlier in the chapter *"The Trap of the Map."* The subjective experience of *jī*, the pivot / mechanism within the acu-point requires self-cultivation. In Western medicine, there is a resistance to and (fear of) subjective experience, in part I think because of a lack of self-cultivation in medical training. This gives the impression that one can stand *outside* what's going on in a patient without affecting (and being affected by) that patient. In reality, no such "outside" truly exists for the cultivated Chinese practitioner. Cultivation however implies clearing all preconceived biases in order to use one's subjective experience of the subtle movements (the *jī*) to guide diagnostic impressions. Nowhere is this more obvious than in pulse-taking. As Zhuāngzi 莊子 says *"Where neither 'this' or 'that' has an opposite is*

---

235 *"There is a difference between grasping the needle and entering the needle. If your posture is correct, breath aligned, patient comfortable, and insertion precise -this is grasping, This is a practice. However, if you abide by and embody the above in a unified principle while capturing the essence of non-duality, and in an instant, align yourself with true illumination of physiology and pathology simultaneously-this is entering. This is guarding the shén* 神 *and jī* 機. *This is a meditation."* Institute of Neijing Research, Instagram post, January 2024.

called the hinge of Dao. And as soon as the hinge is fitted in its socket it can respond endlessly."[236] To celebrate the complexity of each unique moment in its every changing process of transforming, recognizing that we cannot help but be participants in that process is to sense the movement within the *jī* of a point, in order to facilitate change. To do this, we must guard against preconceived beliefs, protocols or ideologies that might get in the way of assessing the *jī* 機. This understanding of reality is in a sense in accord with our current understanding of the so-called "observer effect" in Quantum physics. To be truly objective in order to get a realistic view of what's going on is by its very nature subjective in the sense that subjective implies being relational (and therefore relative to the context) In the realm of complexity theory, it is the emergent properties of the whole that are dependent on the relationships of the parts. One cannot stand outside that complexity and look in if you are to be truly participating in the healing process.

I find chapter 1 of the *Língshū* of particularly crucial importance in treating children. Because their body is still in the primordial process of forming, so too are the channels and holes (*xué* 穴) making them highly sensitive and vulnerable to outside influences. When I am composed and focused and present to take note of the movement of *jī* along their channels, sometimes even simply touching the points (particularly the *yuán* 原 - original points as *Língshū* 1 emphasizes) is enough to affect the condition. Because children are predominantly *yáng* by nature of their intense capacity for growth, they are highly responsive to subtle shifts in whatever we do. To respect this is is to recognize our deep *gǎnyìng* connection. As the *Língshū* says, such is "the Way of *jī*."

---

[236] Zhuangzi, and Graham, *"Chuang-Tzu: The Seven Inner Chapters and Other Writings from the Book Chuang-Tzu,"*pg. 52-53.

Meditations on Channel Theory

Z'ev Rosenberg & Stephen Cowan

"Our heart is not just a simple pump. It is influenced by hormonal and emotional changes, by blood pressure etc; so it is a multivariable system. Which means that it is influenced by a great number of variables. Even breathing increases the variability of the heartbeat. Our heart must be very flexible and able to adapt to all circumstances of our lives. That is why it would be a disaster if the heartbeat was to be regular; it would collapse."

"So we can describe the heart as a complex dynamic system. Only just before a heart disease or cardiac arrest does the fractal dimension decrease and the heartbeat get regular."
- Jan H.T Schroën [237]

Z'ev: Our *zàng* 臟 / viscera (solid organs) are complex systems that pulsate, breathe, expand / contract and respond to multiple internal and external stimuli from hormones, blood flows, breath, fluid densities, toxicity (phlegm, static blood, environmental toxins) while being governed by circadian clocks, solar / lunar cycles and seasonal *qì*. It is the flexibility of the visceral systems, and their communication via the channel system (*tú jīng* 途經) that determines dynamic equilibrium and ultimately health.

Reframing our knowledge of human anatomy, physiology and the constantly evolving information that neuroscience is discovering is a must in Chinese medical energetic science. Specific channels as understood in Chinese medicine are like river basins and their ecosystems, where nerve impulses, blood, interstitial fluids flow through variegated structures that are expressions of the underlying communication system of the channels, including muscles, nerves, arteries, and lymphatic vessels (and fascia). Perverse *qì* also circulates through

---

[237] Schroën,*"Non-Linear Dynamics and Chinese Medicine: An Essay on Research Models, TCM, and Recent Changes in Modern Scientific Philosophy,"*pg. 97.

the channels, aptly described in great detail in the *Sùwèn* 素問 and *Língshū* 靈樞 (see *Sùwèn* 16 on the importance of observing the *qì* of sun and moon and stars, and the eight cardinal turning points of the four seasons). According to Wáng Jūyì 王居易 (1937-2017), the channels are an interwoven communications network (*tújìng* 途徑) that responds to both internal and external environmental changes, pathogens, organic fluctuations, emotions and thoughts. The homeopath Georges Vithoulkas likens this to a supercomputer body/mind intelligence, immediately responsive to all changes. In Chinese medicine, this is one expression of *shén* 神, the self awareness aspect of consciousness expressed in physical form and fully cognizant of the complex changes that are continually occurring.

Stephen: The fundamental idea running throughout the classics is that clear communication implies health. The deeper understanding of this principle is something I think is often missed in the training of many acupuncturists in the West, not to mention of course, most Western trained doctors. As clinicians, the classics tell us that our job is to promote the free flow of communication (*tōng* 通), that anything that blocks the flow of communication will cause suffering. This *tōng* is an important aspect of *shén*/consciousness and must begin with the way we communicate with our patients. The *Shén* doctor follows the principle of *Lǎozǐ* 老子 17: *"vigilant, they are careful in what they say."*[238] Recognizing the power words have to frame consciousness I am acutely aware of the powerful use of western terminology in framing a medical condition being inherently biased towards a rather rigid materialist sense of body function. I have witnessed this fixed language unwittingly interfering with the healing process by missing the potential for change through flow. I am reminded of this constantly in my encounters with patients who have been given a medical diagnosis by their physicians as if it were written in stone. Recently, for the sake of transparency, there has been a mandatory rule of reporting results of laboratory and radiological data directly to the patient *before* the physician has reviewed them. I have seen this generate incredible anxiety in patients, in large part because it is utterly out of context to the specific uniqueness of that patient. This leaves the intimate relationship between doctor and patient completely out of the picture. As Dr. Elizabeth Comen, an oncologist at Memorial Sloan Kettering Cancer Center in New York City, recently commented in a New York Times article about this; *"When information is just given in black-and-white type on*

---

[238] Ames and Hall, *"Dao De Jing: Making this Life Significant: A Philosophical Translation."* Pg. 102

*MyChart, that's not the full expression of compassionate care. Yes, it is immediate care, but it's care out of contex*t."[239]

Recognizing words as medicine that can either promote or prevent flow is one of the four pillars of Chinese medicine (look, listen, ask, touch). Interestingly, *Nàn Jīng* 難經 61 describes these as four levels of clinician skill: the *shén* 神 doctor looks, sage (*shèng* 聖) doctor listens, artisan doctor asks, skilled technician palpates. My sense is that the *shén* doctor has moved through these three other levels, cultivating each until they are fully integrated and spontaneous.

Listening and asking define the qualities of healthy conversation that reflect our relatedness as human beings. This back and forth flow is as much value as actually taking a pulse, which itself is a nonverbal conversation. The rhythm and tone of our language has all the characteristics of a pulse: surging, floating, deep, hard, soft, fast, slow etc. My old teacher Steven Aung taught me that before taking anyone's pulse, one must take one's own pulse, respecting the palpable effect we have on those around us. Carl Rogers[240], the eminent psychologist who radically challenged the status quo in the process of the therapeutic encounter, described the three fundamental requirements for optimizing creative-relationships rather than power-relationships through communication in order to promote healthy transformation as:

- **Positive Regard** - meaning genuine open curiosity on the part of the clinician to the experience. (I have found that this means being open to letting the patient teach *you* something new.)
- **Empathetic Understanding** - meaning ability to stand in the shoes of the other
- **Authenticity** - meaning that your words match your inner feelings. This requires a deep level of trust that your body is a reliable instrument for generating data on what's going on during the encounter. Such trust can only come from self-cultivation and as *Lǎozǐ* 17 says, *"when your trust is sufficient, you will be trusted in turn."*[241]

This deep level of *shén*/awareness of flow is also expressed through the use of metaphoric language which can improve connection and promote flow in a way

---

[239] See Friedman, *"Your Medical Test Results Are Available. but Do You Want to View Them?"*

[240] See Rogers, *"On Becoming a Person: A Therapist's View of Psychotherapy."*

[241] *Lǎozǐ* 17 translation/interpretation S. Cowan.

that analytic data cannot. For example, asking a patient what it feels *like* will enable you to relate to what's going on more openly and empathetically, which serves to put the patient at ease, to feel safe and secure in your presence. This itself promotes flow, but furthermore, such connection will generate a physical response in _you_ the practitioner, that carries valuable information regarding what patterns, channels and points may be involved in that particular moment. Many of the names for acu-points are metaphors generated in this appreciation of navigating the flow of the channels as well.

The system of correspondences is one of the powerful aspects of such analogical reasoning in Chinese medicine. I have had the distinct experience of having many patients' metaphoric descriptions of their symptoms become a more effective guide to treatment than any laboratory results they happen to present. This felt experience does not deny the importance of knowing the channel theories rooted in the classics but rather honors them by keeping to the fundamental principle that relationship in Chinese medicine is primary and context always matters.

Development of Channel Theory in *Sùwèn* 素問 6 and *Língshū* 靈樞 5: *The Architecture of the Three Yáng/Three Yīn Divisions*

Z'ev Rosenberg & Stephen Cowan

調陰與陽，精氣乃光，合形與氣，使神內藏。

"Once yin and yang [qi] are balanced, the essence qi will be luminous. Once the physical appearance constitutes one entity with the qi, the spirit will be retained internally."
- *Língshū* 5[242]

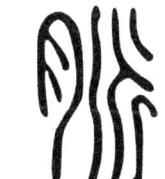

Figure 3.2 - Mài 脈

Z'ev: Our next consideration is the development of the channel system theory, according to the "architectural body" approach/clinical gaze.[243] While developing this book, Stephen and I were discussing one of the difficulties in acupuncture practice that lies in defining *jīng* 經 channels/tracts/conduits including differentiating *mài* 脈/vessels (*fig. 3.2*), from *jīng* 經/channel.

Stephen: Kuriyama devotes a whole chapter to the difference between the *mài (mò)* and *jīng*. According to him, the *mài* seem to indicate the act of palpating the pulsating flow of circulating *xuè qì* 血氣 while the *jīng* are the

---

[242] Unschuld, *"Huang Di Nei Jing Ling Shu: The Ancient Classic on Needle Therapy,"* pg. 123.

[243] Michael Foucault defines the clinical gaze as how the physician fit the patient's story into a medical paradigm. For more information refer to Michel Foucault's *The Birth of the Clinic: An Archaeology of Medical Perception*. Also Rosenberg, *"Returning to the Source: Han Dynasty Medical Classics in Modern Clinical Practice,"* pg. 57-63 & Rosenberg, *"Ripples in the Flow: Reflections on Vessel Dynamics in the Nàn Jing"* pg. 21-25.

channels within which *xuè qì* 血氣 flows.[244] The ideogram *mài (mò)* 脈/shows a flowing stream coupled with the flesh radical. As Kuriyama says, *"the mo were more like rivers than conduits."* The *mò* are further differentiated from the western concept of taking a pulse as merely counting the beats, as Kuriyama insists, *"The grammar of the term thus resists any facile identification of mo with blood vessels. But rendering mo as "pulse" is also awkward."*[245]

Z'ev: The Han dynasty scholar/physicians developed the channel system in such a way that unified different points of reference/gaze into one, by not separating physical/gross anatomy from the "unbroken chain" of unity between heaven, humanity and earth. Since disease states are born out of the unfolding of multiple systems and relationships in the body and natural world, contemporary research on epigenetics acknowledges what has been written about in the texts of Chinese medicine: that the environment we live in influences the expression of our genes as does our situation and actions. The Chinese classics imply that even our thoughts influence who we are, who we become in the future, and even what becomes of our children and grandchildren, thus genes are mutable, and much more than the deterministic view of genetic information they were once thought to carry.

In his book *The Delphic Boat*, Antoine Danchin, defines "information" as viewing the pattern that precedes physical manifestations, and it is the invisible patterns that are primary to their expression in physical form. He states that *"the study of life should never be restricted to objects, but must look into their relationships."*[246] Just as a rowboat has a particular form and design, though over time planks will rot from dampness and need to be replaced, the human being completely changes its cellular components roughly every seven to ten years so that it is completely renewed although the form is the same.[247] Eventually, the original planks are all gone, however, the boat looks exactly the same. The Oracle at Delphi puts forward the question, "but is it the same boat?" Yes, it is recognizable, sitting at the dock. However, nothing remains from the original boat, except for the information that created it. If we examine the planks, we can say they are pine or oak. It doesn't tell us much about the boat itself, since the original planks are gone! According to Danchin the boat is not the material it is made from, but something else, which is far more intriguing. The boat's essence lies in the relationship between the planks, which organizes the material of the planks. Similarly, we should never restrict the study of life to objects, instead, we must look into their relationships. Likewise, the body and mind are not just

---

[244] Kuriyama"*The Expressiveness of the Body and the Divergence of Greek and Chinese Medicine,*"pg. 51.

[245] ibid., pg 51.

[246] Danchin,"*The Delphic Boat: What Genomes Tell Us,*" pg. 1.

[247] Quest Diagnostics, *"Do My Cells Really Change Every 7 Years?"*

the cells, tissues, and viscera, but the relationship of their parts. Observing these relationships is one strength of Chinese medicine, and these observations form the basic theoretical principles of traditional Chinese medicine, such as five-phase theory, viscera bowel theory, etc.

Chinese medicine was perhaps the only medical system to fully embody the unity of expression, pattern, form, mind/spirit and body. Within the Ayurvedic and Tibetan medical systems there is ongoing tension between *chakras* चक्र/ *Nāḍīs* नाड़ी[248] and anatomy.[249] In Greco/Arabic medicine, while there were discussions of "pneuma" and later on "elan vital," medicine was based on a four element humoral theory, and decidedly "physical," although definitely more systems-based than modern biomedicine. And, of course, Descartes arbitrarily separated the mind from the body into separate "universes".

The phenomenon of *qì* in medicine is largely about relationships between systems of function. The material component of human life is constantly changing, but the form stays the same. Just as the principle *lǐ* 理 appears central in Eastern philosophy, a similar idea developed in the West: Aristotle called this *eidos* (εἶδος), the form-giving principle. He defined this principle as something that shapes the embryo, without being changed in the process: "*It contributes nothing to the material body of the embryo but only communicates its program of development…. It does not become part of the embryo, just as no part of the carpenter enters into the wood he works…but the form is imparted by him to the material by means of the changes he effects.*"[250] As it is with the *eidos* of the genome, so it is with medicine. A strength of Chinese medicine is its understanding of relationships *between* phenomena inside and outside the self; it maps exactly how these phenomena are connected and interact with each other. In terms of therapeutics, this translates into combinations of medicinal substances in prescriptions, or combinations of acupuncture points, that interact with the complexity of the human being.

However, just as Aristotle divided the world into parts, classifying them to study it, so the development of science in the West has primarily been reductionist, with a tendency to magnify and focus on the parts. In contrast, the Eastern view accounts for change within a relational structure, and takes advantage of fluid ways relationships can change in order to treat disorders

---

[248] Invisible channels which can be manipulated by yogic practices.

[249] See Gyatso,"*Being Human in a Buddhist World: An Intellectual History of Medicine in Early Modern Tibet,*" where a good portion of the book is devoted to this tension between gross anatomy and the subtle channels/nadis which are "invisible".

[250] Loewenstein, "*The Touchstone of Life: Molecular Information, Cell Communication, and the Foundations of Life* "pg. 337. Quoting Aristotle, "*The Generation of Animals (De generatione animalium)*" (I, 21, 22).

without disregarding the whole system. Western bioscientists have spent several decades gathering micro-data about cellular physiology but do not focus on the relationships between these structures. Wired magazine had a great article about a drug in clinical trials that was designed to transform "bad" cholesterol into "good" cholesterol, but the drug had to be withdrawn due to several patients having heart attacks or dying. It cost the company billions of dollars. According to the author, Jonah Lehrer, the researchers failed to see the entire picture of biological pathways in terms of cholesterol transformation, and designed the drug on incomplete information on the complexities of the body's transformation systems.[251] It will take time, but eventually the public and the scientific community will come to the conclusion that there is great depth and elegance to Chinese medicine and philosophy that was hiding in clear view all along.

In order to practice Chinese medicine at its best, one has to constantly be in a state of awareness rooted in principles (lǐ 理 and theoretical foundations (lǐ lùn 理論). Otherwise, one is caught in the rebound between symptom identification and choosing treatment based on a simplified model of observed symptoms. While this may be adequate for acute conditions, in long-term cases with complex patterns, this is not sufficient. Principle serves as a map that allows one to see the big picture that transcends the limitations of the senses and form in order to synthesize clinical data by applying the appropriate theory to diagnose and treat the whole patient. This may include five phase theory, eight principle diagnosis, six channel classification, or several other problem-solving methodologies embedded in Chinese medicine. Although diagnosis is always based on observation, we must acknowledge that what the patient experiences as health or disease is beyond the flatland of the sense data. The penetrating insight of the physician, based on principle divines the pattern, and chooses appropriate treatment. The more the physician is able to do this, the more he can predict the future development of the pattern, and discern the roots.

In Sùwèn 6 Qíbó 歧伯 responds to Huáng Dì 黃帝 by revealing a tú 圖 / map based on the sān yáng sān yīn 三陽三陰 / three yáng / three yīn differentiations, which differs from Huáng Dì 's understanding of the relationship of calendrical calculations based on heaven / heart, solar / lunar algorithms. Qíbó reiterates the lí hé 離合 / division / unity aspects of the wàn wù 万物 / ten thousand things that arise from the original oneness. He then explains how yīnyáng are differentiated into the six paired channel system.

"When the sages stand facing the South, the front side [of the body] is called broad brilliance (guǎng míng 廣明/); the back is called great thoroughfare(tài chōng 太

---

[251] See Lehrer,"Trials and Errors: Why Science Is Failing Us."

衝)."[252] They then divided the *shàoyīn* 少陰 vessel on the "earth side" of the *tàichōng*, above the *tàiyīn* 太陰 the *tàiyáng* 太陽, The region from the center of the body is called "broad brilliance" The *tàiyáng* vessel is below (behind?) broad brilliance, the *yángmíng* 陽明 is in format of the *tàiyīn*. The *yángmíng* is considered to be *yáng* within *yīn*, outside the *juéyīn* 厥陰 vessel is *shàoyáng* 少陽, the *shàoyīn* is called minor *yáng* within the *yīn*. The text then discusses the nature of the three *yáng* and three *yīn* channels and their relationship to the interior and exterior of the body. *tàiyáng*, *kāi* 開 / opens, *yángmíng* closes, *shàoyáng* is the *shū* 樞 / pivot.

The yin channels are considered to be interior, the *chōng* 衝 / thoroughfare vessel is below, positioned beneath the diaphragm. Behind *tàiyīn* is *shàoyīn*, called *shàoyīn* within *yīn*. The vessel in front of *shàoyīn* is *juéyīn* / ceasing *yīn*. According to Wáng Bīng 王冰, the *yīn qì* is exhausted as it reaches this channel.

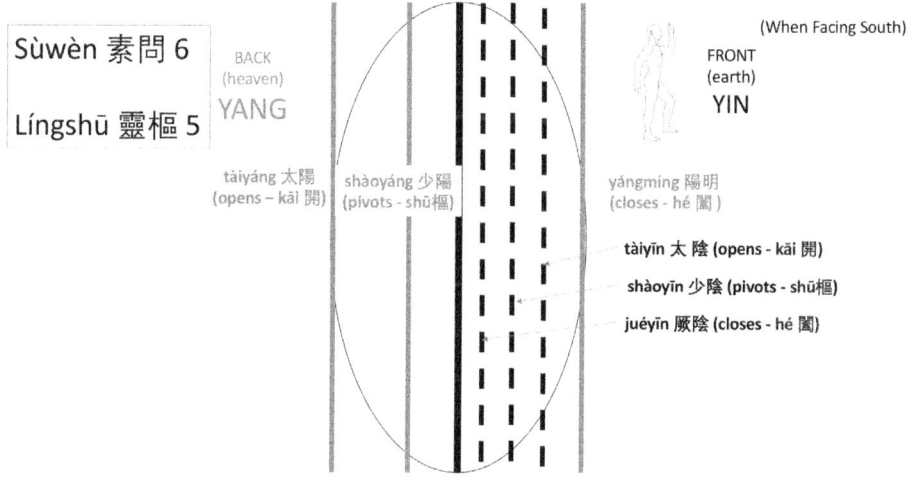

Figure 3.3 - Língshū 5 and Sùwèn 6 Three Yīn/Three Yáng Map[253]

Stephen: It's interesting that in *Língshū* 5 we are given further description of the mapping of the three *yáng*/three *yīn* differentiations of the channels (*fig. 3.3*): For the *yáng* channels: "*tàiyáng kāi* 開/opens, *yángmíng hé* 闔/closes and

---

[252] Unschuld, Tessenow, and Zheng, "*Huang Di Nei Jing Su Wen: An Annotated Translation of Huang Di's Inner Classic - Basic Questions, 2 Volumes,*" pg. 129, quoting Wang Bing's commentary: "*the stomach is in the center of the human body is yang brilliance. Its vessel runs in front of the spleen vessel.*"

[253] This is my (SC) crude attempt at interpreting *Língshū* 5's description of the levels of opening and closing of the *yáng* and *yīn* functions.

shàoyáng, shū 樞/*pivots.*" In pathological conditions "*when the opening is broken, then moats between the flesh sections will be the starting (entry) point for sudden disease.*"[254] *Língshū* 5 goes on to say that for the Yin channels "*tàiyīn* 開 *kāi/opens, juéyīn hé* 闔/*closes and shàoyīn shū* 樞/*pivots.....When the opening is broken, then the granaries have no place where to transport their contents/barrier/flushing.*[255]" This explanation produces a holographic map that is both architectural *and* functional in describing how the channels relate to each other, "move," and can cause/express illness. This causal-relational map would later become the foundation for the "six levels" described in the *Shānghán Lùn* 傷寒論 as how disease progresses within a unified circulatory system.

Z'ev: *Língshū* 5 and *Sùwèn* 6 form a complimentary pair, in which one chapter fulfills the other! In the *Shānghán Lùn*, Zhāng Zhòngjǐng 張仲景 adapted this six channel model of *kāi* 開/opening, *hé* 闔/closing and, *shū* 樞/pivoting to a depth/regional/positional model suitable for tracking symptom patterns that correspond to specific herbal formulas that treat *zhòng fēng* 中風/wind strike, *shānghán* 傷寒/cold damage and *wēn bìng* 溫病/warm disease.

There is a similar model in *Sùwèn* 31,*Treatise on Heat/Rè Lùn* 热論, where the progression of exterior evils passes through the six paired channel complex, within the context of heat diseases. As Huáng Dì states , "*Now, as for heat diseases, they are all of the type 'shānghán', harm caused by cold.*" Here we see that terminology can have subtle differences in different contexts, and that one has to take a medical text as a holistic entity, lest one superimpose one therapeutic system upon another. The therapeutic system delineated in the *Shānghán Lùn*, differs from those described in acu-moxa texts such as the *Língshū*, *Sùwèn* and *Nàn Jīng* 難經. We must always be aware of these subtle differences when discussing medicine.

Stephen: In Chinese language, context *always* matters. The meanings of characters have the flexibility/adaptability to change based on their relationship with the characters around them, sometimes functioning like verbs; the *mò/mài* being one example, which can be thought of as both verb (pulsation) and noun (river-like vessel). This quality of language is what, I think, makes Chinese medicine so innately "holistic" in contrast to Western medicine that is caught in the constant dichotomy of either/or (either noun OR verb, either structure OR function, either mind OR body etc.). Indeed there is interesting research in child development that has shown how culturally, in the past, East Asian children were traditionally taught verbs first (e.g walking, sitting, eating etc.) while Western children tend to learn nouns first (e.g. daddy,

---

[254] Unschuld, "*Huang Di Nei Jing Ling Shu: The Ancient Classic on Needle Therapy*" pg. 113.

[255] ibid., pg. 115.

ball, cup) and this prioritizing verb over noun seems to encourage deeper attention to context[256] and adaptability to change in a novel holistic way.[257]

What I find so striking about the progression from the basic channel mapping in *Sùwèn* and *Língshū*, towards the unified circulatory concept in *Nàn Jīng* is how this principle opened the door for Zhāng Zhòngjǐng to formulate the revolutionary ideas in the *Shānghán Lùn*. To see the *liù jīng* 六經 / six channels as a unified system that functions as both noun *and* verb at the same time has profound implications in the treatment of active (verb) disease progression. A door opens in order to function as a door, likewise it pivots and closes. This is how the flowing circulation of the *"ring without end"* is preserved.

Z'ev: Further discussions in other Han dynasty texts complete the body architecture by front and back, upper middle and lower burners, left and right, interior and exterior, completing a blueprint of the body and its channel pathways as both noun and verb. To the regular channels, we add the *bié mài* 別 脈 / divergent vessels, *luò mài* 絡脈 / network vessels and the *qí jīng bā mài* 奇經八 脈 / eight extraordinary vessels, being the pre-natal foundation for the rest of the channel system and body. as we will see, they represent the underlying blueprint based on the relationship of heaven and earth, the influence of the celestial spheres and constellations, and the very formative forces of human life.

---

[256] See Masuda and Nisbett, *"Attending Holistically versus Analytically: Comparing the Context Sensitivity of Japanese and Americans."*

[257] See Imada, Carlson, and Itakura, *"East–West Cultural Differences in Context-sensitivity Are Evident in Early Childhood."*

The Sinew Channels in *Língshū* 靈樞 and *Nàn Jīng* 難經: *A Discussion of Zàng Xiàng* 臟象/*Visceral Manifestation and How the External Body Reflects the Internal Organs*

Z'ev Rosenberg & Stephen Cowan

知調者利，不知調者害。

"To know how to achieve a balance is beneficial. Not to know how to achieve a balance causes harm."
- *Língshū* 靈樞 33[258]

五運主病 木火土金水 順則皆靜 逆則變亂 四時失常 陰陽偏勝 病之源也

"As for the wǔ yùn 五運/*five movements governance of disease: when wood, fire, earth, metal, and water all move in sequence then each is calm; when there is rebellion, then they transform into chaos, the four seasons lose their constancy, yin and yang lose balance and are conquered. This is the source of disease."*[259]
-Zhāng Yuánsù 张元素 (1151–1234), (*Yīxué Qǐ Yuán* 医学启源)

Z'ev: The Han dynasty medical classics, specifically (for our discussion here) the *Língshū* 靈樞, have provided the foundation for the practice of Chinese medicine for two thousand years, up to and including the 21st century. The advent of modern biomedicine in early 20th century China, and the importation of TCM to the West, brought disruptions to this continuous trend. In most Western countries, the paucity of quality translated work, and the pervasive "reductionist scientific" mindset of biomedicine, has led to a reframing and restructuring of Chinese medicine that has often obscured its original practice. Thanks to such translators as Paul Unschuld, the core medical classics of China are now readily available in academic standard translations which help define the radical body-mind maps conceived by the Han physicians.

---

[258]Unschuld, *"Huang Di Nei Jing Ling Shu: The Ancient Classic on Needle Therapy,"* pg. 363.

[259] Welden, *"To Bring Order out of Chaos: Literati Medicine of the Jin Dynasty (1115-1234),"* pg. 247.

Língshū 靈樞 13 discusses the *jīn jīng* 筋經/sinew (or tendino-muscular) channels, their pathways, diagnostics and clinical applications. For example, the map of "*The sinew of the foot major yang [conduits] (tàiyáng* 太陽) *starts from the little toe. It ascends and connects3 with the knuckle. From there it extends diagonally further upward to the knee. Downward it follows the outer edge of the foot and connects with the heel. It ascends along the heel and links up with the hollow of the knee.*"[260] This chapter also discusses channel divergences, and treatments for swelling, cramping and pain along these channels. For example: "*A swelling and pain extending from the little toe into the heel. The hollow of the knee is cramped; the spine is bent backward. The sinews in the nape are tense. The shoulders cannot be lifted.*"[261] For treatment the text continues by saying "*to achieve a cure, an aggressive 7 piercing with a hot needle is to be repeated until an effect can be seen.*"[262] This is just one example of the wealth of diagnostic and treatment strategies for what we call today "musculoskeletal" (or orthopedic) disorders.

Stephen: As we have been saying, one of the central ideas of "*a ring without end*" is that human beings exist as a unity with celestial and earthly circulatory cycles. To see the body-mind-spirit as landscape is central to understanding how the Chinese conceptualized a unified circulatory system centuries before the West. The *Nàn Jīng* authors were clearly trying to extrapolate from the all-important *Língshū* 12 "stream waters chapter *Jīng Shuǐ* 經水," corroborating this with their empirical observations in order to understand the basis of nourishing life (*yǎngshēng* 養生). *Língshū* 12 contains a detailed discussion of dissection that could have easily been taken from Leonardo Da Vinci's notebooks. As an artist, Leonardo naturally observed the body as a landscape. However, unlike the Western renaissance artists who based their observations on Greek theories, the Han Dynasty medical authors present a greatly expanded idea of anatomy as a reflection of the realms of spiritual ecology. It is no accident to me that *Língshū* 12 Stream Waters *jīng shuǐ* is positioned between *Língshū* 11 called *jīng bié* 經別 (diverging channels) and *Língshū* 13 *jīng jīn* 經筋 / the sinew channels. This series: *jīng bié, jīng shuǐ* and *jīng jīn* offer an understanding of how the circulatory system branches and flows throughout the whole body. To think of tendons as channels may seem like a radical view but consider that mountain ranges are also called "*mài* 脈" in Chinese landscape paintings! Observing the body as a landscape, one naturally sees any part of the body as a series of communicating *jīng* 經/passages. Thus *jīng jīn* could be more literally translated as "the passages through muscles and tendons." In both *Língshū* 11 and 13 Unschuld translates *bié* 別/divergences from the point of view of a

---

[260] Unschuld,"*Huang Di Nei Jing Ling Shu: The Ancient Classic on Needle Therapy,*" pg. 225.

[261] ibid., pg. 226.

[262] ibid., pg. 226.

coherent circulatory system that the *Nàn Jīng* 難經 is repeatedly emphasizing , and so *bié* might just as accurately interpreted as "branching off."[263]

On inspection, the muscles and tendons contain bundles of vessels (nerves, veins, arteries, capillaries, fascia, and lymphatics) that all provide nourishment (*yíng qì* 營氣) to function properly in life. One might be tempted to say that the *jīng*-passages through muscle/tendon are what *Língshū* 13 is referring to as branching off from the central *yíng*-circulatory system. However, from the point of view of spiritual ecology, the muscles and tendons themselves may be seen as passages, that connect to each other just the way mountains form ranges that carry streams and vegetation in the form of networks. This wider perspective of circulation that includes nerve bundles, fascia and muscles as well as blood vessels is to me one of the keys to understanding *qì* flow throughout the body-mind-spirit. Essentially *every* part of the body-mind functions as a conduit of communication! This is why *Nàn Jīng* 24 stresses the importance of understanding how anything that blocks or "cut's off" the flow of communication is the cause of internal disease, be that muscle spasms, sprains, tics, clots, impactions or anxieties.

We can see the importance of understanding the blocks in the flow of communication though the story of Cook Ding (Páodīng 庖丁) in the *Zhuāngzǐ* 莊子 Ch. 3 and approach to dissecting the ox. His method symbolizes one's mastery of mindful awareness, skillful adaptability and effortless flow. He carefully assesses challenges, acts with precision and works patiently until everything naturally falls into place.

> *"Whenever I come to a complicated place, I size up the difficulties, tell myself to watch out and be careful, keep my eyes on what I'm doing, work very slowly, and move the knife with the greatest subtlety, until — flop! the whole thing comes apart like a clod of earth crumbling to the ground. I stand there holding the knife and look all around me, completely satisfied and reluctant to move on, and then I wipe off the knife and put it away."*
> - Zhuāngzǐ 莊子[264]

In *tàijí* 太極 practice, there is a central principle of healthy *tǐ yòng* 體用/form and function, that there must be "no breaks, no twists, no starts and stops, no

---

[263] When we asked Paul Unschuld about this possible interpretation he agreed that within the context of circulation "branching off" could be considered.

[264] Watson,"*The Complete Works of Chuang Tzu,*" pg. 51.

protrusions and no hollows" for there to be balance, flow and internal power (*jìn* 勁).

> "*We may say that the Earth has a vital force of growth, and that its flesh is the soil; its bones are the successive strata of the rocks which form the mountains; its cartilage is the porous rock, its blood the veins of the waters*".
> - Leonardo da Vinci[265]

As a true artist, always curious, Leonardo da Vinci stands in contrast to Vesalius and the other Renaissance anatomists in picturing the flow of streams through mountains as akin to the passages of vessels in the body. However, it was the *Nàn Jīng* authors who present a true appreciation for the notion of what Elizabeth Hsu calls the "body ecologic" which "*highlights the idea of mutual resonance between macrocosm and microcosm and the continuities between the inside and the outside of the physical body.*"[266] It is this fundamental principle that led to the conceptualizing of a single continuous circulatory system of *yíng qì*, that Western doctors are forever missing as they try to fix the parts but miss the whole.

Z'ev: *Língshū* 靈樞 47 discusses how to examine and view the external body in order to understand the shape, size, strength, location and functional qualities of the five internal *zàng* 臟 / viscera. In Chinese medicine, this is the fundamental principle known as *zàng xiàng* 臟象, or visceral manifestation. The *Sùwèn* 素問, (the companion volume of the *Huáng Dì Nèijīng* 黃帝內經 tells us that "the internal state of the viscera can be viewed in outward signs".

In *Língshū* 47, for example, it lists the following:

- The heart: when small, it is at peace, and evil *qì* cannot harm it. It is easily harmed by sadness.
- When the heart is big, sadness cannot harm it. It is easily harmed by evil *qì*.
- When the heart is elevated, it fills the chest (with the lung). Such people suffer from vexation and tend to be forgetful. They find it difficult to open their hearts and speak.

---

[265] See Capra, Fritjof. "*What We Can Learn from Leonardo.*" - an essay adapted from lectures delivered by Fritjof Capra at the Center for Ecoliteracy's seminar "*Sustainability Education: Connecting Art, Science, and Design,*" August 16–18, 2010.

[266] Hsu, "*The Transmission of Chinese Medicine,*"pg. 80.

- When the heart has sunken into the depth, the viscera lose their *qì* to the exterior and suffer *shānghán* 傷寒/cold damage. They are easily made to fear by someone else's words (When the heart *qì* is depleted, fears are generated).
- *Shǎoyīn qì* 少陰氣 resonates with *tàiyáng qì* 太陽氣, which governs the exterior of the body. Then cold and wind evils can easily penetrate the interior. This is why a strong heart *qì* is important to prevent even exterior contraction disorders.

Many Western practitioners of acupuncture/moxibustion focus on what is categorized as *wài kē* 外科/external medicine, which includes musculoskeletal disorders, along with skin disorders and *dài xià* 帶下/vaginal discharge. While one can practice anatomically-based insertions of needles without even examining external signs of internal organ function as described in *Língshū* 靈樞 47, or palpating the vessels, this is quite limiting from a Chinese medical perspective, completely ignoring *zàng xiàng* 臟象. The *Língshū* provides sophisticated maps that reveal a unique perspective to musculoskeletal disorders that is often not obtainable from a biomechanics/orthopedic approach. The *Língshū's* discussion of the *jīn jīng* 筋經/tendino-muscular channels offers a systematic approach to diagnosis and treatment that does not exclude the important relationships of the internal viscera and their associated external tissues/structures to each other. The *jīn jīng* 筋經/sinew (tendino-muscular) channels are dependent upon and reflect the internal condition of the *zàngfǔ* 臟腑/viscera/bowels. Each of the five yin viscera is reflected in an associated tissue; the *gān* 肝/liver specifically with the sinews, *xīn* 心/heart with the blood vessels, *shèn* 腎/kidney with the bones, *fèi* 肺/lungs with the skin, and *pí* 脾/spleen with the *ròu* 肉/flesh. Each of these tissues is nourished by the *jīng* 精/essence of these organs, so if excessive effort is given to building muscle mass and sinew strength alone, this will come at the expense of the liver and the kidneys. The "bulking up" of muscle mass, so popular today in extreme weight lifting or gym workouts, draws on the essence stored in these viscera in order to supply them resulting in predictable imbalanced in the relationships with the other organs.

If one uses insertion techniques into ligaments/tendons/trigger points, one is utilizing draining technique. If the pain, stiffness and discomfort that the patient feels is the result of unintentional over working a region of the tendino-muscular system, and you simply relieve the pain discomfort or stiffness, by using a draining, or strong technique, you are actually weakening the associated *zàng* 臟; specifically, the liver and kidneys. With strong needling, you are enabling the patient to get "back in the game," but at the potential cost of limiting their ability to compete, work out, or improves one's longevity. This illustrates one of the primary differences between a scholar physician and technician; a scholar physician takes into account all factors, and makes the patient aware of tradeoffs from different aspects of one's lifestyle. The technician simply fulfills the immediate demands of the athlete/patient to get them "back in the game/gym."[267]

This is not to say, of course, that in acute injury, one cannot use these techniques as part of one's tool box; but with the awareness gained by seeing the body/mind as a whole entity of multiple interdependent relationships, not a mechanistic series of parts. If you observe patients over many years, you will see exactly what the tradeoffs do in terms of their health. Treating the zàng 臟 with herbs after weakening them through acupuncture is akin to compensatory/allopathic medical treatment, i.e. treating "side effects". It is no different than giving mega doses of vitamin C for colds, which is cold in nature, and in turn weakens the spleen, causing tàiyīn 太陰 issues (digestion and assimilation). Língshū 靈樞 47 states:

> "When cold and warmth harmonized, then the six short-term repositories (fŭ 腑) transform the grain (gŭ 穀) and no wind blockage-illness sets in. The conduit vessels are freely passable. The limbs and joints are all in peace. That is man's regular, healthy condition."[268]

Here we must look at the concept of tensegrity[269] and bio- tensegrity. Several years ago, my colleague Ken Rose had reintroduced me to the work of Buckminster Fuller, who was a pioneer of science and whole systems theory. He built his domes and other architectural marvels based on this principle. In bio-tensegrity, the various tissues and structures of the body are maintained through a system-wide "gravity" which holds these structures in place, maintaining their separate orbits of influence so that they do not interfere with each other. When one stimulates an external component of that mega-structure, it influences the entire system.

---

[267] For more information on the *Technician and Scholar Physician* see Chapter 5 of Rosenberg, *"Returning to the Source: Han Dynasty Medical Classics in Modern Clinical Practice,"* pg. 65-70.

[268] Unschuld, *"Huang Di Nei Jing Ling Shu: The Ancient Classic on Needle Therapy,"* pg. 448.

[269] *"Tensegrity."* https://en.wikipedia.org/wiki/Tensegrity.

The *Nàn Jīng* 難經 chapters dealing with five phase dynamics, specifically 31-35, provide a framework for how external and internal stimuli impact the entire system, leading to bias and imbalances. Just as perverse *qì* can impact the entire system, careful, judicious treatment with acupuncture, moxibustion and herbal medicine can restore the balance with minimal interference in the whole system.

One of the main issues I have with dry needling as a technique for just treating local tendo-muscular issues is that every message given by a needle insertion, adjustment or moxa, create *"ripples in the flow"*. Therefore, we must be cautious when needling local pain or tension as the entire body-mind system will respond accordingly to this stimulus, and as a result, this can lead to long-term problems, even as they relieve tension or pain in the short term. This is why the map-makers of the *Língshū* conceived of the channel system and recognized the connections between internal viscera and bowels with associated tissues and their associated channels. Every illness, trauma, pain, tumor and infection is the result of imbalances in the relationships which permit perverse *qì* to lodge in weakened areas, either by exterior invasion of wind, cold or damp, traumatic injury, areas that are biased by our posture, lack of movement or lack of *shén* 神 awareness or by internal emotional imbalances that can *also* impact the entire body-mind system.

Nàn Jīng 50 discussed the five *"xié* 邪/evils" that can afflict the body-mind: depletion evils, repletion evils, robber evils, weakness evils and *zhèng* 正/"correct" evils that can distort the entire channel system by deregulating the five phase relationships of the channels, and *zàngfǔ* 臟腑. Wherever we are blocked, stuck or compromised, illness can take hold. This reveals the true wisdom of the *Nèijīng* 內經 and *Nàn Jīng*: that everything is inter-connected in very precise ways that the authors of these texts observed directly. These classics offer the practitioner detailed maps of the channel system that reflect the universal heaven/human/earth paradigm.

This is the problem with using excessive force in treatment. Medical treatment begins with the careful examination of the whole body-mind in all its complexity, using these maps to generate diagnostic acumen and strategies for treatment. When a physician fails to see systematically in the way the *Nèijīng* and *Nàn Jīng* train the mind to view local lesions, the more likely that force will be applied. Unfortunately, this in turn will lead to transferring the local perverse *qì* to another, usually more internal domains in the body-mind. These domains are defined by what Elisabeth Hsu calls "the tripartite body,"[270] the sentimental body, ecological body, and architectural body.

In Chinese medicine, every symptom, every lesion has an original set of interrelated causes; either internal, external, or neither internal or external. Utilizing the subtle diagnostic methods of vessel (pulse), abdominal, palpation, tongue, allows us to confront complexity through the patterns of relationships from which we can deduce the origin of a majority of presenting symptoms and pathologies. Using the channel system maps, we can comprehend why these symptoms appear in a particular location or side of the body. The normative, dynamic equilibrium-seeking intention of the human body-mind, (what Chinese medicine calls *yuán qì* 原氣), is, as previously stated, akin to what Dr. George Vithoulkas (homeopathic physician) calls the "supercomputer intelligence" of humanity and nature. We have an endless supply of self-correcting mechanisms that just need a gentle stimulus or reminder in order to be awakened.

---

[270] Hsu, *"Pulse Diagnosis in Early Chinese Medicine: The Telling Touch,"* pg. 14-15.

Língshū 靈樞 11: Meditations on the Bié Mài 別脈 Maps of the Underground Rivers and Aquifers

Z'ev Rosenberg, Stephen Cowan & Brian Kirbis

Zev: In *Nàn Jīng* 難經 27 and 28, we have succinct descriptions of the *qí jīng bā mài* 奇經八脈/eight extraordinary conduit vessels. In *Nàn Jīng* 27, it states "*the sages [of antiquity] devised and constructed ditches and reservoirs and they kept the waterways open in order to be prepared for an extraordinary [situation].*"[271] Lǐ Jiōng 李駉 comments: "*In times when the rainfloods rushed wildly through the ditches and into the reservoirs, the sages just listened to their flow. They did not [have to] make any further plans [to prevent a catastrophe].*"[272] Huá Shòu 滑寿 goes on to states: "*the eight singular-conduit vessels are not included in the sequence (of the main conduits and network vessels. The singular-conduit (vessels) serve (as additional ditches and reservoirs) in the case of an overfilling of the network vessels.*"[273]

Stephen: Our latest research concludes that the terms "channel," "collateral," "divergence" and "branch" which first appear in the Inner Canon and describe the size and depth of the vessels, derive from analogies used to describe the length, depth and size of waterways. It is, I think important to keep in mind that the word "divergence" doesn't imply a separate pathway independent of the whole circulatory system.

Z'ev: In Difficulty 28, it states "*Similarly, when the [conduits and network vessels] of man are filled [to overflowing, their surplus contents] enter the eight [single-*

---

[271] Unschuld (2016), "*Nan Jing: The Classic of Difficult Issues,*" pg. 275

[272] ibid., pg. 275

[273] ibid., pg. 275

conduit] vessels – where they are no longer part of the circulation"[274] From the perspective of *A Ring Without End*, we propose that it is impossible for any part of the human vessel to be disconnected from the overall circulation of *xuè* 血 / *qì* 氣.

I was thinking about last winter's flooding rains and snows that hit California after many years of drought. The rain and snowmelt flooded the Central Valley, the "breadbasket of California," which relies on the underlying aquifer and centuries of accumulated water, flowing down from mountains via rivers and streams. These sudden, excessive rains and snowmelt restored an ancient lake, flooded much farmland, but also helped to recharge the aquifer as the excessive water percolated down through the topsoil. The transport of water via rivers and streams to the valley floor led to the attempt of the earth to absorb this excess precipitation by absorption into aquifers and underground rivers.

So, based on a unified view of circulation in the human organism, how could it be possible that there would be any perceived separation between the *bié mài* vessels, *qí jīng bā mài*, and the regular *jīngluò* 經絡 channel system? The ancient Chinese philosophers saw the human entity as a conduit between heaven and earth, and a unity of flow of *qì* and blood!

Stephen: Yes, if we consider the whole water cycle that includes the atmosphere (heavens) as well as the ground (earth), we would not say that floodwaters are "sequestered" or "cut off," though they may be temporarily held in one place until evaporative transfer back into the natural circulatory system of water from ground to sky and sky to ground. When we consider the human being as a microcosm of that whole cycle, this distinguishes Chinese medicine from Western medicine.

Z'ev: Referencing Péng Ziyì 彭子益's *"Circular Dynamics of Chinese Medicine"* we see this movement as an "unbroken chain," eternal and pervasive, he states:

"Those who would like to study Chinese medicine must first understand the reasoning for the names of the twelve meridians. in order to understand the reasoning

---

[274] ibid., pg. 276-277.

In conversation with Brian Kirbis, he notes that *sàn* 散 can be translated as "dissipates," or "scatters". This does not necessarily mean that the *qìxuè* 氣血are no longer part of the circulation in the *bié mài*.

for the names of the twelve meridians, one must first understand the principles of yin and yang, five elements and six environmental factors; in order to understand the principles of yin and yang, five elements and six environmental factors, one must first understand the 24 solar terms as the circular movement of the heat from the sun as it strikes the surface of the earth and descends, stores, rises or expands."[275]

I've always felt that the Chinese were pioneers in irrigation, and one of the earlier civilizations based on the cultivation of grains. Clearly, the *Língshū* in its five phase categorizations states that grains and beans are the major food category. This stands out from other more nomadic civilizations that relied on animal husbandry, such as the Tibetan and Mongolian civilizations, which had different metaphors for their medicine, until their later contacts with China during and after the Mongol conquest. At this point, Chinese influences on both Tibetan and Mongolian medicine were quite apparent.[276] It is interesting that agrarian societies such as Korea and Japan, where there is little pasture land for animal husbandry were quick to adapt the Chinese medical system to their cultures. This is another important observation by Paul Unschuld.[277]

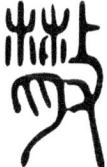

Figure 3.4 - Sàn 散

Stephen: Yes the character *sàn* 散 comes to mind here (*fig. 3.4*). *Sàn* 散 can mean "to disperse, scatter, disseminate." It's a common word in Chinese medical therapeutics. The ideogram is related to the thrashing of grain- It shows a hand holding a stick beating the flesh of a plant. Lǎozǐ 老子 uses the term as a way of understanding the act of dispersing. As he discusses in chapter 64:

其微易散

---

[275] McMahon, *"Circular Dynamics of Ancient Chinese Medicine I."* pg 2.

[276] Hsu, *"A Hybrid Body Technique: Does the Pulse Diagnostic Cun Guan Chi Method Have Chinese-Tibetan Origins?"*

[277] See *"Medicine in China"* series for more details Unschuld, *"Medicine in China: A History of Ideas."* & Unschuld,*"Medicine in China: Historical Artifacts and Images."*

What is subtle is easy to <u>disperse.</u>[278]

How water/blood disperses, disseminates to all the various potential spaces in the body seems to be the point *Nàn Jīng* is making in understanding health and disease processes as it applies to divergent and collateral channels.. Recognizing the way nutrients enter the blood stream and likewise how pathological agents of disease can spread throughout the body are both essential to understanding how to heal and nurture life through *yíng/wèi* 營衛. The *Nàn Jīng* tells us that there are no breaks in circulation and therefore we must be mindful of the whole when treating the parts.

Brian: I love this idea of thrashing. It's the way Shén Nóng 神農's treatment of medicinal substances is treated as well. How we describe this releasing of vital principle from material form. I'm thinking of the "descending and dispersing" relationship between lung and kidney as a fundamental aspect of the relationship between the channels and their divergents. One piece that fascinates me as how they work as *jīng* 經/aqueducts but also function in relation to pathogens and sickness.

Stephen: Exactly, from a circulation perspective a better word for *sàn* might be "perfusion."

Brian: Stephen, this is what I've been holding in mind from the beginning of this conversation. The perfusion is like the fibrous roots of plants that both "terminate" or "perfuse" in the earth and are responsible for uptake.

Addressing this issue seems to require acknowledging the pedagogy at the heart of generation of medical knowledge, vis-a-vis, internal cultivation. I don't believe that pulse or other observational methods are sufficient to "locate" something like the divergent channels unless a meditator hadn't already experienced them within their own body. Similar to Shén Nóng's "mirror-like" stomach in relation to herbs.

Stephen: Yes, the subtlest little hairs of the roots on one end of a plant buried in the soil soak up the subtlest nutrients and water that perfuse the soil. This kind of inner/outer cultivation (*xiūxíng* 修行) of the subtle is one of the keys to healthy growth. I'm thinking here about membranes and the way vital nutrients cross through these lipid bilayers according to the principle of higher and lower concentration, that could be considered an example of *yīnyáng* 陰陽

---

[278] *Lǎozǐ* 64 translation/interpretation S. Cowan.

dynamics.. Further along, *Lǎozǐ* 64 says: *"The giant tree grows from a tiny shoot."*[279] This kind of nourishment from the subtle is something often missed today. Likewise, from the perspective of treating disharmonies *before* they manifest into pathologies, Western medicine often waits until disease is an acute emergency and then demands instant relief, (a form of instant gratification,) and so requires extremely powerful drugs like steroids, immunosuppressants and psycho-pharmaceuticals to get the job done quickly. The problem with this heavy-handed approach, in my opinion, is that it has no subtlety or specificity. Because there is nowhere that circulation does not reach, these drugs tend to hit the whole body all at once, sort of like "acceptable *collateral* damage" when dropping bombs. This is why the list of adverse reactions and side effects are so long with many western drugs.

Chinese herbal medicine, and for that matter acu-moxa, aim at generating much subtler effects that over time have the power to transform disease patterns and support one's healthy destiny. There are Chinese herbs that disperse (*sàn* 散) accumulation rather than suppressing symptoms and this seems to be one of many distinctions from biomedicine.

Z'ev: The idea of *sàn* 散 as "dispersion" and "perfusion" is an accurate description of how Chinese herbal medicine works. While the concept of *tōng jīng* 通經/penetrating or targeting channels was adapted by Zhāng Yuánsù 張元素. During the Jin dynasty period, the core idea was that herbal formulas were both systemic *and* targeted to specific areas at the same time. Each formula had guiding medicinals to bring the *jūn* 君/sovereign or most "active" ingredients to specific areas. Concurrently, the formula was always designed to protect the spleen and stomach, which was the first *zàngfǔ* 臟腑 region to "receive" the medicinals and metabolize them, and each formula was a harmonious ecosystem in and of itself.

Stephen: As in Chinese medicine, self-cultivation practices (*xiū yǎng* 修养) such as *tàijí* 太極 or meditation focus on the examination of subtle changes within body-mind, observing how patterns manifest, shift and transform. This offers a deep observation of our true nature <u>as</u> Nature. Such cultivation practices however require time and patience, curiosity and caring. Now isn't that exactly what the Chinese medicine practitioner is doing when they look, listen and take a pulse to assess the subtle roots of suffering?

---

[279] *Lǎozǐ* 64 translation/interpretation S. Cowan.

The Mother of Qì: *Thoughts on the Xuèqì* 血氣 *Couple*

Stephen Cowan & Z'ev Rosenberg

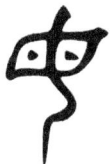

Figure 3.5 - Mǔ 母 [280]

天下有始
以為天下母 既得其母
以知其子 既知其子
復守其母 沒身不殆

Everything in the world begins through the world-mother.
Find the mother and you'll understand its children.
Once you understand the children, go back and safeguard the mother and your life
will be unharmed.
- Lǎozǐ 老子 52[281]

Stephen: Let us look more deeply into what it means to be a microcosm. This seems to be a pivotal question that distinguishes Chinese medicine's ways of nourishing life (*yǎngshēng* 養生) in contrast to the Western medical model of treating disease. To be a microcosm means that we echo (*yīng* 應) the cosmic forces of the universe. This is an idea that even Quantum physicists still struggle to see.

---

[280] *Mǔ* 母 – mother, pictogram of a woman with breasts.

[281] *Lǎozǐ* 老子 52 translation/interpretation S. Cowan.

Sùwèn 素問 25 states *"For all piercing to be reliable, one must first regulate the spirit."*[282] and in *Sùwèn* 26, *Discourse on the Eight Cardinal [Turning Points] and Shenming*, Qíbó 岐伯 advises Huáng Dì 黃帝 that *"all laws of piercing require an observation of the qi of sun and moon and stars and of the eight cardinal [turning points] of the four seasons."*[283] As we've stated previously, these statements reveal to us that not only is it important for the practitioner's body-mind to be calm and concentrated in the healing process but that one's awareness of the cycles of moon, sun, and stars, also has a powerful effect on knowing how to effectively treat a person. This spirit-connection was how the *shén* 神 doctors practiced but it is now often dismissed as "old wives tales" by modern Western medicine and even by some practitioners of TCM medicine.

Z'ev: I would add that this is not only a lacuna of modern biomedicine, it is also an underlying cause of illness for modern Western society. The loss of connection of our patients with circadian rhythms, essential nutrients, contact with unblemished soil, clean air or water has led to an epidemic of sleep disorders, gastrointestinal malfunction, chronic fatigue, and emotional/psychological issues. As new illnesses appear, reflecting the loss of communication of vital human systems/channels/viscera, the treatments in turn become more toxic, extreme and even paranoid in their scope. A patient I advised today on post-chemotherapy and breast cancer was put on three antidepressants, two tranquilizers along with the aromatase inhibitors. The patient still has sleep problems, along with severe constipation, dry mouth, and *zàng zào* 脏躁/visceral agitation.

Stephen: As for "old wives tales," when I was a young pediatrician on call for neonatal deliveries at the hospital, those old midwives all knew that on full moon nights we were going to be VERY busy with women going into labor. Despite conflicting research refuting and proving this empirical data,[284] it only took me a few sleepless on-call nights to realize that truth.

Z'ev: During my formative years as a scholar/physician, I also closely aligned with pediatrics. I had two assistants, both lay midwives, who invited me to births, and many referrals for obstetric and postpartum care with Chinese

---

[282] Unschuldand Tessenow, *"Huang Di Nei Jing Su Wen: An Annotated Translation of Huang Di's Inner Classic - Basic Questions, 2 Volumes"* pg. 428.

[283] ibid., pg. 433-434.

[284] See Marco-Gracia,*"The Influence of the Lunar Cycle on Spontaneous Deliveries in Historical Rural Environments."* & Matsumoto, and Shirahashi, *"Novel Perspectives on the Influence of the Lunar Cycle on the Timing of Full-Term Human Births."*

herbal medicine and acupuncture. I was able to observe firsthand the importance of harmonizing with seasonal, lunar and solar cycles in this realm. It was truly a blessing to take part in this budding branch of Chinese medicine unfolding in the West. One lesson I learned was that it is essential to take part in all stages of pregnancy as a practitioner, with regular treatment, herbs, diet and lifestyle recommendations, rather than just assisting at births for the best results. I always told my pregnant patients that "seeking acupuncture or herbs at or just before birth is like inviting a friend to a movie in the last fifteen minutes".

One case that comes to mind is a woman who was given a due date for her birth and pressured to deliver, otherwise, she would be induced. Of course, this pressure actually makes it more difficult to do so. I felt her pulses and found that the left *guān* 關 / gall bladder pulse was extremely wiry and replete, indicating that the *dài mài* 帶 脈 and gall bladder were both congested. As it turns out, she had a lot of suppressed anger with her husband, who was widowed just a year before their marriage, and all of her photos, furniture and other belongings were still in their home (along with his two sons from the previous marriage). We addressed those issues, and then I needled *wài guān*外關 / outer pass (TB 5), *zú lín qì* 足臨泣 / foot governor of tears (GB 41), *yáng líng quán* 陽陵泉 / yang mound spring (GB 34), Du 20 (*bǎi huì* 百會 / hundred meeting (Du 20), and *hé gǔ* 合谷 / joining valley (LI 4). After twenty minutes, she asked me to remove the needles, and returned home with her midwife. A half hour later, I got a phone call, "it's a girl"!!

Z'ev: In a sense, the practitioner dances with one's needles and moxa. What comes to mind is Biǎn Què 扁鵲 (407 310 BCE) with needle in hand (*fig. 3.6*), like the shamanic image of piercing evils with sharpened stones.[285]

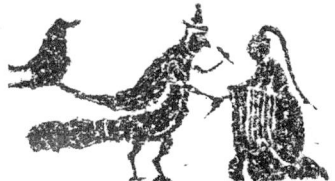

Figure 3.6 - Rubbing of Biǎn Què 扁鵲 [286]

---

[285] A legendary doctor who lived during the Warring States period who was said to have uncanny diagnostic & treatment skills.

[286] Unschuld, "*Medicine in China: Historical Artifacts and Images,*" pg. 97. - Rubbing of Biǎn Què 扁鵲 from a tomb relief dating to the Han Dynasty.

Stephen: In *Sùwèn* 26 Qíbó goes on to say: *"At the time of beginning of the crescent moon, xuèqì* 血氣 *originates as essence (jīng* 精*) and the guard qi (wèi qì* 衛氣*) begins to move."*[287]

For the Han Dynasty practitioners, place, position and timing matter for accurate diagnosis and effective treatment. Our intimate connection with the cyclic movement of the cosmos is one aspect of what it means to be a microcosmos. The other is our connection to the earthly influences. Qíbó goes on further to say:

> *"The fact is, for nourishing the spirit, one must know whether the physical appearance is fat or lean and whether the camp and the guard [qi], the blood and the qi, abound or are weak. Blood and qi, [they are] the spirit of man; it is essential to nourish them carefully."*[288]

Acumoxa therapy is largely concerned with being in the right place at the right time. This echoes what is stated in *Sùwèn* 1 *"The people of high antiquity, those who knew the Way, they modeled [their behavior] on yin and yang and they complied with the arts and the calculations."*[289] The practitioner tunes themself through meditation, qigong/yoga, taking care to regulate their sleep-wake rhythms. daily activity, diet, and refining the herbal formulas they take to fit the ever changing context they happen to be in. To navigate the complexities of modern life, Qíbó is telling us that as practitioners we must develop the sensitivity to "tune in" to this *xuèqì* aspect in our patients, and to always keep in mind that the seasonal *qì*, circadian rhythms and solar/lunar cycles affect the circulation of *xuèqì* which is the resonating (*yīng* 應) spirit of each of us. Qibó's statement: *"Xuèqì is the spirit of the human being."* is a powerful message in treating the whole person. It implies that Blood and Qì are an intimate couple that are inseparable partners indispensable for life's physiological activities to function properly.

---

[287] Unschuld,and Tessenow, *"Huang Di Nei Jing Su Wen: An Annotated Translation of Huang Di's Inner Classic - Basic Questions, 2 Volumes,"* pg. 443.

[288] ibid., pg. 443.

[289] ibid., pg. 30.

There is an often quoted saying by Chinese medical practitioners and *tàijí* 太極 masters that *"Blood is the Mother of Qì and Qì is the commander of blood."*[290] While there are hints at this quote in *Língshū* 靈樞 18 & 30, Ted Kaptchuk claims the source of this famous quote originated with Gōng Tíngxián 龔廷賢 (1581–1616) in his discussion of *qì* and blood in *Shòu Shìbǎo Yuán* 壽世保元/*Preserving Vitality in Life* (1615).[291] What does it mean to be the *mother* of *qì*? For that matter what does it mean to be a mother? As a pediatrician, it is eminently clear to me that one must care for both mother *and* child as a functioning unity to successfully nourish life and promote health. This may seem obvious when caring for a newborn but I find it is also what takes finesse in all pediatric care.

In the delivery room, which is the holiest place I know, we get an opportunity to bear witness to the powerful transformation that happens at the time of a birth. Long ago, midwives taught me to wait until the umbilical pulsations have stopped before cutting the cord because this extra blood contains valuable information for the baby: an added dose of maternal oxygen-breaths and an extra store of iron that supports hemoglobin as well as placental stem cells that have a protective value to the health of the baby. This waiting for me became a powerful meditation in the delivery room. Back in the '80s, the majority of OBs disregarded this notion in their rush to clamp the cord and surgically separate infant and mother. It has only recently been shown that delayed umbilical cord clamping improves iron stores in infants up to 6 months of age.[292] It also offers an extra dose of stem cells (a form of *yuán qì* 原氣) provided from mother to child.

Immediately following the intense, often violently painful labor, once the infant is dried and warmed and placed on the mother's chest to suckle, I sense the room filled with a powerful light. It is this warmth and lightness that has the feeling one gets after a big storm has passed and the sun breaks through the clouds.. I find it also similar to that surge of energy one sometimes feels after a long illness has passed. This lightness of being is a picture of resilience and

---

[290] *Xiě wéi qì zhī mǔ, qì wèi xuè zhī shuài* 血為氣之母，氣為血之帥 - This common saying can be linked to Yú Shù 虞庶 (1064-1067)'s commentary in *Nàn Jīng* 難經, 32 *"The heart controls the blood; the blood represents the camp [qi]. The lung controls the qi;the qi are the guard [qi]. The flow of the blood relies on the [movement of the] qi; the movement of the qi depends on the [flow of the] blood. Blood and qi proceed [through the organism] in mutual dependency."*- Unschuld (2016), *"Nan Jing: The Classic of Difficult Issues,"* pg. 300-301

[291] Kaptchuk,*"The Web That Has No Weaver: Understanding Chinese Medicine,"* pg. 54.

[292] See KC, et al, *"Effects of Delayed Umbilical Cord Clamping vs Early Clamping on Anemia in Infants at 8 and 12 Months."*

recovery. It is the quality of *shénmíng* 神明, the light of the sun and moon and stars within us. I get the chance to bear witness to such *shénmíng* whenever I am present for the transformation of a woman into the mother, who is after all born *with* her child. In fact one might say the child gives birth to the mother!

Xuèqì as a mother-child unity is an interesting example of microcosmic thinking: It reflects the great *yīnyáng* cycles of day-night, heaven-earth relationship. The mother is *yīn* to her *yáng* child. The circulation of this cosmic couple is of principle importance in our medicine. Without appreciating it, we are mere mechanics. The fact that the blood *carries* the *qì* the way a mother *carries* her baby in utero and after birth is powerful imagery for me. One aspect of this is to consider the oxygen-carrying capacity of blood.While the Han dynasty physicians certainly had no concept of Oxygen, they did recognize the life-giving qualities carried in blood. Of course, I want to shy away from making too literal a correlation here. When we look at the *yīnyáng* unity of Blood/Qì as a reflection of Earth and Heaven respectively present in a human being we have a clear image of the trilogy presented all through the medical classics.

Z'ev: A beautiful summation of the heaven/human/earth trilogy in Han dynasty as applied to human health and medicine. I do find, however as you do, that in hospitals and medical offices that the environment often works against true healing. Florescent lighting, sterilizing chemicals, horrendous food, closed windows with no air circulation all work against a nurturing, healing environment which is so essential to recovery. I refuse to have my clinical practice, teaching or any other professional activity in an environment that makes me feel ill. For many years I got to observe what Business Week magazine called 'sick building syndrome', where many of my patients were constantly ill with cold damage from recycled, chilled air in closed buildings made of synthetic materials unable to properly conduct *qì*. Many of the classrooms I taught in were either old, poorly lit, or in industrial parks that were the antithesis of the message being presented in the teaching materials. One of the issues plaguing our profession is this obsession with "fitting in," wearing white coats, working in these sterile environments and trying to fit into what is an unhealthy paradigm.

Stephen: *Nàn Jīng* 難經 22 states that *qì* refers to the quality of a warm breath, *xuè* refers to the quality of moistening.We can see this moistening and irrigating effect as the blood side of the *xuèqì* couple when we witness a mother suckling her child. The hydration and nourishment (*yíng* 營) provided is essential for the infant's growth and immunity. But what of the intimate warm feelings experienced by mother and child that we know comes from oxytocin secretion in response to the infant's cry? Is this not the *qì* side of the *xuèqì* couple, that *moves* the mother into action by inducing the letting down of her milk and generating the loving warmth of bonding? As with everything in our practice of Chinese medicine according to the classics, in considering *xuèqì* as a unity, the whole is *always* greater than the sum of the parts. This is the true meaning of emergence.

Z'ev: I love the idea here of the dialogue, the *yīnyáng* communication between *xuè/qì*. This is the veritable "music of the spheres" at work. This quote reminds me of what was said of Linnaeus: "*wherever he walked, the plants died before him.*" In his mechanistic, devitalized analysis and categorization of plants, any sense of intelligence or life force was lost.

> "*When there is some magic about the way things operate it means that the interconnection of things is so subtle that the functioning requires that everything is in the right place and goes at the right pace. Our trouble is that we want to understand how things work, but in so doing we destroy the movement itself. So many explanations are just in order to rebuild what has been destroyed by this single act of an analysis of life.*"[293]

Stephen: This seemingly magical sense of wonder we witness at the moment of birth, gives us a direct experience of the *xuèqì* couple as an emergent property, the whole being remarkably greater than the sum of the parts and this reality is no less *scientific* than the linear-logic approaches proposed by reductionist perspectives. Indeed, as noted neuropsychologist Richard L. Gregory has states:

As *Sùwèn* 26 tells us, this same phenomenon of emergent properties that arise from *xuèqì* unity, is likewise reflected in the *yíngwèi* 營衛 couple. The unity of couples gives us the ability to generate a diversity of harmonics that define our changing relationships. As *Lǎozǐ* 42 famously says:

> "*Out of the Dào* 道 (*process*) *comes one/yī* 一 (*unity*), *out of oneness comes two/èr* 二 (*yīnyáng* 陰陽), *out of two comes three/sān* 三 *and out of three comes a myriad of diversity/wàn wù* 萬物"[294]

---

[293] Larre, Rochat de la Vallée, and Root, "*Essence, Spirit, Blood and Qi*," pg. 83

[294] *Lǎozǐ* 老子 42 translation/interpretation S. Cowan

It's interesting that in complexity theory, one of the simple rules for emergence to take place is, as Neil Theise says, *"Rule # 1: Numbers Matter. There must be sufficient numbers of interacting parts to form a complex system."*[295]

Indeed, how is it possible, for example, that a human being (or any mammal for that matter), can produce tens of millions of different antibodies, a number far greater than the number of structural genes in the mammalian genome? In reality, a small number of genetic segments is used, but the diversity is generated during the development of the embryo by something far greater than just the sum of the genes. This is seen in the science of complexity and "self-organization" where Francois Jacobs noted that this generation of a multitude of antibodies operates at three levels.[296] And as we know from Chinese medicine three is a magic number! Such is the miraculous emergence of *yíngwèi within xuèqì* that is the focal point for much of the *Nàn Jīng* 難經 discussion on circulation.

Z'ev: In the work of the great scientist Francisco Varela, he speaks of autopoesis, or *"the property of a living system (such as a bacterial cell or a multicellular organism) that allows it to maintain and renew itself by regulating its composition and conserving its boundaries."*[297] He redefined the immune system as lacking a distinct central "processor" organ, but as an intelligence that responded uniquely to all sorts of external and internal threats, what Chinese medicine has considered as *xié qì* 邪氣 / perverse *qì*. This body / mind intelligence is of course intrinsic to Chinese medical physiology, which recognizes functions such as *sānjiāo* 三焦 / triple burner which is 'function without form' according to the *Nàn Jīng*, and crosses over several systems and viscera of the body. Varela largely rejected the "search and destroy" metaphor applied to the immune system as biomedicine understands it. Rather, as Stephen points out above, immune mechanisms emerge from the body / mind "super-intelligence" that we call *yíng / wèi*. In an interview on Edge.org, Varela talks about autoimmunity stating *"(in an) autoimmune condition, the system eats itself up. From my point of view, the right approach is first to understand the nature of this global regulation. One hint on how to do this is to look for ways to reconnect the system. In this regard, autoimmune diseases are seen as a deregulation, a condition that calls for more connectedness."*[298]

---

[295] Theise,*"Notes on Complexity,"* pg. 24

[296] See Jacob, *"The Possible and the Actual"*

[297] Merriam-Webster Online Dictionary.

[298] See Varela, *Chapter 12 "The Emergent Self."*

This is exactly what acupuncture/moxa is designed to do, reconnect broken connections in the channel system, *bié* 別/separations that do not allow *xuèqì* to flow unimpeded. On one level the channel system is a communications system that binds all phenomena, tissues, viscera/bowels and functions together in a whole.

Stephen, you had described *A Ring Without End* as a circle. Han and pre-Han dynasty philosopher/physicians were masters of pattern differentiation and correlative thinking. They looked at the night sky, observed the turning of the sphere and saw cycles that influenced movements in the body. Eclipses were seen as perturbations, chaos in these cycles. So in the human being; counter-flows, vacuities, repletions, *bì zhèng* 痹症/impediments, *dú* 毒/toxins were all perturbations in the harmonious flow in the channel system, the *"ring without end."*

Elisabeth Hsu points out that Han and pre-Han dynasty physicians applied synchronous correlation, i.e. correlative thinking to their diagnoses and treatment. This is described by Hsu as correlative cosmology[299] in terms of *wǔxíng* 五行/five phases, siting the *Mǎ Wáng Duī* 馬王堆 manuscripts as an early source. In *Sùwèn* 素問 69-77, a highly developed doctrine, *wǔ yùn liù qì* 五運六氣/five movements six *qì* was developed and added by Wáng Bīng 王冰, which tracked changes in sixty year cycles, five phases times twelve, to track diseases alongside the nature and character of each year and season, also based on a circular, repetitive movement of the heavens.

Stephen: When a child comes into our life, the challenge is how to contain all the moment to moment, day to day chaos generated by change. It is this *xuèqì* mother-child relationship that generates respectively the consistency and momentum for change, and with it, the potential for harmony and growth amidst the disruption of routines and habits, the fears of making terrible mistakes, the uncertainty generated by too much information and the immense responsibility parents naturally feel. *Nèijīng* and *Nàn Jīng* medicine tells us again and again that it is the need to safeguard one's *xuèqì* relationship in order to avoid the depletion caused by externally and internally induced agitation. This is the key to promoting healthy circulation of *yíngwèi* in nourishing

---

[299] Hsu, *"Pulse Diagnosis in Early Chinese Medicine: The Telling Touch,"* pg. 23.

life. Understanding the power greater than the sum of the parts is the essence of what is meant by "relational health."[300]

Zev: Loss of relationships in the body/mind is what generates illness. Loss of the circulating communication in the brain/gut/vagus nerve axis generates emotional/psychological and neurological disorders. The five *zàng* 臟 when they lose communication with each other generate multiple pathologies. When human pathology becomes widespread to large groups of people, when "we sell our mother earth (Crazy Horse)" we begin to distort the seasons, essential elemental substances of life on which we all depend: soil, air, water. We dam the rivers, causing blockages in essential flows that kill fish, animals and destroy the life of native communities that rely on clean water flowing and nurturing fish, life and crops. We destroy the fabric of heaven/earth, and humanity at the center dynamic becomes estranged. Communities are broken, navigation of life/essence is lost, loneliness and despondency are the result.

We are now witnessing climate change, where the extraction of yin fire (petroleum products) from the inner earth, and then combustion of these raw materials brings *yáng* fire into the atmosphere. Native Americans warned us to not dig up these essences from the earth, that this would destroy us. How tragic that we have built our entire civilization on this yin fire!

Stephen: Lǎozǐ 老子's prescription at the beginning of this chapter *"to safeguard the mother"* for nourishing life seems like timely advice for all of us today. In Macrocosmic terms, the Earth represents the yin aspect of our mother-child unity and we, her children. As the Earth heats up with excessive *yáng qì*, we are bound to deplete our resources, impairing the very mother that irrigates us with her nourishment.

For the beginning practitioner faced with a patient who presents with mixed symptoms of excess and depletion, one must always keep in mind this intimate *xuèqì* relationship. This requires a wider appreciation for the context/environment that they are simultaneously treating, not just the individual human being. This environment-human continuity is the classical Daoist

---

[300] "Relational health" is a term coined by the American Academy of Pediatrics in a policy statement - See Garner, and Yogman, *"Preventing Childhood Toxic Stress: Partnering with Families and Communities to Promote Relational Health."*

Note: This mother-child relationship of *xuèqì* is perhaps a slightly different spin on circulation from Ed Neal's idea that circulation in the channels primarily meant blood circulation in the classics.

perspective of the sage (*shèng* 聖). Likewise from a Confucian perspective, the *jūnzǐ* 君子 (refined practitioner) always includes treatment of the family relationships in that patient's life. Too often we focus on boosting *wèi qì* 衛氣 and disregard *yíng qì* 營氣.

On a more simple practical level, I have found that when I have a loved one hold the hand of the patient during a treatment, I get a much more powerful effect than when that patient is left alone in a room. Even more powerful, I have placed needles in both mother *and* child and had them then hold hands creating a living Manaka ion pump cord to reinforce the mother-child unity of *yíngwèi* 營衛 *xuèqì* 血氣. This is particularly effective in cases of autism where a child is experiencing being cut-off from their surroundings, an apt metaphor for the times we live in.

Too often we think acupuncture is about *qì* and not blood circulation. Likewise, too often Western doctors focus on the blood and disregard the *qì*. This is a lopsided treatment that treats the parts but not the whole. Each time we pierce an acupuncture point, we must keep in mind this mother-and-child reunion.

As Paul Simon so aptly says:

> *"No, I would not give you false hope*
> *On this strange and mournful day*
> *But the mother and child reunion*
> *Is only a motion away"*[301]

---

[301] Paul Simon. *Mother and Child Reunion.*

Nàn Jīng 難經 **30:** *Traveling Hand-in-Hand*

Stephen Cowan

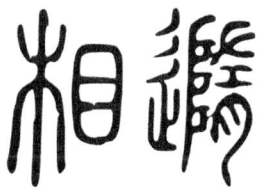

Figure 3.7 - Xiāng Suí 相隨 [302]

"The marvel lies in how the two qi separate, Yin and Yang transform and give rise to billions, while simultaneously gathering together and carried as one"
-From the *Tàijí* 太極 Classics[303]

The third volume of the *Nàn Jīng* 難經 is dedicated to the *zàngfú* 臟腑 relationship, the organ networks that function, as everything does, as a microcosm of *yīnyáng* 陰陽. It is no accident that this follows volume 2 which examines the nature of flow through the channels. Volume 3 begins with *Nàn Jīng* Difficulty 30 from which our book derives its title.[304] It asks a fundamental question: *"How do yíng qì* 營氣 *and wèi qì* 衛氣 *travel together?"* As we discussed in the previous chapter, this *yíngwèi* couple resonates with the two aspects of *xuèqì* 血氣: the circulation of irrigation and warm flow.

---

[302] *Xiāng suí* 相隨 meaning "to accompany each other" *xiāng* 相 – an image of a tree and eye meaning mutual/each other as a concept of interdependence (see discussion in the forward of Afterglow). *Suí* 隨 composed of *chuò* 辵 – to travel and *suí* 隋 - an image of city wall + left hand (helper hand) over moon/flesh meaning to follow, listen to, submit, accompany

[303] *The Song of Form and Function* (*tǐ* 體/体 & *yòng* 用) by Cheng Man-ching, translated by Ed Young

[304] See MindNode in *Appendix II: Blueprints and Charts from Z'ev's Notebook* pg. 291.

In *Nàn Jīng* 30, the difficult question hinges on the phrase *xiāngsuí* 相隨 meaning *"to accompany each other, to go hand in hand."* How do the *wèiqì* and the *yíngqì* follow each other through the body-mind, how do they relate to each other, or better yet, how do they *listen* to each other? There is, I think, love in this question. How are the immune protective aspects of our circulation *devoted to* the nourishing growing aspects? Western medicine would *never* ask such a question in such poetic terms.

From a Western reductionist biomedical perspective, the immune system and the digestive system function as two independent systems. At least that was the way it was taught in medical schools until very recently. It wasn't until 2007 when the National Institutes of Health initiated the Human Microbiome Project (HMP) that Western medicine began to appreciate the intimate relationship between immunity and gut health.[305]

Nàn Jīng 30 begins to answer this question of *yíngwèi* circulation with the line:

經言人受氣於穀

"The scripture (Nèijīng) states: Man receives his qi from the grains."[306]

This line comes from *Língshū* 靈樞 18 and is where the *Nàn Jīng* authors creatively jump off from.

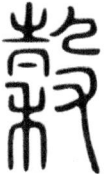

Figure 3.8 - Gǔ 穀

Gǔ 穀 ideogram (*fig. 3.8*) containing the images of a hand holding a sickle that is threshing grain. 穀 represents all foods as a product of the digestive process. 穀 in modern Chinese uses the 谷 ideogram meaning valley, which reminds me of the line from *Lǎozǐ* 老子 6:

---

305 See National Institutes of Health, *"The Healthy Human Microbiome."*
306 Unschuld (2016), *"Nan Jing: The Classic of Difficult Issues,"* pg. 286.

谷神不死

"The Valley Spirit never dies"

Gǔ shén 谷神 was the name of the harvest God in early Shang dynasty, marking its transition from hunter-gatherer society to a new agrarian culture. The fertile valley represents the birth of civilization in all cultures. In China, this "central plain" (*zhōngyuán* 中原)[307] around the middle and lower regions of the Yellow river was associated with the color yellow (*huáng* 黃) of ripening grain, Yellow being associated with the Earth phase related to the spleen/stomach (the organs of the central position).

穀入於胃，乃傳與五藏六府

"The grains enter the stomach from which they are further transmitted to the five zang and six fu."[308]

In the *Nàn Jīng*, the middle warmer has the central role of cooking food and transforming what we eat into *gǔ qì* 谷氣. During the process this *gǔ qì* separates into the clear and the cloudy portions, which serve as the origin (*yuán* 元) of *yíng* 營/*wèi qì* 衛氣.

其清者為榮，濁者為衛

"The clear (qīng 清) [portion] turns into camp [qi]; (yíng qì 營氣), Turbid (zhuó 濁) [portion] turns into guard [qi] (wèi qì 衛氣)"[309]

The *Nàn Jīng* authors present a radical conceptualization of the *sānjiāo* 三焦 as a unified processing system that only recently has Western biomedicine begun to accept as the *Neuro-gastro-immune-hormonal complex*, which flies in the face of the way Western subspecialty medicine is actually practiced today. Typically, the gastroenterologist does not speak to the neurologist much less the psychiatrist. Nor does the immunologist speak with the

---

[307] *Zhōngyuán* 中原 can be literally translated as the "central or middle source" I am reminded of the *yuán* -source points that are considered Earth points on the Yin Channels.

[308] Unschuld (2016), *"Nan Jing: The Classic of Difficult Issues,"* pg. 286

[309] ibid. pg. 286

gastroenterologist. Even more absurdly, the gastroenterologist isn't really trained to speak to patients about *food* even though there is mounting evidence that this multidisciplinary understanding is essential for the treatment of any chronic disorders, particularly those pertaining to conditions of chronic inflammation.[310] And even though research has documented the microbiome is of central importance in proper neuro-gastro--immune function.

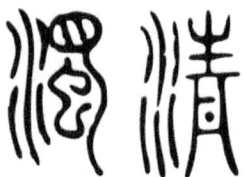

Figure 3.9 - Qīng Zhuó 清濁[311]

It's interesting that the ideogram *zhuó* 濁/turbid (*fig. 3.9*) shows tiny microorganisms in dirty or cloudy water. *Nàn Jīng* implies that the *wèi qì* 衛氣 aspect of circulation functions as immune surveillance, acting to fight off invasion of infectious agents. Perhaps we might extend the analogy to say that one fundamental function of the *sānjiāo*/neuro-gastro-immune complex is to support *wèi qì function by way of supplying* turbid *zhuó* aspect of food containing microorganisms critical for a healthy microbiome.

From the standpoint of the "Hygiene Hypothesis," we know that children exposed to environments that are too clean will have reduced immune resilience and heightened risk for atopic and autoimmune conditions[312] in contrast to children raised in rural areas where they are exposed to dirt, and have lower risks of allergies. Not only is exposure to "dirt" important in developing *wèi qì*, research has shown that in families with a strong history of food allergies, the introduction of high allergen foods early in babies will reduce

---

[310] Hughes, et. al., *"Immune Activation in Irritable Bowel Syndrome: Can Neuroimmune Interactions Explain Symptoms?"*

[311] The Clear ((*qīng* 清) and the Turbid (*zhuó* 濁) ideograms: *Qīng* 清 clear water: shows image of water plus image for green/nature/natural. *Zhuó* 濁 shows image of cloudy or muddy water shows image of water that has organisms in it

[312] The hygiene hypothesis was first proposed in 1989 by D.P Strachan, Examining the higher risk of allergies and eczema based on excessive hygiene. See Strachan*"Hay Fever, Hygiene, and Household Size."*

their risk of food allergies.[313] This gives us a picture of the *yíng-wèi* couple working hand in hand to help us grow and thrive through what we eat. From the standpoint of Han dynasty thinking, it is important to realize that "turbid" does not have the same negative connotations that it has in the modern Western sense of the word colored by Germ theory.

The *Nàn Jīng* presents a radical perspective of the circulation of *yíng/wèi qì* throughout the body/mind. *Nàn Jīng* tells us that the *yíng qì* travel within the blood of the blood-vessels while the *wèi qì* travel *outside* of the vessels. This "outside" again might be considered to be the microbiome which exists in many surfaces of the "outside of the body (gut mucosa, skin, respiratory mucosa) and contains the community of "outsiders," the non-human organisms and are said to be part of *sānjiāo* function, (it is no accident, I think, that following the discussion of *yíng/wèi qì* circulation in *Nàn Jīng* 30, *Nàn Jīng* 31 explores ideas about *sānjiāo* functions.)[314]

To extend this idea of the separation of *qīng* 清 and *zhuó* 濁 (*fig. 3.9*) further, the *Nàn Jīng* authors must have seen how blood clots , separating out into a clear yellow serum part above and the thicker blood part below. While the *Nàn Jīng authors couldn't have known that* serum, which constitutes 55% of total blood volume is composed of 90% water, salts, lipids and hormones and is rich in proteins: albumin, immunoglobulins, clotting factors and fibrinogen, they certainly had an empirical awareness of these two aspects of blood. Today in Western medicine we use a simple test that requires no advanced technology, the Erythrocyte Sedimentation Rate (ESR) as a way of measuring the degree of inflammation. The ESR depends on gravity, placing a blood sample in a capillary tube and waiting for it to settle out into its two layers. Inflammation will cause the heavier turbid immune elements to clump and fall more quickly to the bottom of the tube causing the clear liquid serum portion to rise. If there is no inflammation, the red blood cells will settle more slowly.

Of course, as we have repeatedly stated, there is always a danger when making too direct or literal a translation of these texts into western medical terms. However, we can marvel at how the ancients sensed all this without the use of modern instruments like microscopes and centrifuges. They understood

---

[313] The first study was done on 2015 looking at preventing peanut allergy in children with strong family. Multiple studies have subsequently shown that most high allergy foods when introduced early can lower the risk of food allergy. See Chipps, "*Randomized Trial of Peanut Consumption in Infants at Risk for Peanut Allergy.*"

[314] See MindNode in *Appendix II: Blueprints and Charts from Z'ev's Notebook* pg. 291 & 292.

qīng 清 and *zhuó* 濁 because they followed the principle of *yīn-yáng*. They looked to Nature (heaven-earth) for their model and knew that blood, being the life-giving substance, must contain *both* heaven (air) and earth (food).)

其清者為榮，濁者為衛

"The clear (qīng 清) [portion] turns into camp [qi]; (yíng qì 營氣), Turbid (zhuó 濁)
[portion] turns into guard [qi] (wèi qì 衛氣)"
-Nàn Jīng 30[315]

Herein lies the difficult question asked in *Nàn Jīng* 30. How is it that the lighter clear *qīng* 清 which is considered *yáng* in nature turns into the *yíng qì* which is considered more yin while the turbid *zhuó* 濁 which is considered more *yīn* in nature turns into the *wèi qì* which is considered more *yáng*.

The answer lies in their intimate relationship. Just as we saw in the last chapter, *xuèqì*/ blood and *qì* have a mother-child relationship, here too it is essential to remember the principle described in the *Tàijítú* 太極圖 , the map of *yīnyáng* dynamics (*fig. 3.10*), that the dots represent their mutually generating relationship. *Yīn* is always in the process of turning into *yáng* and *yáng* is always turning into *yīn*.

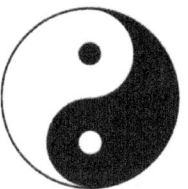

Figure 3.10 - Tàijí 太極 Symbol

The *Tàijítú* tells us that *yīn* cannot exist without *yáng*, so too, the *xuèqì*, and the *yíngwèi* couplets cannot exist apart. As *Nàn Jīng* 30 tells us, they travel hand in hand"!!! This is the key to understanding the dynamic nature of transformation. Thus just as *yīn* gives rise to *yáng*, so too the more *yīn* turbid (*zhuó* 濁) gives rise to the more *yáng* wèi qi. Likewise, the more *yáng* clear (*qīng* 清) gives rise to the more *yīn* yíng qi. *Nàn Jīng* 30 answers this difficult question like this:

---

[315] Unschuld (2016), *"Nan Jing: The Classic of Difficult Issues,"* pg. 286.

陰陽相貫 如環之無端

"The yin and the yang [conduits] are tied to each other like a ring without end."[316]

It is this dynamic relational principle that establishes the idea of a complete and open-ended circulation of *yíngwèi* without beginning or end that is the key to what it means to be alive as opposed to being dead.

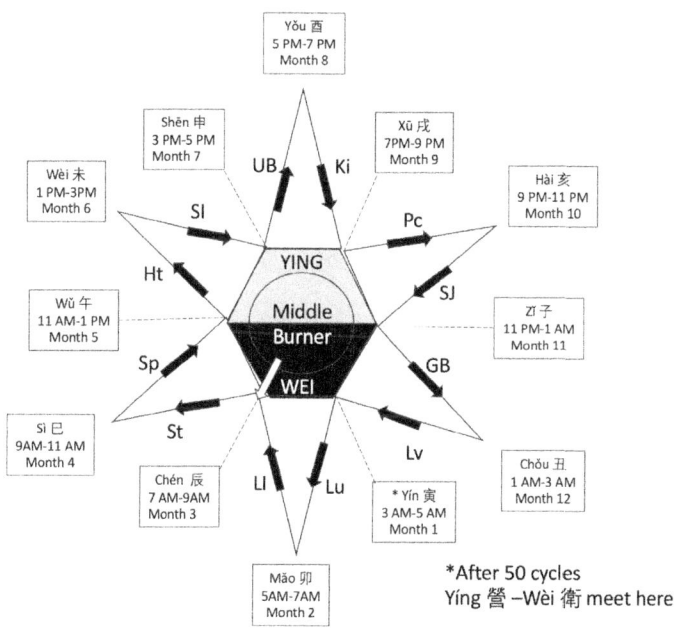

Figure 3.11 - Nàn Jīng 30 Map

Zhàng Shìxián 恨世賢 created a detailed space/time map of *Nàn Jīng* 30 (*fig. 3.11*) to illustrate these profound ideas. He explains how the circulation of *yíngwèi* which has its source (*yuán* 原) in the middle burner is dependent on digestion (diet/microbiome etc.), and travels (hand-in-hand) through all 12 organ-networks in a sequence that resonates with the heaven-earth circadian rhythms of time of day and month of year. This revolutionary understanding of Macro/Microcosmic synchrony then becomes a practical guide for practitioners to orient themselves when called to treat complex illness.

---

[316] Unschuld (2016), *"Nan Jing: The Classic of Difficult Issues,"* pg. 286

Zhàng's circadian map serves as an excellent guide to understanding where interruption in the circulatory flow might be in a patient. For example, an 11 month old girl was brought to see me last winter because, for the past month, she had been waking every night around 4 AM with symptoms of agitation, intense itching, and shortness of breath. When examined by her pediatrician, he said her lungs were clear, there were no rashes and tests for infections were negative. The child's mother was told that there was nothing wrong and to seek out a sleep trainer. Frustrated with this advice, the child's mother, who was quite experienced, having had two other children, trusted her own intuition and was seeking my advice.

The child appeared shy and somewhat listless (she had been up since 4 AM that morning). Her mother said she had become extremely clingy over the last month and cried every time her mother left the room. She had also become an extremely picky eater recently, preferring pasta and bread to anything else and this had been a source of tension between mother and child, her mother trying to provide healthy diet for her children.

Developmentally she had only just begun crawling. There had been no recent history of trauma. On examination, her complexion was somewhat pale as was her tongue with a thin white coat and a bright red tip. Slightly enlarged non-tender cervical lymph nodes were noted bilaterally. Her belly was mildly distended though soft and non-tender. When asked about this, her mother said she had noticed the distention began after a prolonged cold she had had last month. When she mentioned this to her pediatrician, he said it was not related. Careful examination of her skin revealed distinct dry patches on the outer surface of her elbows and knees. Because of her small size, the child's pulse was somewhat difficult to differentiate but appeared to be tight (*jǐn mài* 緊脈) on the left side relative to the empty (*xū mài* 虛脈) pulse on the right hand. The examination confirmed what Zhàng's map had suggested: that there was a relative block in the circulation between Liver and Lung networks (4 AM). A diagnosis of relative liver *qì* stagnation and lung *qì* deficiency was tentatively made.

Treatment was aimed at improving the circulation of *yíngwèi* between the lung and liver by strengthening the lung and reducing the liver *qì* stagnation. Acupuncture points selected were *tài chōng* 太沖 / great rushing (Liv 3), *gān shū* 肝俞/liver shu (Bl 18), *nèi guān* 內關 / inner pass (PC 6), *bǎi huì* 百會 / hundred meeting (Du 20), *hé gǔ* 合谷 / joining valley (LI 4), *liè quē* 列缺 / broken sequence (LU 7), *sān yīn jiāo* 三陰交 / three yin intersection (SP 6) and *zú sān lǐ* 足三里 / leg three mile (ST 36). *Xiǎo chái hú tāng* 小柴胡汤 / Minor Bupleurum Decoction was prescribed twice a day. Diet was discussed in detail, along with a probiotic to improve her digestion and support immune resilience. Her mother was taught to gently massage *nèi guān* 內關 / inner pass (PC 6), *tài chōng* 太沖 / great rushing (Liv 3) and *zú sān lǐ* 足三里 / leg three mile (ST 36).

We had a lengthy discussion about the developmental implications of this pattern. As a child begins to develop greater independence (crawling, walking) there is a natural tension that occurs between safety and exploration, order and change. Depending on the temperament of the child and the context of their life, this can express itself as "separation anxiety" and "stranger danger" that extends all the way to distrust of various foods, many children becoming extremely picky eaters. From a five phase perspective, this tension is a metaphor for the metal-wood *kè* 剋 relationship with the earth caught in the middle.

According to Zhàng map, the middle burner is the central driver of circulation through the organ networks. The time of night is a clue to where (when) the disharmony lies. The examination (looking, listening, asking, palpating) confirms the diagnosis. This child did quite well and within a week was back to sleeping through the night. Had we not treated, she might have gone on to develop eczema, asthma or excessive tantrums later in the spring.

Unlike the western biomedical model that waits for things to break before fixing them with powerful pharmaceuticals, when you treat *relationally* as the *Nàn Jīng* maps tell us, you are able to see subtle patterns of impaired communication within the particular context and treat much earlier by improving the circulation of *yíngwèi* to ensure they are traveling *hand in hand* before things harden into fixed pathologies. To paraphrase Lǎozǐ 老子 64:

為之於未有, 治之於未亂

"Deal with the situation before it becomes obvious , Treat it before it gets out of control."[317]

---

[317] *Lǎozǐ* 老子 64 translation / interpretation S. Cowan.

Part IV:
Ring

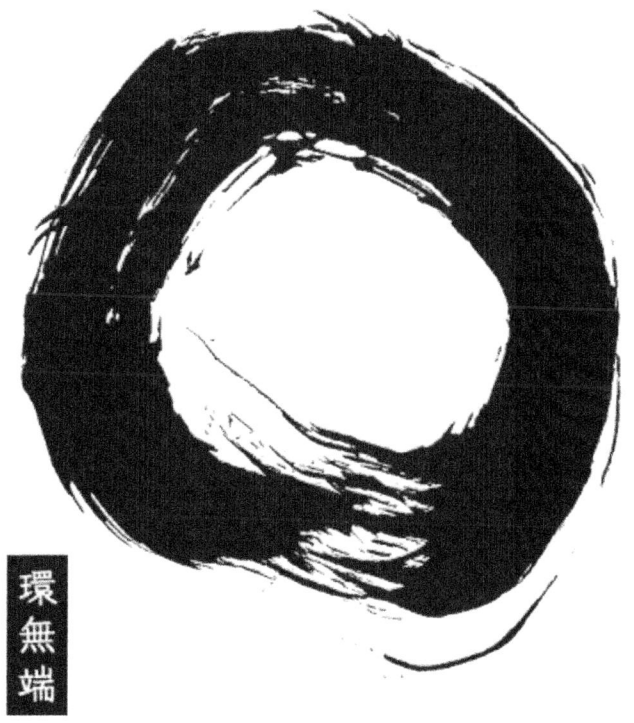

環無端

318

Thoughts on Repairing (Mending) the Broken Vessel (Ring): *Acupuncture Channels as a Communication System*

Z'ev Rosenberg

In *Ripples in the Flow: Reflections on Vessel Dynamics in the Nàn Jīng*, I discussed how chapters 1-23 of the *Nàn Jīng* 難經 systematically developed and taught the *cùn* 寸/*kǒu* 口 vessel diagnostic system, by establishing the mind/body domain and differentiating this by *yīnyáng* 陰陽 and *wǔxíng* 五行 categorization. The deeper vessel diagnoses read the *yīn*/internal realm of the body/mind, the more "superficial" reading the *yáng*/external realm. The *cùn* 寸/inch position read the *yáng* portion and upper body, the *chǐ* 尺/foot position read the yin, lower portion. The *guān* 關/gate position was the separation and interface of *yīn* and *yáng*, above and below. In *Nàn Jīng* 18, the five phase dynamic was applied to *cùn guān chǐ* 寸關尺 positioning, and in doing so unified channel theory with *zàngfǔ* 臟腑 theory, allowing for both physiology and spacial orientation of the body/mind to be addressed. As we have previously discussed, the *Sùwèn* 素問 established the "architectural body," mapping upper middle and lower, front and back inside and outside, and established depth and location of the acupuncture channels based on an informational, blueprint model. This by no means excluded a more physiological, *mài* 脈/vessel based approach to *qìxuè* 氣血, but emphatically expressed that there was more than one way to view the human organism, both the visible and invisible, consciousness/emotionally based aspects.

A Ring Without End, emphasized so much in both the *Nàn Jīng* 難經 and *Língshū* 靈樞, is an "unbroken chain" that maintains the form, health and psyche of a human being, and resonates in an interdependent cosmos with astronomical, heavenly and earthly rhythms. Due to the life/death cycle of created beings, with its eventual decay, inherited *jīng* 精/constitutional issues, and free will-based violation of natural law, the free flowing channel system can easily be disrupted by poor diet, lifestyle, lack of balance in rest/activity, emotional and psychological traumas. Also, our interactions with a world we have systematically poisoned, absorbing noise, toxic chemicals and overwhelming media input has had its effect as well.

Largely as a result of the Covid epidemic, I deepened my studies of classical acupuncture texts and adjusted my practice to restoring the "unbroken chain" of the channel system. What I discovered was a profound shift, both physiologically and psychologically / emotionally in my patients when I focused on repairing communication in the channel system. Using the tools of the *Nàn Jīng*, including five phase acupuncture, extraordinary vessels, *wǔ yùn liù qì* 五運六氣, I crafted treatments to repair the channels, which in turn enhanced native immunity to the pandemic, repaired damage to those who were infected (long COVID).

There are basically two major qualitative analyses that must be done in vessel diagnosis:

1) Reading the interactions of *yīnyáng, yíngwèi* in the vessel flow and dynamic. An example of *yīnyáng, yíngwèi* out of sync is the "shifting rug" pulse image (*mài xiàng* 脈象), which feels like two snakes coiling around each other, unable to merge into a single unified flow.

2) Reading and measuring the interface of *xié qì* 邪氣 / perverse *qì* and *zhèng qì* 正氣 / correct qi. We need to establish what is the correct *qì* of the patient, based on constitution, condition, and the supply of *jīng* 精, *qì* 氣, *xuè* 血 and fluids available, then measure the degree, phase, advancement and tenacity of the *xié qì*.

Then we can develop a treatment strategy that addresses whether we:

a) Drain or expel *xié qì*
b) Strengthen *zhèng qì* to keep *xié qì* in check or
c) *Hé fǎ* 和法 / harmonization to maintain physiological / psychological balance. (to be continued with case histories)

Repairing the Ring: *Strategies & Reflections*

Z'ev Rosenberg

We now move our focus to engaging with the channel system itself with our tools; acupuncture needles, moxa in its various forms, palpation and guiding *qì* flow. We will first tune our bodies and minds, beginning with studying the medical classics, and training ourselves to envision the channel system as a living, breathing entity in resonance with the natural world in which we are swimming, the *dà hǎi* 大海 / great sea. Continuous study of the *Nèijīng* 內經 and *Nàn Jīng* 難經 allows us to access the multiple layers of the channel system, and view the flow of *xuèqì* 血氣. We begin with vessel (pulse) diagnosis, described in great detail in my previous book, *Ripples in the Flow: Reflections on Vessel Dynamic in the Nàn Jīng.* We are tapping the streams, rivers, lakes and underground rivers and feeling them flow under our fingertips. We then feel anomalies in body temperature with our hands, palpate the abdominal cauldron and individual channels, and note the tone of voice, skin colorations, scents, and constitutional signs.[319]

We earlier pointed out Francisco Varela's theory of autoimmunity, and the need to repair what he reframed as "immune networks" rather than targeting specific molecules or substances that circulate within those networks. Stephen and I feel that acupuncture / moxibustion is one of the primary modalities for repairing the channel system. By observing broken links, connections channels, blockages, depletions of *xuèqì* 血氣 or repletions of *xié qì* 邪氣 vacuous, we can restore the flow, restore the continuity of the *"ring without end"* Then the source qi of all healing and equilibrium in the body and mind can restore itself, bringing spontaneous recovery.

Extraordinary Vessel Treatment Strategies:

When I treat the extraordinary vessels, I always visualize them as underground rivers (as described in, and aquifers, and use the master / couples plus points along those vessels to direct these flows deep inside the body. For example, for treating the *dài mài* 帶脈 / belt channel, I will choose *wài guān* 外關 /

---

[319] See *Língshū* 靈樞 47, for correspondences between body imaging and internal viscera, such as the position of the sternum revealing the depth and angle of the physical heart.

outer pass (TB 5) with *zú lín qì* 足臨泣 / foot governor of tears (GB 41), and add points along the *dài mài* trajectory such as *zhāng mén* 章門 / cycle gate (Liv 13), *dài mài* 帶脈 / girdling vessel (GB 26), *wéi dào* 維道 / linking path (GB 28) or *jū liáo* 居髎 / stationary crevice (GB 29). Very effective for a variety of abdominal complaints, stagnation and tightening of the abdominal muscles, diaphragm, gynecological and genitourinary disorders.

Nàn Jīng Five Phase Treatment and Transportation Holes:

In *Nàn Jīng* 10, five evils and ten variations are described . A unique treatment system employs the five transporting points to harmonize the *zàngfǔ* 臟腑. We first determine by the pulse in each position if the *qì* associated with different phases and viscera / bowels (wiry for liver / gall bladder, hairlike for lung / large intestine, etc.) appears in a different position. For example, if a wiry pulse is felt in the left *cùn* 寸 position, the child phase (wood) has "invaded" the mother, and we should choose the wood point on the heart channel *shén mén* 神門 / spirit gate (HT 7), or the fire point on the liver channel *xíng jiān* 行間 / moving between (Liv 2) to harmonize and or drain the repletion. One's pulse taking skills must be very refined in order to practice this method, as it is based on an internal cycle of evil *qì*, here defined as the correct space and position of each phase and associated viscera / bowel being violated by five types of internal evils.

Branching Vessel Treatment Strategies:

Língshū, 11 gives the pathways of the *bié mài* 別脈, but not any in depth treatment descriptions. Later scholar physicians attempted to fill in these gaps. I use treatment strategies developed by Dr.'s Miki Shima and Chip Chace in their book *The Channel Divergences.*[320] My treatment goal is to utilize the channel system to direct *qì* to the internal viscera and bowels. For example, when wanting to access the kidneys, I will choose *yīn gǔ* 阴谷 / yin valley (Ki 10) and / or *tài xī* 太溪 / supreme stream (Ki 3), *shèn shū* 腎俞 / kidney shu (Bl 23), and *dà zhù* 大杼 / great shuttle (BL 11) (the he point of the bones). When treating the gall bladder, I will choose *tóng zǐ liáo* 瞳子髎 / pupil crevice (GB1), *yáng líng quán* 陽陵泉 / yang mound spring (GB 34), and *qiū xū* 丘墟 / mound of ruins (GB 40). When treating the liver I'll choose *tai chōng* 太沖 / great rushing (Liv 3), *qū quán* 曲泉 / spring at the crook (Liv 8), usually either with either the gall bladder or kidney divergences. I find this produces a very powerful and strengthening treatment for patients with depletions of the internal viscera.

---

[320] Shima, and Charles, *"The Channel Divergences: Deeper Pathways of the Web,"* pg. 35.

Regular Channel Treatment Strategies Applying Japanese 'Master/Couple' Points, Abdominal and Mu points, Back Shu points (*Sùwèn* 素問 63):

A method I learned from Japanese schools of acupuncture that I use widely in practice, is to use distal points unilaterally on opposite sides on the limbs as a form of "master/couple" treatment similar to the extraordinary vessel treatment strategies. And sometimes the chosen points overlap. For example, to treat the *yángmíng* 陽明 channel in a broad fashion, I will combine *yáng xī* 陽谿/ yang stream (LI 5) with *jiě xī* 解谿/stream divide (ST 41). If I want a more draining treatment, I will combine *sān jiān* 三間/third space (LI 3) with *xiàn gǔ* 陷谷/sunken valley (ST 43). Sometimes I will choose the *yuán* 原 points on a channel at hands and feet, such as combining *yáng chí* 陽池/yang pool (TB 4) with *qiū xū* 丘墟/mound of ruins (GB 40). Other times, I will harmonize the channel by utilizing five phase dynamics, for example to harmonize the *shàoyīn* 少陰, heart and kidney, I will choose *rán gǔ* 然谷/blazing valley (Ki 2) (the fire point on the water channel) with *shào hǎi* 少海/lesser sea (HT 3) (water point on the fire channel).

Length of Treatment, Circadian Rhythms and Timing:

The *Nàn Jīng* and *Língshū* 靈樞 both discuss the concepts which one needle retention. *Nàn Jīng 23* discusses the measurement of the channels with the number of breaths. *Qì* and blood move through the vessels at the rate of 6 *cùn* 寸/ for each complete inhalation and exhalation. The total length of the channels and collaterals equals 1620 *cùn*. 1620 divided by 6 equals 270. Thus 270 breaths are required for *qì* to make one complete cycle through the body. The exact retention time could then vary based on the individual's breath rate, though Lǐ Jiōng 李駉 in his commentary gives us an idea of how many breaths one take within the 24 hour period.

> *"The circulation of the camp and guard [qi] through the entire body has its meeting point at the [qi opening of the] hand major yin [conduit]; it follows the passage of heaven and amounts to 13,500 breathing periods [each twenty-four hours]."*[321]

Based on this calculation of 13,500 breath per 24 hour period, one would have approximately 9.375 breaths per minute. Taking what is in the outlined in the *Nàn Jīng* of 270 breaths required for a complete circulation by 9.375 we have 28.8 minutes for retention time.

Língshū 12 Qíbó 岐伯 explain how long to retain needles by the number of breaths.

---

[321] Unschuld (2016), *"Nan Jing: The Classic of Difficult Issues,"* pg. 249.

足陽明刺深六分，留十呼。 足太陽深五分，留七呼。 足少陽深四分、留五呼。 足太陰深三分，留四呼。 足少陰深二分，留三呼。 足厥陰深一分，留二呼。

"The foot yang brilliance [conduit] is to be pierced 6 fen deep. [The needle] is to remain inserted for ten exhalations.
The foot major yang [conduit] is to be pierced 5 fen deep. [The needle] is to remain inserted for seven exhalations.

The foot minor yang [conduit] is to be pierced 4 fen deep. [The needle] is to remain inserted for five exhalations.
The foot major yin [conduit] is to be pierced 3 fen deep. [The needle] is to remain inserted for four exhalations.
The foot minor yin [conduit] is to be pierced 2 fen deep. [The needle] is to remain inserted for three exhalations.
The foot ceasing yin [qi conduits] is to be pierced 1 fen deep. [The needle] is to remain inserted for two exhalations."[322]

In *Língshū* 15 & 18 we see the discussion of the complete circulation of *qì* through the channel system.

五十營備，得盡天地之壽矣
When 50 circulations are completed, the longevity of heaven and earth can be taken full advantage of.
-Língshū 15[323]

營在脈中，衛在脈外，
營週不休，五十而復大會，
陰陽相貫，如環無端．

"The camp [qi] are in the vessels. The guard [qi] are outside the vessels. They circulate without a stop. After 50 [circulations] a grand meeting happens. Yin and yang [qi] penetrate each other's realm. This is like a ring without end."
-Língshū 18[324]

Since 24 hours equals 1440 minutes, one can divide 1440 by 50 to get the calculation of 28 minutes and 48 seconds. This is where we get the guideline for approximately 30 minutes of needle retention for treatment.I try to leave the needles in for at least this length of time. I always consider time of day in choosing points and channels (*tàiyáng* 太陽 in the morning perhaps, *shàoyáng* 少

---

[322] Unschuld, *"Huang Di Nei Jing Ling Shu: The Ancient Classic on Needle Therapy,"* pg. 221.

[323] ibid., pg. 247.

[324] ibid., pg. 260.

陽 in the afternoon, *shàoyīn* in the evening), lunar cycles, and seasonal *qì* as well. This is a more complex discussion, and will be addressed in a later text.

Wáng Lètíng 王樂亭 (1894-1984) Acupuncture for Qì Transformation:

Wáng Lètíng was a mid-twentieth century acupuncturist who was famous for using gold needles. He based his treatments on Lǐ Dōngyuán 李東垣's spleen stomach theories, translating formulas such as *bǔ zhōng yì qì tāng* 補中益氣湯 / tonify the middle to augment the qi decoction, *shí quán dà bǔ tāng* 十全大補湯 / all inclusive great tonifying decoction, and *tiáo zhōng yì qì tāng* 調中益氣湯 / regulate the middle and augment the qi decoction into acupuncture point formulas, assigning herbal qualities to specific acupuncture points. For example, he'd choose..

Acupuncture Point	Chinese Herb
Nèi Guān 內關 / Inner Pass (PC 6)	*Fú Líng* 茯苓 / Poria
Zhōng Wǎn 中脘 / Middle Cavity (Ren 12)	*Rén Shēn* 人參 / Ginseng Radix
Hé Gǔ 合谷 / Joining Valley (LI 4)	*Huáng Qí* 黃芪 / Astragali radix
Zú Sān Lǐ 足三里 / Leg Three Mile (ST 36)	*Bái Zhú* 白朮 / Atractylodis Macrocephalae Rhizoma
Sān Yīn Jiāo 三陰交 / Three Yin Intersection (SP 6)	*Bái Sháo* 白芍 / Paeoniae Radix alba
Yáng Líng Quán 陽陵泉 / Yang Mound Spring (GB 34)	*Ròu Guì* 肉桂 / Cinnamomi Cortex
Qū Chí 曲池 / Pool at the Crook (LI 11)	*Chuān Xiōng* 川芎 / Chuanxiong Rhizoma
Zhāng Mén 章門 / Cycle Gate (Liv 13)	*Rén Shēn* 人參 / Ginseng Radix
Zhōng Wǎn 中脘 / Middle Cavity (Ren 12)	*Gān Cǎo* 甘草 / Glycyrrhizae Radix
Taì Chōng 太沖 / Great Rushing (Liv 3)	*Bái sháo* 白芍 / Paeoniae Radix alba

He'd then choose ingredients from Lǐ's main formulas listed above and combine points as in an herbal prescription. When I am working with metabolic disorders focused on spleen/stomach issues, *tàiyīn* 太陰 and *yángmíng* 陽明, I will combine some of these points with distal points on the *tàiyīn* and *yángmíng* channels. combining with abdominal points after palpation. These combinations can treat constipation or diarrhea, issues with appetite, obesity or weight loss, and bloating. An example treatment I would use is the following:

I wold treat the *yángmíng* and *tàiyīn* 太陰 channel distal points opposite limbs unilaterally: Drain *sān jiān* 三間/third space (LI 3) and *xiàn gǔ* 陷谷/sunken valley (ST 43), then palpate to choose either *shǒu sān lǐ* 手三里/arm three mile (LI 10) or *qū chí* 曲池/pool at the crook (LI 11). Then regulate or supplement: *yáng xī* 陽谿/yang stream (LI 5) and *shǒu sān lǐ* 手三里/arm three miles (LI 10) and *jiě xī* 解谿/stream divide (ST 41) (opposite side). Followed by supplementing spleen (*tàiyīn* 太陰) with *jiān shǐ* 間使/intermediate messenger (PC 5) and *zhōng fēng* 中封/middle seal (Liv 4) or *shāng qiū* 商丘/shang mound (SP 5). Or combine *chǐ zé* 尺澤/cubit marsh (Lu 5), *yīn líng quán* 陰陵泉/yin mound spring (SP 9) and *fù liū* 復溜/returning current (Ki 7). Which is a great combination I learned from reading Wáng Jūyì 王居易's (1937-2017) treatment strategies.

Then I'd palpate and needle abdominal mu points such as *zhāng mén* 章門/cycle gate (Liv 13), *zhōng wǎn* 中脘/middle cavity (Ren 12), *shàng wǎn* 上脘/upper cavity (Ren 13), *shí mén* 石門/stone gate (Ren 5), *qì hǎi* 氣海/sea of qi (Ren 6), *tiān shū* 天樞/heaven's pivot (ST 25) or *dà héng* 大橫/great horizontal (SP 15), some of these with moxa on the needles.

In some cases, I might consider utilizing back shu points, such as *dà zhuī* 大椎/great vertebra (Du 14), *gāo huāng shū* 膏肓俞/vital region shu (Bl 43), *gé shū* 膈俞/diaphragm shu (Bl 17), *sānjiāo shū* 三焦俞/sānjiāo shu (Bl 22), *dà cháng shū* 大腸俞/large intestine shu (Bl 25). If the bowel is sluggish, I'd add *shàng jù xū* 上巨虛/upper great shuttle (ST 37). If spleen is damp, *yīn líng quán* 陰陵泉/yin mound spring (SP 9). If kidney are vacuous, *yīn gǔ* 阴谷/yin valley (Ki 10) or *fù liū* 復溜/returning current (Ki 7).

Regulating the *Yuán Qì* 元氣 and Ministerial Fire:

As discussed in *Afterglow: Ministerial Fire and Chinese Ecological Medicine*, the goal of Chinese medical treatment is to restore the normal function of source *qì*, which is the true, spontaneous healing power of the body/mind. In turn, the connection of ministerial fire with source *qì* is significant in acupuncture and moxa treatment, as the warmth of ministerial fire *qì* circulates throughout the body, via the *shàoyáng* 少陽 channels (gall bladder/triple burner), to enable all metabolisms of the body (water, food, transformation of blood). The ministerial fire also enters *juéyīn* 厥陰 to warm the blood, which also must circulate freely to warm, nourish and maintain normal visceral function. In turn, the defense *qì* is an expression of the warmth of ministerial fire. Without the free flow of ministerial fire, *qì* transformation is impossible. Specifically, the gall bladder governs the movement of ministerial fire throughout the body, so needling and warming the *shàoyáng* 少陽 channels is of extreme importance. To do so, we can choose channels and points that are blocked to restore the flow of not only the *xuèqì* 血氣, but the ministerial fire as well. I will often combine (unilaterally on opposite limbs) *jiān shǐ* 間使 / intermediate messenger (PC 5) with *zhōng fēng* 中封 / middle seal (Liv 4), along with *qiū xū* 丘墟 / mound of ruins (GB 40) with *yáng chí* 陽池 / yang pool (TB 4) as distal points, then choose points along these channels where palpation indicates blockages. I will then combine with abdominal points such as *dài mài* 帶脈 / girdling vessel (GB 26) (which also opens the *dài mài* 帶 脈 / belt channel), *zhāng mén* 章門 / cycle gate (Liv 13), or *qì chōng* 氣沖 / rushing chong (ST 30). *Nàn Jīng* 難經 66 is devoted to the source points on the channels, which are needled to access the source qi of the five yin viscera and six bowels. The text describes the triple burner is the special envoy that transmits the original *qì*. In the commentary by Lǐ Jiōng 李駉 he states "*The Triple Burner sends its qi from this rapids [hole] to penetrate [the entire organism]; also, this rapids [hole] is the place where [the qi of the Triple Burner] stop and rest*"[325] I will often use these points in a treatment, as I mainly practice internal medicine, and wish to apply deep treatment and adjustment to the internal viscera.

Sānjiāo 三焦 Resonant Holes and Treating Three *Jiāo* with Distal Points:

In *Nàn Jīng* 難經 62, the resonant holes of the upper, middle and lower burner are discussed: *shān zhōng* 膻中 / chest center (Ren 17) for the upper burner, *zhōng wǎn* 中脘 / middle cavity (Ren 12) for the middle burner, and *guān yuán* 關元 / gate of origin (Ren 4), *shí mén* 石門 / stone gate (Ren 5), *qì hǎi* 氣海 / sea of qi (Ren 6) for the lower burner. These are the 'dividing lines' that separate the upper body from the middle burner, and in turn the lower burner. In addition, the *yáng* channels have source points that access the *sānjiāo*, and on the *yīn* channels the wood points, and here we can influence the *sānjiāo* directly, which means we are able to regulate the ministerial fire. An example of how I would apply this to treatment is by needling front mu points corresponding to the upper middle or lower burners (see above), and accessing yuan points on the *yīn* and *yáng* channels. I also will sometimes choose points directly on the hand *shàoyáng* 少陽 channel as well.

Modern patients have sometimes a deep lying complexity of stasis of cold blood phlegm and / or dampness influenced by long-term pharmaceutical treatments (such as baby aspirin which erodes the stomach lining when taken long term), procedures (such as inserting IUD's), hormone replacement therapy or birth control pills, toxic drugs used for autoimmune disorders, chemotherapy

---

[325] Unschuld (2016), "*Nan Jing: The Classic of Difficult Issues,*" pg. 479.

and/or radiation. This must always be considered when diagnosing via tongue, vessel/pulse or palpation, and in one's treatment strategies.

The Secret Circulation

Stephen Cowan & Z'ev Rosenberg

"While living, people are supple and sift,
but once dead, they become hard and rigid cadavers.
While living, the things of this world and its grasses and trees are pliant and fragile,
but once dead, they become withered and dry."
-Lǎozǐ 老子 76[326]

Stephen: The "difficulties" that *Nàn Jīng* 難經 writers tackle in their attempt to correlate their empirical observations and measurements with the principles laid out in the *Nèijīng* 內經 canon, enabled them to map out a complete circulatory system that reflects the geographical landscape of hills, valleys, rivers and streams found in nature. This correlative thinking is perhaps one of the most important principles that distinguishes Chinese medicine from Western reductionist medical philosophy.

Z'ev: "The body as landscape" is a central metaphor of Chinese medicine and philosophy.

Stephen: Several *Nàn Jīng* chapters (25, 31, 38, 39, 66) are dedicated to what commentator Huá Shòu 滑寿 (1361 CE) calls the "secret circulation" of the *sānjiāo* 三焦 / Triple Warmer in the body.[327] In their process of mapping human physiology, the *Nàn Jīng* authors were aware of a hidden physiological movement of warmth circulating throughout the body-mind. As with many chapters in the *Nàn Jīng*, the "difficulty" they were trying to sort out comes from the *Língshū* 靈樞 statement that the *sānjiāo* *"emits qi in order to warm the muscles and flesh and fill the skin."*[328]

---

[326] Ames, and Hall,"*Dao De Jing: Making This Life Significant: A Philosophical Translation*" pg. 195.

[327] See MindNode in *Appendix II: Blueprints and Charts from Z'ev's Notebook* pg. 292 & 293.

[328] Unschuld, "*Huang Di Nei Jing Ling Shu: The Ancient Classic on Needle Therapy*," pg. 384.

From one perspective, the whole of the *Nàn Jīng* can be thought of as an in-depth discourse on the dynamic movement of life that enables the practitioner to determine the state of health and disease within a person. Thus one of the important difficult questions that is brought up by the *Nàn Jīng* authors in their endeavor to create a complete map of the functions of the human being is why the *Nèijīng* says there are five *zàng* 臟 organs and six *fǔ* 腑? This first appears in *Nàn Jīng* 25 and then again in *Nàn Jīng* 38. In their analogic correlative thinking, there must be a sixth *zàng*, that is the complement to the *sānjiāo* and they designated the *xīn zhǔ* 心主/ *the Heart/Mind Master* partner to the *sānjiāo*. But anatomically speaking, they ask, *where* is this *sānjiāo/xīn zhǔ* couple?

The problem that the *Nàn Jīng* is trying to work out is how the body maintains its thermodynamic regulation of warmth. This is hundreds of years before Western medicine was able to conceptualize thermoregulation. It really wasn't until the experiments with thermoelectricity by Becquerel and Breschet in 1835 that Lefevre was able to measure the "thermal topography" of the body.

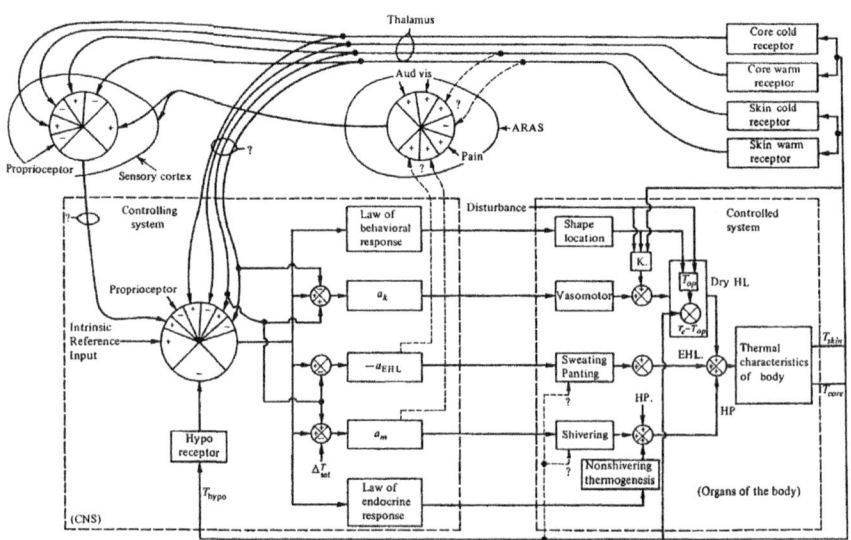

Figure 4.1 - Western Mechanistic View of the Regulation of Internal Body Temperature[329]

Nàn Jīng 23 revisits *Língshū* 靈樞 15, mapping out the structural measurements of the 12 vessels, carefully defining anatomic calculations of length and correlating these empirical findings with the *Yìjīng* 易經 movement of the sun through the day, season and years. To get a better understanding of

---

[329] Cooper, "*Some Historical Perspectives on Thermoregulation*," pg. 1720.

the contrast between the Western mechanistic view (*fig. 4.1*) and the Chinese mandalic map of how body temperature is regulated to provide thermodynamic stability, take a look at how the movement of *yáng* lines in the twelve tidal hexagrams progress through the seasons. (*fig. 4.2*).

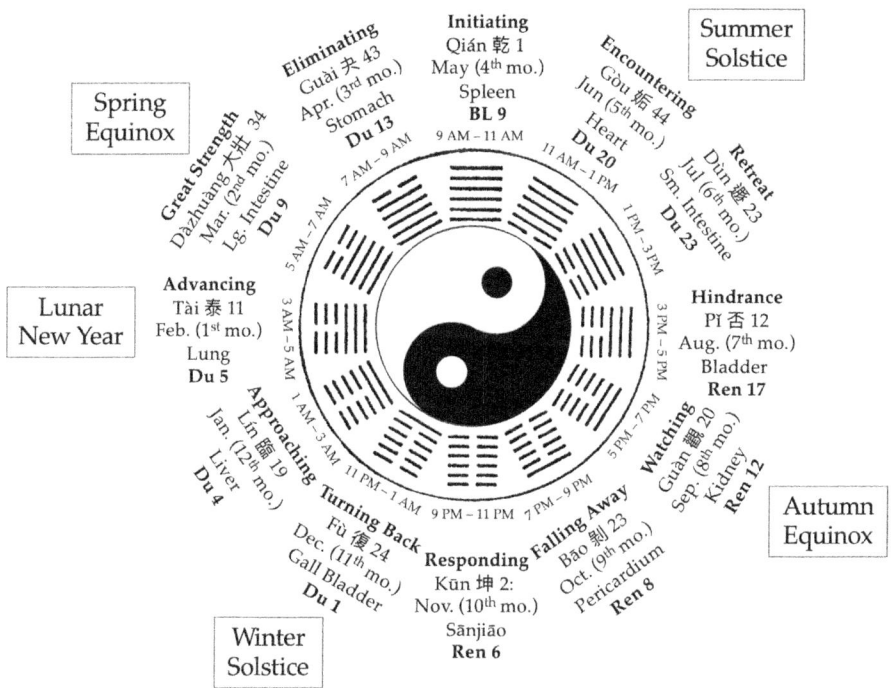

Figure 4.2 - Circulation of Yuan Qì Through the 12 Tidal Hexagrams[330]

The modern western map resembles the electrical wiring circuitry in your house, reflecting Western culture's mechanistic logic of how things work whereas an understanding of the Chinese biological maps reflect the non-linear eco-logical reality that our nature is fundamentally a microcosm of circadian cycles in Nature, that is, that we are warmed the way the Earth is warmed by the movement and cycling of the sun.

Z'ev: The Western chart reads like a "flatlands" two dimensional view of the body / mind; sophisticated engineering, with tremendous detail in mapping mechanisms, molecules, structures and substances (hormones,

---

[330] S. Cowan distillation of material discussed in Liu, "*Classical Chinese Medicine,*" pg. 330.

neurotransmitters, but without a conclusive gestalt to tie all of this information together into a useful diagnostic or clinical strategies. It is as if biomedicine, for all of its sophisticated technology within these limits, is yet to discover quantum mechanics, complexity theory, or other dimensional approaches. I discuss thermoregulation in *Returning to the Source: Han Dynasty Medical Classics in Modern Clinical Practice* and *Afterglow: Ministerial Fire and Chinese Ecological Medicine*. The "Picasso Principle" discussed in chapter 4 of *Returning to the Source*[331] like the Zen monk/judge that listens to the multiple perspectives of the defendants and witnesses that observed a feudal lord being murdered in the forest, the physician must engage multiple perspectives in order to arrive at a comprehensive diagnosis. To this end, he does a complete history, skillful questioning, vessel diagnosis, abdominal palpation and other tools. This is the *yuán wù bǐlèi* 援物比類/grasping the cause, making an analogy principle discussed in *Sùwèn 76*.

Stephen: We can visualize living organisms as thoroughly integrated beings within the thermodynamic cycling of the planet itself in this illustration that I have adapted from Kleidon's recent map (*fig. 4.3*) predicting climate based on nonlinearity and so-called randomness below. As stated in Kleidon's schematic, we can see:

"the planetary hierarchy of free energy generation, transfer and dissipation (solid lines), and associated effects (dotted lines), and the different layers are associated with different forms of free energy and gradients associated with disequilibrium. For instance, motion is associated with gradients in momentum and represents kinetic energy. Hydrological cycling is associated with gradients in chemical potential, and geo-potential is associated with potential and chemical free energy."[332]

---

[331] See *The Picasso Principle* in Rosenberg, *"Returning to the Source: Han Dynasty Medical Classics in Modern Clinical Practice,"* pg. 57-64.

[332] ibid., pg. 1022.

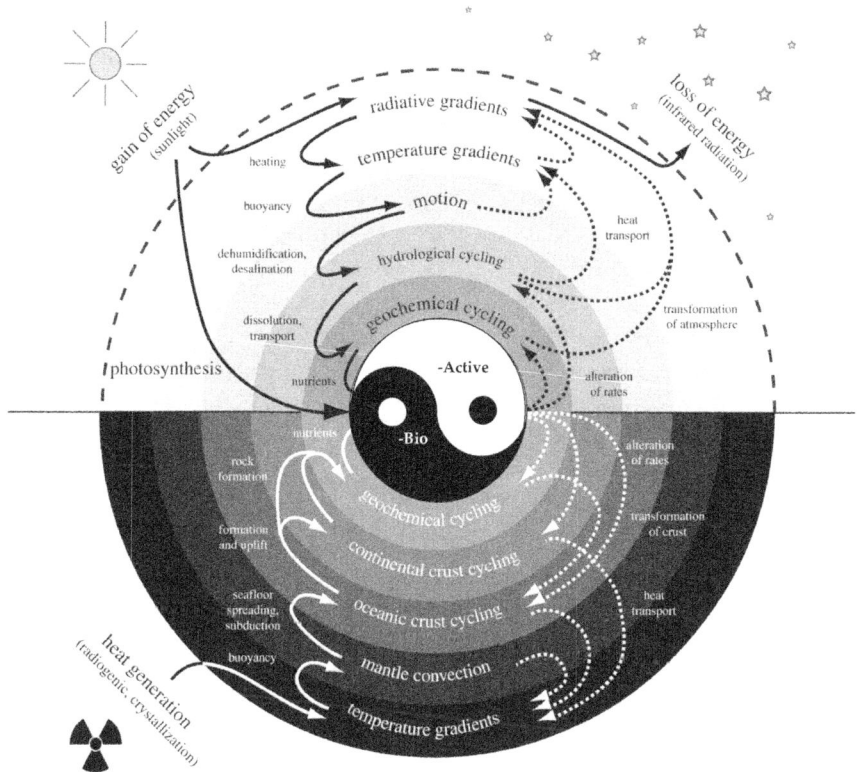

Figure 4.3 - Schematic of the Planetary Hierarchy of Free Energy Generation[333]

I have, superimposed the *tàijí* 太極 map in the center that, for the sake of this context, I've labelled as "bio-active" to denote one aspect of the intimate inter-dependent *yīnyáng* relationship. This enables us to look back at the sequence of hexagrams in the above map *(fig 4.2)* and notice that, as we saw in Zhāng Shìxián's map of *Nàn Jīng* 23 *(fig. 2.19)* and *Nàn Jīng* 30 *(fig. 1.3)*, our physiologic thermodynamics mirror the seasonal cycles and revolves around the spleen (soil) and triple warmer (*sānjiāo*). It is noteworthy, I think, that, as with Zhàng's maps, the Spleen is positioned in association with the first hexagram *Qián* 乾 (double heaven trigram ☰ "Initiating") and the sixth *fǔ* 腑, *sānjiāo* corresponds to the second hexagram *Kūn* 坤 (double earth trigram ☷ "responding"). All prenatal (*yuán* 原) and postnatal *qì* begins with digestion.

---

[333] Image adapted from Kleidon, *"How Does the Earth System Generate and Maintain Thermodynamic Disequilibrium and What Does It Imply for the Future of the Planet?"* pg. 1022

The *Nàn Jīng* authors were aware of the fact that there are physiologic functions beyond the bounds of anatomical structure. The *sānjiāo*, as a hidden sixth *fǔ* 腑, often described as a "cauldron," is a remarkable clinical observation. It is the repository of warming *qì* even though it is said to have no form (in both *Nàn Jīng* 25 and 38)[334]. In commentaries on *Nàn Jīng* 31, we can see the *Nàn Jīng* empiricists debating whether the *sānjiāo* is a function or a structure, as they try to work out the relative domains of the three warmers in order to understand their functions and disorders.

I am struck by this idea of a cauldron. In early Chinese history, Roger Ames notes, *"the Chinese "stew pot" has a possible etymological source of the character, hé* 和 *'harmony'. According to archeological data, the proto-Chinese staple was kang, a millet broth or stew similar to the popular chou (Cantonese joke.)"*[335]

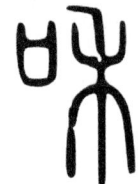

Figure 4.4 - Hé 和

The ideogram (*fig. 4.4*) depicts grain being placed in the mouth. Ames goes on to state *"the Lǚ Shì Chūnqiū Yìndé* 呂氏春秋引得 *(ca. 250 B.C.) describes the culinary art of the stewing pot:

"In the business of proper flavoring and seasoning, there must be sweet, sour, bitter, acrid and salty, and there must be an order in the mixing and proper proportion. Blending these together is extremely subtle and they must be self-expressive. The variations within the cooking pot are so delicate and subtle that they defy words and conceptualization."[336]

This cooking metaphor seems to me to be a perfect depiction of the *sānjiāo* function as a "cooking pot." To "defy words and conceptualization" seems to be the difficulty the *Nàn Jīng* authors are grappling with as they map the human body.

---

[334] See MindNode in *Appendix II: Blueprints and Charts from Z'ev's Notebook* pg. 289.

[335] Ames, *"Putting the Te Back into Taoism,"* pg. 118.

[336] ibid., pg. 118 referencing *Lu-shih ch'un-ch'iu pen-wei-pien* (*Lǚ shì chūnqiū* 呂氏春秋/ *Master Lü's Spring and Autumn Annals*).

The hidden "metabolic" functions that circulate in the body are further defined in *Nàn Jīng* 66 where the *sānjiāo* is given the unique role of "special envoy" to the *mìng mén* 命門 which transmits original/source *qì* (*yuán qì* 原氣) throughout the body. *Nàn Jīng* 66 states that "origin" is an honorable designation" for the *sānjiāo*.[337] As practitioners we have access to this "secret metabolic circulation" at the *yuán xué* 原穴 source points along all the channels. Given the important position associated with *Kūn* 坤 (double earth trigram ☷ "responding" (or receiving), the *sānjiāo* functions in maintaining thermodynamic health, providing all parts of the body access to *yíng/wèi* nourishment and protection. The *sānjiāo* is furthermore in charge of the movement of fluids throughout the interstitial spaces along the fascia and membranes of the body. The *sānjiāo* is invisible for the very reason that, for the living being, it's always working in the background to harmonize the relationships of the various organ networks to ensure that there is smooth flowing communication between them. It's no accident then that the *sānjiāo* is paired with the "sixth *zàng* 臟/" that goes by two names: *xīn zhǔ* 心主 (heart/mind master) and *xīn bāo lùo* 心包络 (heart/mind envelope-net). The triple warmer/pericardium couple functions as the membranous tissue/function that maintains healthy warm relations within the living body-mind by way of the thermodynamic functions of digestion and water metabolism. Noting that the *Kūn* 坤 hexagram lies at the very deepest yin position, during the month just before Winter solstice, in this regard, the *sānjiāo* is responsible for keeping the ministerial fire (*xiāng huǒ* 相火) on a low simmer even when the sun is nowhere in sight. As Z'ev has noted in *Afterglow: Ministerial Fire and Chinese Ecological Medicine*[338] this "cooking pot" metaphor is of primary importance in understanding the role of ministerial fire (*xiāng huǒ* 相火) in maintaining health and managing chronic illness, particularly at a time in our history where there seems to be a breakdown in healthy relationships and an abundance of "cold" influences related to Western diet.

Z'ev: In the writings of Zhèng Qīnān 鄭欽安, he discusses how each of the six conformations/stages of *shānghán* 傷寒/cold damage are describing the strength or weakness of ministerial fire. At the *tàiyáng* 太陽 stage, the main issue is to harmonize *yíng qì* 營氣 and *wèi qì* 衛氣. At *yángmíng* 陽明 stage, the ministerial fire is flaring strong, trying to eliminate cold by 'burning out' the pathogen. In the *shàoyáng* 少陽 stage, there is an oscillation of heat effusion and

---

[337] See MindNode in *Appendix II: Blueprints and Charts from Z'ev's Notebook* pg. 293

[338] Rosenberg, "*Afterglow: Ministerial Fire and Chinese Ecological Medicine*," pg. 71-74.

chill, the "flickering" of ministerial fire as it periodically rises and falls in the *sānjiāo* 三焦 and gallbladder channels. In the yin stages, the ministerial fire is weak, and cold evils can penetrate the yin viscera causing internal damage.

Stephen: For the practitioner, this mandalic map can be extremely helpful whenever there are pathological conditions that involve temperature instability, immune dysfunction, or fluid imbalances. By incorporating *yuán xué* 原穴 / source points as part of the treatment whenever there is a breakdown in communication between the organs, between ourselves and others, between ourselves and Nature, seek the *sānjiāo* for healing relationships and ensuring healthy circulation. If we, as earthlings, are a reflection of, and resonate with, the dynamic flow of our planet, it should come as no surprise then that as the planet heats up, causing floods and fires, we are witnessing political turmoil, epidemics, autoimmune disease, and surges in neuropsychiatric disorders. All these are disturbances in the original *qì* of our planet and an uprising in ministerial fire that stems from a failure to care for the "secret circulation."

Z'ev: Confucian scholars always recognized the interplay and relationship between order and chaos, to "go with the flow," and *nì* 逆 / counterflow. Steering counterflow, separations of *yīn* and *yáng*, restoring ministerial fire to its proper position in the lower burner are all essential strategies in the practice of medicine, but also in healing our home planet ecologically. In our reading of Chinese medical philosophy, as an ecological medical system. Stephen and I see restoring the position of humanity as conduits and expressions of heaven and earth *qì* are essential in restoring both the health of humanity and the planet.

Mapping the Unnamable

Stephen Cowan & Z'ev Rosenberg

無名人曰：汝遊心於淡，合氣於漠，順物自然，而無容私焉，而天下治矣

"Let your mind wander in simplicity, said No Name, "blend your qi into the boundless, follow occurrence appearing of itself in things, and don't let selfhood get in the way. Then all beneath heaven will be governed well."[339]
-Zhuāngzǐ 莊子

Stephen: The "secret circulation" of the *sānjiāo* discussed in the previous chapter reveals that there is something missing from anatomical maps (East and West) that I think is important to consider here though it is difficult to put into words. It is a deep self-cultivation that dates back at least to *Lǎozǐ* 老子 and *Zhuāngzǐ* 莊子 and probably before that, which I sense has implications for how the Eastern sage-physicians of the late Han dynasty perceived the human body in contrast to our modern Western perspective.

The radical perspectives in the *Nàn Jīng* 難經, as Unschuld states, "mark the end of the formative epoch (of the *Huáng Dì Nèijīng* 黃帝內經), because it discarded all the irrelevant ballast of the past and concentrated - in a most coherent manner - on nothing but the most advanced concepts of systematic correspondence."[340] My personal sense is that the *Nàn Jīng's* emphasis on unifying coherent holistic systems-thinking reflects deep self-cultivation practices (*xiū shēn* 修身) that were certainly a part of contemporary culture. The contemplative practices found in the *Huáinánzi* 淮南子 texts of the early Han dynasty highlighted "mirror-like knowing," that defines a quality of health of the body-mind as a reflection of relationships found in Nature.

---

[339] Hinton, and Zhuangzi. *Chuang Tzu. The Inner Chapters,"* pg. 107.

[340] Unschuld (2016), *"Nan Jing: The Classic of Difficult Issues,"* pg. 8.

Z'ev: Chip Chase in his "Extraordinary Vessels" text called this the "Inner Gaze."[341] Being able to see one's internal channels and viscera by looking inward. A fully conscious human being feels one's body as mindful awareness. When I was at school, one of my teachers, Daniel Santos, in our first acupuncture class, had us visualize the channels internally before teaching us their "official" locations in textbooks. Amazingly, nearly all the students were able to visualize the channels correctly.

Stephen: Such deep ecological perspectives would later emerge as the "Dark Mystery School" (*xuán xué* 玄學)[342] that followed the fall of the Han dynasty during the Six Kingdoms period (220-589 CE) and had a major influence in cultural circles of the time. A few of the noteworthy scholars of that school were Wáng Bì 王弼 (226-249 CE) and Guō Xiàng 郭象 (252-312 CE) who's commentaries on the *Yìjīng* 易經 and *Lǎozǐ* 老子 were part of the so-called Neo-Daoist movement that unified ideas and practices of Daoism with the ethical/educational doctrines of Confucius.[343] This meditation on *xuán* 玄 (dark mystery) refers back to several passages in *Lǎozǐ* 老子. For example, chapter 56 which describes a sequence of cultivation (the order varies depending on the source) as follows:

> "*Stop the banter, Shut the gates, Turn down the lights, Blur the sharp edges, Dissolve the parts, Unite the dust. This is called xuán tóng,* 玄同"[344]

This *xuán tóng* 玄同, I interpret here as "dark reunion" though there are certainly many other translations of this interesting pair of characters. *Dark Reunion* implies a deep meeting like looking around in a room with all the lights out, where the conventional labels and demarcations between things disappear and a different, hidden reality emerges. In this practice, the metaphoric mind is born.

---

[341] See Chace, Shima, and Li,"*An Exposition on the Eight Extraordinary Vessels: Acupuncture, Alchemy, and Herbal Medicine.*"

[342] Often referred to as so-called "Neo-Daoism" in outdated and inaccurate Orientalist constructions of Daoism.

[343] See Chan, and Lo, "*Philosophy and Religion in Early Medieval China*" & Hall & Ames, "*Thinking from the Han: Self, Truth, and Transcendence in Chinese and Western Culture.*"

[344] *Lǎozǐ* 老子 56 translation/interpretation S. Cowan.

Zhuāngzǐ says *"No other and no self, no self and no distinctions, that's almost it. But I don't know what makes it this way. Something true seems to govern, but I can't find the least trace of it. It acts, nothing could be more apparent, but we never see its form. It has a nature but no form."*[345]

There's a worrisome trend I am seeing in many children these days, perhaps due to the excessive dependence on screens, where they can no longer use their imagination to visualize stories and thus are unable to see hidden connections between things. I developed a game to play with children in my office that I call the "This-and-That game" to help stimulate their metaphoric mind. I have them choose any two objects in the room and then they have to come up with three ways that the two objects are the same. For some kids (and their parents too) they get so caught up with how objects are *different* that they get stumped. This reflects a dominance of the analytic mind and is often a subtle sign of their alienation which can present as a host of pathological conditions. And yet as they learn to relax their mind-body, softening the edges between things, in order to look deeply, they discover that seemingly different objects have characteristics or uses in common, and new shared connections and meanings emerge that were not obvious just minutes before. In fact, *everything is related*! This is "deep reunion, *xuán tóng*." It is the root of analogic thinking which the *Nàn Jīng* authors found so essential to perceiving the multiple meanings within the human form as intimately related to the world.

While strictly Confucian ideals of family order and bureaucratic hierarchy tended to influence the way the body was perceived and organized as a kingdom, throughout the *Nàn Jīng*, we can see attempts to combine these views with the Nature-based perspectives related the *Huái Nán Zi* texts: the idea that we are resonant with and reflect the self-organizing (*zì rán* 自然) principles found in nature. The five phase relationships combine both Confucian and Daoist analogic thinking: the heart (fire) as emperor with its four ministers and at the same time the five phases as components in the unending seasonal cycle of growth and death.

In the *Nàn Jīng* there are a number of chapters where we see the authors tackling the "difficult" questions of how to *analogize* the anatomic findings they were seeing empirically in the human body in order to correlate them with the natural landscape. For example, in *Nàn Jīng* 41, the authors ask:

---

[345] Hinton, and Zhuangzi. *"Chuang Tzu. The Inner Chapters,"* pg. 19.

肝獨有兩葉，以何應也

"Only the liver has two lobes. What does this correspond to?"[346]

The question and answers given demonstrate this deep investigation into analogic thinking: what is this *like* in Nature? In other words: *how is this like that?* In this particular way, Chinese medicine stands in radical contrast to the mechanical maps made in Western medicine that imagine the human form as an utterly separate machine with no correspondence to its natural surroundings. *Nàn Jīng* 41 proposes the meaning of the liver's physical form by explaining that the liver corresponding to the Wood phase because it's green, and therefore associated with the Spring season which is positioned between Winter and Summer, Water and Fire, which in turn is why we find the liver anatomically located in the space *between* the kidneys and heart. *Nàn Jīng* 41 states this is the reason why the liver appears to have two lobes, or "two hearts," one still close to its mother winter (kidney) and one leaning towards its child, summer (heart). This reference to an intimate circulation of *xuè qì* 血氣 between the kidney and heart mediated by the liver has some interesting modern implications in terms of blood flow.

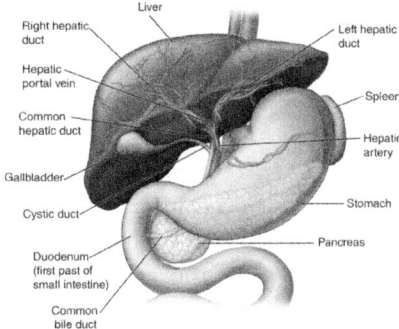

Figure 4.5 - Anatomy of the Liver[347]

Gazing at the anatomic illustration above (*fig. 4.5*) through the ecological eyes of a Han Dynasty sage, we see the "streams" that flow through the liver communicating with the spleen and stomach (and kidneys) below and the heart above. The *Nàn Jīng* authors conclude that the liver's two lobes correspond to

---

[346] Unschuld (2016), *"Nan Jing: The Classic of Difficult Issues,"* pg. 345.

[347] *"Liver: Anatomy and Functions."* Johns Hopkins Medicine, November 19, 2019. https://www.hopkinsmedicine.org/health/conditions-and-diseases/liver-anatomy-and-functions.

the leaves of a tree. Zhàng Shìxián 慔世賢's map (*fig. 1.21*) indeed is a drawing of the liver as if it were leaves.

We now know that one of the liver's many functions is that of a detoxification system for the blood. When the liver has broken down toxic substances, these by-products are excreted into the bile or blood, the bile excreted through the intestines, the blood by-products filtered out by the kidneys, leaving the body in the form of urine.

Z'ev: The *Nàn Jīng* discussed that each of the five yin viscera has its position, *qì*, qualities, and function, and interacts with the other phases and viscera in a healthy or unhealthy way, via the generating (*shēng* 生) and control (*kè* 剋) cycles. When the *qì* of a phase overwhelms another due to imbalance (physiological or emotional)—or seasonal violation disrupts the normal order— this is considered to be a form of internally generated evil *qì*. Accordingly, in the description of the liver in *Nàn Jīng 41* we see that the liver has "two lobes," or "two hearts:"

> *"Only the liver has two lobes. What does this correspond to? The liver is [associated with the] East and [with the phase of] wood. Wood [corresponds to] spring. [During this time of spring] all things come to life, they are still young and small. In their sentiments they are not [yet] close to anything. [The period of spring] moves away from the major yin [of winter] and it is still near to it. It is separate from the major yang [of summer], but is not far away from it. It appears to have two hearts. Hence, [the liver] has two lobes. This also corresponds to the leaves of the woods."*[348]

The springtime is the season between winter and summer. The *shàoyáng* 少陽 is the small *yáng*, the new growth of springtime when the buds are just breaking through their shells, putting out two young leaf sprouts. It is a delicate and tenuous time, reaching for the summertime season of flourishing growth, associated with *tàiyáng*, but still longs for its mother, *tàiyīn*, that dwells in the winter time. For this reason, we say that "the liver has two lobes". It reaches in two directions, backwards and forwards. For this reason, the liver is associated with time and transition. It coordinates the rhythmic flow of *qì* throughout the body, and is connected with regular movement of blood. A healthy liver insures healthy emotions. *Sùwèn* 素問 2 tells us not to punish ourselves in the springtime. Instead, we should loosen the hair and clothing, wake early with the dawn, and walk in the courtyard in the early morning to get the *qì* flowing.

---

[348] Unschuld (2016), *"Nan Jing: The Classic of Difficult Issues,"* pg. 345.

The springtime is a tenuous, unstable time. It is marked by shifting weather and frequent winds, as winter grasps for it's final appearance. As the sun warms the air, the *qì* of summertime begins to predominate. All beings respond to the increase in light and warmth with increased activity, new development and plans. One clears out the old to generate the new. Chapter 1 of the *Jīn Guì Yào Lüè* 金匱要略/*Prescriptions from the Golden Cabinet*, cautions us about extreme weather imbalances during these shifts, and how it can lead to illness by stating:

> Question: "There are [times when a given season] has not yet arrived, but [its qì] arrives; when [a given season] arrives, but [its qì] does not arrive; when [a given season] arrives, but the previous season's qì fails to leave; [and when a given season] arrives and [its qì is] excessive. What does this mean?"

> The Master says: "At midnight of the jiǎ-zǐ day after the winter solstice, lesser yáng rises. At the time of lesser yáng, yáng begins to be engendered and the weather becomes warm and congenial. If the weather becomes warm and congenial before jiǎ-zǐ, this is a case of qi arriving before its season. If jiǎ-zǐ has already arrived, but the weather has not become warm and congenial, this is a case of qì failing to arrive in time for its season. If the time of jiǎ-zǐ has arrived but severely cold weather fails to resolve, this is a case of the season arriving and [the previous season's qì] not leaving. If the weather at the arrival of jiǎ-zǐ is warm as in the height of summer in the fifth and sixth months, this is a case of [the season] arriving and [the qì] being excessive."[349]

Each of these situations can create an imbalance in the body's natural ability to adapt, which can lead to illness. This why one need to be mindful of these shifts and adjust their habits, clothing, and even diet accordingly to stay in balance with the seasonal shifts.

Nàn Jīng 41 uses metaphor to express empirical findings when it states that the springtime is the season between winter and summer. The *shàoyáng* is the small *yáng*, the new growth of springtime when the buds are just breaking through their shells, putting out two young leaf sprouts. It is a delicate and tenuous time, reaching for the summertime season of flourishing growth, associated with *tàiyáng*, but still longs for its mother, *tàiyīn*, that dwells in the wintertime. For this reason, we say that the liver has two lobes. It reaches in two directions, backwards and forwards. For this reason, the liver is associated with time and transition. It coordinates the rhythmic flow of *qì* throughout the body and is connected with regular movement of blood.

---

[349] Zhang, Wiseman, and Wilms, "*Jin Gui Yao Lue Essential Prescriptions of the Golden Cabinet: Translation and Commentaries,*" pg. 16-17.

Stephen: Yes, as we have been saying throughout this book, the *Nàn Jīng* authors observe the body with an ecological eye, that is, seeing the body as an analogy for landscape, in this case, the liver as a tree, the meanings and functions of the various organs are found through their relational positioning and its metaphoric correspondence with relationships found in Nature. These relationships define an organ's meaning and function.

Z'ev: Biomedicine simply lays out the anatomy on the table. It never asks how or why the body is arranged in this way. Sonya Pritzker several years ago stating that modern TCM has also moved in that direction, i.e. this is where this channel is located, this is the definition of the spleen *zàng* 臟, this is what kidney yin vacuity "is". The education is based on this Western education influenced model, but a medical model based on metaphor cannot stand on its own with such limited quantitative analysis. In other words, medicine requires metaphor in order for the human entity to have meaningfulness beyond that of being merely a machine.

Stephen: One of the difficult challenges, I think, Chinese medicine practitioners face today is how to maintain such an analogic perspective when confronted with the powerful influence that Western medical labels and diagnoses exert on our reality. It takes tremendous discipline not to fall under the spell of reductionist materialist maps. There is a perception that somehow the Western body map is *more* factual than the rather poetic metaphors and correspondences Chinese medicine utilizes. As we've stated previously, many practitioners may be tempted to treat Western diagnoses with Chinese medicine but this runs the risk of limiting the true power of the medicine that comes from seeing through *Nàn Jīng* eyes. When we utilize *xuán tóng* as part of our clinical gaze, to soften the edges, unify the dust in order to see the deep hidden connections to the natural world, we find solutions that go unseen in the Western doctors, solutions that have stood the test of time and have the capacity to unlock creative solutions to the current health crises we are facing today.

Z'ev: Seeing the world through *Nàn Jīng* eyes requires training in Chinese natural philosophy and an immersion in language and culture. In many TCM schools, half the education is given over to matching *zàngfǔ* 臟腑 patterns to biomedical disease entities in an entirely arbitrary fashion and leaving graduates grasping for deeper meaning in their practices, and embracing artificial substitutes. A true Chinese medical education cultivates the "clinical gaze," aligning perception to match the principles outlined in the classical texts.In order to do so, we must train our minds "against the grain" of the materialist philosophy and separation of phenomena into discrete objects. Only a mind trained by dedicated study, reflection and application, will be able to practice effectively.

Stephen: Likewise, like the *Interstitium* discussed in previous chapters, the "secret circulation" flowing through the fascia, the discovery of a *Glymphatic system* went unrecognized in western medicine until very recently.

> *"Throughout the body, lymphatic fluid movement supports critical functions including clearance of excess fluid and metabolic waste. The glymphatic system is the analog of the lymphatic system in the CNS. As such, the glymphatic system plays a key role in regulating directional interstitial fluid movement, waste clearance, and, potentially, brain immunity."*[350]

And yet, remarkably, the Chinese medical classics, seeing through the relational lens of *yīnyáng*, recognized this complete circulation two millennia ago, and understood one of the *shàoyáng* functions as a pivot (*shū* 樞) in the body, between the *tàiyáng* and the *yángmíng* 陽明, that is fundamental for promoting the flow of *xuè qì* 血氣 and clearing toxins from the body-mind.

Sùwèn 素問 8 states that *"The liver is the official functioning as general.Planning and deliberation originate in it.The gallbladder is the official functioning as rectifier. Decisions and judgements originate in it"*[351] The use of metaphor is no less scientific for when we look, we can see the "scientific" functions of liver / gall bladder detoxification embedded in the glymphatic system just as clearly as we can appreciate the *sānjiāo* 三焦 function of irrigation and master of the waterways within the *interstitium*, two organ-systems until recently utterly unseen by Western medicine. That the Han dynasty physicians observed the dissected organs of the body is of no doubt. How else would they know that the liver has two lobes yet to see with *Nàn Jīng* eyes is to see that we are a network of relations and from this, creative solutions to the difficulties of our times can be found.

---

[350] Hablitz and Nedergaard.,*"The Glymphatic System: A Novel Component of Fundamental Neurobiology."*

[351] Unschuld, Tessenow, and Zheng, *"Huang Di Nei Jing Su Wen: An Annotated Translation of Huang Di's Inner Classic - Basic Questions, 2 Volumes,"* pg. 156.

Thoughts on the Gall Bladder Channel: *Running the Rapids*

Z'ev Rosenberg & Stephen Cowan

Z'ev: In a recent conversation, I had asked Stephen what he had thought about the gall bladder channel as illustrated, where it zig zags in two locations; along the sides of the trunk, and on the head. He compared the flow of the channel to a rapid running stream descending a mountainside, over rocks, sudden drops, rushing to and fro. I mentioned mountain canyons in the San Jacinto Mountains of Southern California, where the roads down from the mountains have cut deep canyons, and follow the course of streams through them, winding with sharp curves, barreling through all obstructions over time. He also noted that as an extraordinary *fǔ* 腑 / bowel, it had qualities of both *yīn* and *yáng*, storing essence. *Shàoyáng* 少陽 *qì* has something of this aggressive fast moving nature, and if we read the life stories of major rivers, whether in China, Tibet, or North America, we find their "biographies" to tell of rapid descents, deep gorges, diversions of flow, until finally they hit plains and flat lands, rich soil, broad, lazy flows, deep channels, and in some cases filled with soil, and cloudy.

Shàoyáng qì is the governing *qì* of spring (*chūn wēn* 春温), and like melting snow, it wants to expand and flow. Just as the liver has "two lobes," *shàoyáng* qi can be constrained either from "behind" (*tàiyīn* 太 陰 winter cold / damp qi) or "after" (*tàiyáng* 太 陽 summer heat). In a recent Zen talk, the teacher pointed out that we are living in a time of turbulence to the left and the right. When traveling in a boat down a canyon with rapids, the key is to maintain the exact middle course between the two extremes, to avoid capsizing.[352] As in daily life, so in our health, we navigate *shàoyáng* qi by maintaining our center, managing our ministerial fire so it warms the *xuè qì* 血氣, without "burning out" through over activity, and preserving our *wèi qì* 衛氣 / defense *qì* by dressing flexibly and avoiding over exposure to the wind.

---

[352] See Roshi, Murphy. *"Earth as Koan, Earth as Self – with Susan Murphy Roshi."*

A few days ago, my wife and I were returning from synagogue when a very cold wind, very unusual for Southern California in April hit our backs. It was strong enough to penetrate through my sweater and scarf. I returned home, but about the time I went to sleep I had a sudden attack of wheezing, coughing up copious phlegm, sneezing and chill. Ginger tea and a hot water bottle helped, but it took a hot bath and sweating plus *chái hú guì zhī tāng* 柴胡桂枝湯/ bupleurum and cinnamon decoction to overcome the effects of the over-riding cold/damp *qì* delivered by wind. Before that, we had a warm spell, and the warmth caused stagnation of liver/gall bladder *qì*. I (and many of my patients) felt body heaviness, irritability, dream filled sleep, aches and pains, and abdominal bloating and discomfort. I suggested (and took for myself) *chái hú shū gān tāng* 柴胡疏肝汤/bupleurum soothe the liver decoction, which worked wonders in small doses.

Z'ev: Again, the role of time, pattern, *wèi qì* 衛氣/*xié qì* 邪氣 interfaces of which *Nàn Jīng* guides us. Michael Broffman taught me this decades ago. Lǐ Dōngyuán's 李東垣 described how internal spleen vacuity/space into which *wèi qì* collapses (yin fire) and *xié qì* proliferates. I would like to see his ideas become the basis of the next "earth phase" book.

Stephen: Yes, if we take these ideas plus Varela's and apply them to herbs (as also having circular cognition) we begin to see how Chinese medicine treatments are geared at reducing the so called "edge of catastrophe" where viruses thrive!

Chinese commentators have interpreted this passage as an exhortation to flexibility, i.e., to always adapt one's theoretical book knowledge to the real and ever changing situations one is confronted with, as we see with Wú Kūn 吳昆 (1552–1620?) Who wrote:

"The Nèijīng 內經 believes that by drawing on facts and comparing the likes, the knowledge of things, can be lifted to a theoretical level. Hence, Sùwèn 素問 76 states: [they] drew on the facts, compared the likes and transformed them into mysteries."[353]

---

[353] Unschuld, Tessenow, and Zheng, "*Huang Di Nei Jing Su Wen: An Annotated Translation of Huang Di's Inner Classic - Basic Questions, 2 Volumes,*" pg. 659.

Mapping the Space-Time Between

Z'ev Rosenberg & Stephen Cowan

Z'ev: The *qì* at the time of the writing of this book is a Wood Dragon year. According to five movements *wǔxíng* 五行 / theory, it is the *shàoyáng* 少陽 *qì* of spring that can be easily overwhelmed by the *tàiyīn* 太陰) damp *qì* of winter. In California, for the first time in decades it has been unusually cold, especially at nighttime, and the rainy / snowy season which usually is winding down continues. The cold and damp *qì* has been mobilized by the normal wind characteristic of springtime, leading to chronic cough, excessive phlegm, aching and heavy joints. If there is cold (damp) *qì* in the third and fourth months, the *yáng qì* is still weak, and will be easily damaged by the cold.

This core concept of host (*zhǔ qì* 主氣) and guest *qì* (*kè qì* 客氣) is essential for the Chinese scholar / physician in predicting epidemics and seasonal illnesses. Springtime as a major transitional season is a time where one has to be both cautious and flexible in adapting to changing conditions. Coordination may be difficult in the springtime, as one is pulled in two directions, concurrently towards the quiet repose of wintertime, and forwards to the full burgeoning of summertime. We are swept up in the *shàoyáng qì*, and it can be turbulent. This can lead to a loss of direction, along with weakening of our resistance to external contractions of *xié qì* 邪氣.

The defense *qì* is often weakened in springtime. The rising *shàoyáng qì* easily opens the pores to emit sweat, and wind-cold can easily enter the *còu lǐ* 腠理 / interstices. This is also the season of chūn wēn 春温 or spring warmth disease, when wind cold contracted in the wintertime transforms to heat in the *shàoyīn* 少陰 channel, if there is weakness of kidney *jīng* 精 / essence. This fragile, changeable season can lead to *shí bìng* 时病, a seasonal disease. Many colds and flus strike when cold snaps follow warm spells, a very common scenario in springtime. Chinese medicine has many prescriptions that are useful for such spring-warmth epidemics depending on the pattern, such as *bái hǔ tāng* 白虎湯 / White Tiger Decoction, *zhī zǐ chǐ tāng* 梔子豉湯 / Gardenia and Prepared Soybean Decoction, and *huáng qín tāng* 黃芩湯 / scutellaria decoction.

The liver is the viscera of memory and prediction, corresponding to that Wood moment that lies between the past and the future. Therefore, the liver exists in the true present, but a present that is constantly in motion. If we don't flow with the ever-moving now, than the liver *qì* stagnates. Spring is the season of transition. Just as *juéyīn* 厥陰 / reverting yin is the end of *yīn* and beginning of *yáng*. To flow is to transform winter to spring, darkness to light. Illness in *juéyīn* is the separation of *yīn* and *yáng*.

The *Nàn Jīng* 難經 was written in a time when humanity lived closer to nature and its cycles, and the text reflects the rhythms of seasons, crickets, breath, and transformations in plants, animals, river flows and snow melt. It requires a discerning mind, observing eye, and listening ear, one that can hear the sound of one's own blood pulsating in one's head. The eye observes the changing motions, expressions and colors in the face as thoughts pass through, as words are spoken, as feelings are processed. The face turns red, then pale, the breathing gets stronger, then weaker, the voice increases in pitch and timbre. The Chinese physician responds to the moment by inserting an acupuncture needle, a carefully chosen herbal formula (the *chái hú tāng* 柴胡湯 bupleurum family is especially important at this time of year, and *xiǎo chái hú tāng* 小柴胡 湯 / minor bupleurum decoction has many modifications for the constantly changing illness patterns), or perhaps just with carefully chosen words. Here the synchronicity of the *Nàn Jīng* lies in the response to what is observed in the patient-healer encounter. In applying the teachings of five movements / six *qì* to modern conditions and location(s), we begin by reading the environmental *qì* where we live.

For example, Santa Fe, New Mexico (my home away from home) lies between two mountain ranges to the east and west, on an elevated plateau above the Rio Grande. The mountain range to the east (Sangre de Cristo) blocks much of the cold *qì* of the northern Rockies, and many of the heavy snowstorms. Santa Fe is where the high desert, low desert, Rocky Mountains and Great Plains meet, bisected by a major river. It is an ideal region for more artistic and meditative concerns, but its poor soil, lack of water, high winds in springtime and cold nights are not ideal for a large population or intensive economic activity. As one can have cold *qì* at almost any time of year, along with intense high altitude sunlight, Santa Fe is not an area where damp, tropical illnesses or warm diseases proliferate. However, wind damage, desiccation, and invasions of cold are common.

If we observe patterns of where the Chinese (and other cultures by extension) historically have developed their cities and civilization centers, we find that the mapping of terrain according to the four directions is at the core of these determinations, historically these choices were not at random or merely the result of economic activity. In the West, Hippocrates *On Airs, Waters and Places*[354] goes into detail about ideal environmental and climatic settings for a healthy, flourishing society. In this book, Hippocrates determines the physical

---

[354] Hippocrates, *"The Internet Classics Archive: On Airs, Waters, and Places by Hippocrates."*

constitution of local inhabitants, and their tendency to seasonal illnesses based on a geomantic understanding of local regions considering the soil, prevailing winds, balanced or imbalanced seasonal *qì* and related factors According to David White

> *"Observing the natural divisions and geographical patterning of the environment around us gives wonderful insight into core classical physiology. One such observation the ancients took into account was the dividing range, and one of China's primary east-west watersheds, the Qinling / Zhongnan mountains. Qinling (秦岭 - literally the "Qin Ranges"), held the responsibility of thermal regulation of the cold qi /air that could impose on the south and the damp qi / air that could invade the north, not dissimilar to the functioning of the ge 膈 / diaphragm and its relationship to that of southern fire and northern water in the body. It created the drainage basin of the Yangzi and yellow river systems."*[355]

Here we see that landscape, and reading the landscape, precedes human culture, and was essential in the development of Chinese and other civilizations in terms of health, longevity, economic activity, governance, agriculture and human activity. In ancient Greek civilization, the same concerns were a core concern of the Hippocratic medical system.

In Daoist cosmology and practice, there is what is called the central microcosmic orbit, containing the flows in the *dū mài* 督脉 and *rén mài* 任脉. Along this central channel, we have dual expressions of *jīng* 精 containing glands which mirror the extraordinary fu/bowel of the gall bladder. This includes the thymus, pituitary, and pineal glands (third eye, walnut shaped) along the central channel (although we can say the pineal gland is bifurcated in its shape and form, having "lobes" like the liver, and responsible for secreting melatonin and regulating sleep and circadian function). As is the thymus, which is also bifurcated like a walnut, and with a major role in immunity (and decreases in size and function at adulthood). The thalamus is a paired gray matter structure of the diencephalon located near the center of the brain. All information from your body's senses (except smell) must be processed through your thalamus before being sent to your brain's cerebral cortex for interpretation. The thalamus also plays a role in sleep, wakefulness, consciousness, learning and memory. The pituitary also has two lobes, and is related to the hypothalamus, which governs complex hormonal and central nervous system functions.

The paired glands include both the ovaries (called *wài shèn* 外肾 / outer kidneys in Chinese medicine), gonads, adrenal glands, and thyroid. In Chinese medicine, we can consider these to be governed by the gall bladder, which

---

[355] White, (instituteofneijingresearch), *"Observing the Natural Divisions and Geographical,"* Instagram, April 8, 2024, https://www.instituteofneijingresearch.com/.

governs all the extraordinary fu / bowels including the bone marrow, brain, mai / vessels, uterus and bones. As discussed in the previous chapter, the gall bladder is also *zhōng jīng zhī fǔ* 中精之腑, the bowel holding the central essences. All of the ductless glands store and transmit *jīng* 精 / essence, and can be considered to be expressions of gall bladder qì (*shàoyáng* 少陽 qi), including the *sānjiāo* 三焦 / triple burner transmit essence throughout the body, and are tied to the *mìng mén* 命門 / life-gate fire, which stores *xiàng huǒ* 相火 / ministerial fire.

Stephen and I were discussing the heart and *xīn bāo* 心包 / heart "wrapper" (pericardium) as a paired or lobed single viscus, as the pericardium wraps itself around the heart and is not necessarily seen as a separate *zàng*.

It says in *Língshū* 36 The Separation of the Five Jin / Ye Liquids: *"when the jin and ye liquids of the five types of grain find together, they will generate a paste. Internally this paste will seep into the hollow spaces in the bones and supplement the brain with (bone) marrow, and it descends to flow into the inner side of the thighs (genital organs)."*[356] The eyes themselves are paired along the central channel, and the *Sùwèn* 素問 states that the eyes are where the *mìng mén* resides. They are also, as Elisabeth Rochat expresses it, *"the culmination of all the refined essences brought to it by the network of circulation. What is in the heart is in the brain and also in the eyes. The body fluids of the zàngfǔ* 臟腑 *rise to filter in the eye."*[357] Also *"the heart is the quintessence of the five zàng, the eye is its orifice."* The *luò* 絡 channel branches off from the hand *shàoyīn* 少陰 into the brain as well.

Stephen: I am struck by the Han dynasty clinicians' innate trust in Nature's relational logic to provide a deep ecological understanding of how to navigate change in order to promote healing in people. This idea of mapping transitions which carries within it the central idea of change (*yì* 易) and transformation (*huà* 化) so important in Chinese thinking in contrast to Western anatomic mapping that reduces the body to a static form of "this" OR "that." The *tǔ* 土-soil phase is often associated with transitions between the seasons (and between the organs). I think our society tends to minimize the importance of the soil, of these transitions in our busy life. Careful examination of the transitions between states of well-being and states of disease enable the practitioner to act "before things happen" as *Lǎozǐ* 老子 advises.

Z'ev: In his famous work, The Canon of Medicine (*al-Qānūn fī aṭ-Ṭibb* القانون في الطب,), Ibn Sīnā ابن سينا, one of the preeminent philosopher and physician during the Islamic Golden Age, noted that in the autumn season, phlegm

---

[356] Unschuld, *"Huang Di Nei Jing Ling Shu: The Ancient Classic on Needle Therapy"* pg. 385.
[357] Rochat de la Vallée, *"The Double Aspect of the Heart,"* pg. 30-31.

disorders tended to increase, as the body did not throw off superfluous fluids out through the skin as in the summer season of expansiveness. Rather, the tendency of autumn is contraction and consolidation, so that waste fluids will tend to congeal in the interior of the body / mind system.

Stephen: Z'ev's comments above regarding the vulnerabilities to wind-invasion during the tenuous transition of Springtime rings true to my own experience treating children. In pediatrics every year, we see a second burst of colds and flu infections in March which has a different nature from the flu of deep winter months. Fevers are not as high, runny noses and rashes are more prominent, and generally the illness typically do not last as long unless one is not supporting the child properly. Likewise, in October, as the air begins to cool, pediatricians prepare themselves for a rise in respiratory symptoms. Autumn and Spring are transitional times that carry their own precarious dangers and while modern Western medicine tends to focus on which particular strains of viruses occur during these times, they often fail to notice the multitude of other environmental and physiological factors at play during these times. Interestingly, recent research has demonstrated that variations in humidity and temperature are important drivers in the seasonality of human respiratory viruses, a remarkable observation that, as Z'ev noted, was clear to the *Nàn Jīng* authors 2000 years ago. While advances in Western science have focused on *"the conditions that increase virus stability and transmissibility created by indoor environments conducive to virus transmission and a dampening of host cell immune response,"*[358] they fail to appreciate the greater macrocosmic meanings of seasonal cycles and transitions taking place on (and in) our body-mind. Chinese medicine at its core is rooted in the *yīnyáng* polarity described in the *Yìjīng* 易經. This *tàijí* 太極 map has been called the "tu par excellence"[359] because of its function as a cosmological map meant to help us prepare for and guide us through transitions. At its very basis, the *Yìjīng* maps the transitions between seasons as a function of the shared continuum that exists between polar opposites. For example, the *Xiāntiān Yìjīng* 先天易經 pre-heaven map arranges Mountain (*Gěn* 艮 / ☶) and Stream (*Duì* 兌 / ☱) diagonally across from each other (*fig. 4.6*).

---

[358] See Neumann, and Kawaoka, *"Seasonality of Influenza and Other Respiratory Viruses."*

[359] See Lackner, *"4. Diagrams as an Architecture by Means of Words: The Yanji Tu."*

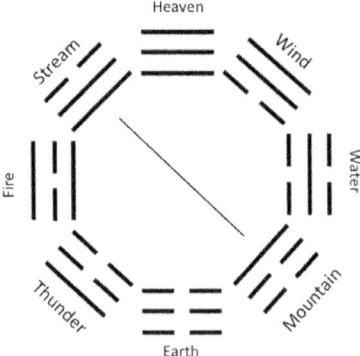

Figure 4.6 - Bāguà 八卦 - Mountain (Gĕn 艮/☶) & Stream (Duì 兑/☱) Arrangement

The *bāguà* 八卦 map (*fig.4.6*) illustrates the apparent opposite nature of mountain (two *yīn* below one *yáng*) and stream (two *yáng* below one *yīn*). However, the *Yìjīng* tells us that in Nature, the mountain needs the stream to be a "living" mountain as much as the stream needs the mountain to be a living stream. Likewise, water-fire exist on a continuum as do wind-thunder and of course heaven-earth.

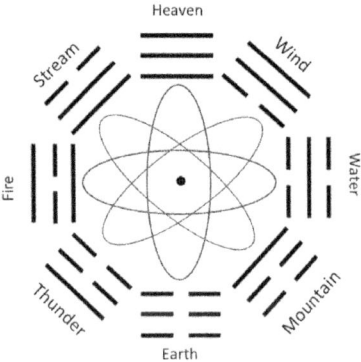

Figure 4.7 - Bāguà 八卦 Inter-Related Polarities

This relational perspective stands in stark contrast with the either-or dualistic lens through which Western science views Nature (e.g. us or them). As we have seen throughout this book, the process of change is reflected in the currents and rhythms of qì generated by these inter-relationships. This is the open-ended process called *Dào* 道. It's circulation has no beginning or end as the classics tell us.

The experienced clinician always considers the continuum between polar opposites, remaining attentive and adept at interpreting the dynamic rhythms and pulses of theses space-time transitions, recognizing the intrinsic interconnectedness and interdependence of *yīnyáng* aspects in all life. In this ecological way, we are able to navigate the changes in order to skillfully ride the waves and get the most out of what life offers us.

Z'ev: Each chapter of the *Nàn Jīng*, along with much of the *Sùwèn* and *Língshū*, traces these fascinating pathways, resonances and connections within and between the channels, network vessels, and their connections with internal viscera and structures. By studying deeply these connections, we can observe a complete system of physiology that is an "unbroken chain" woven together by the channel system. Stephen and I have produced *A Ring Without End* with the desire and hope that our colleagues and students can be inspired to become "archeologists" of texts and case histories in order to uncover the beautiful symmetry and depth of the Chinese medical classics, and apply in their own clinics. Both of us in our long professional careers have seen the results of such deep study and application. It is our wish to share with the reader our experience and years of study in order to inspire deeper, more individualized practice of our noble medicine, and to strengthen confidence in the generational transmission of these timeless principles.

Afterword: *Translation and Transmission in the Art and Science of Medicine*

Brian S. Kirbis

> *It should be such that this [knowledge] is to be transmitted to subsequent generations, and it must be such that these laws are elucidated. It should be such that nothing ever is lost and that [their transmission] continues for long without interruption. To see to it that they are applied easily and are difficult to forget, they should be laid down in commonly valid structures. They should be worded in separate paragraphs, distinguishing outer and inner, and creating a complete set from beginning to end.*
> -The Spiritual Pivot (*Língshū Jīng* 靈樞經)[360]

A Ring Without End is an artfully composed treatise on the development of channel theory proceeding from nature-based metaphors of the human body, through the emergence and development of an orthodox Chinese medical canon, and nearly two millennia of historical revisionism as this ancient wisdom tradition enters into global circulation. It is based on the combined efforts of the two authors in their mutual dedication to the art of healing, agility in character and textual analysis, and desire to pass on a distillate of critical, clinical, and practical experience to future generations of practitioners.

This project extends back to May 2022 and to several pages of notes by Z'ev Rosenberg that, true to his nature, begin with a musical epigraph by Charles Mingus:

> *"What I'm trying to play is very difficult, because I'm trying to play the truth of what I am. The reason why it's difficult - it's not difficult to play the mechanics of it - it's because I'm changing all the time."*

In medicine as in music, the challenge is to convey something of the ever-changing stream of awareness emerging from the hidden source to flow through and around us. *This book, like Mingus' music, has soul!*

---

[360] Unschuld, *"Huang Di Nei Jing Ling Shu: The Ancient Classic on Needle Therapy,"* pg. 36

This lyrical journey came to fruition over three years - three cycles of birth, growth, proliferation, consolidation and storage. It is a continuation of Z'ev Rosenberg's previous work, *Afterglow: Ministerial Fire and Chinese Ecological Medicine*. This time, rather than single authorship, we are graced by the presence of longtime friend and collaborator Stephen Cowan. Where *Afterglow* is the softly burning candle illuminating the interior, this current work details a journey of exploration by these two sage physicians and soul brothers through the depths and breadth of a Chinese imaginal landscape.

An intimate tone persists throughout the book, situated within an otherwise rigorous methodology. Our two scholar-practitioners alternate between unlocking individual seal-form characters and maneuvering obscure passages, the latent power activated within the archaic script illuminating the text in new and revealing ways. The source material is derived primarily from translations by Paul Unschuld, with whom Z'ev Rosenberg maintained a correspondence throughout the duration of the book's creation.

To understand something of the requisite dedication and the immensity of a project such as this, consider this question originally posed by François Jullien in *The Book of Beginnings*: *what is it to enter into a way of thought?* In response to his own inquiry:

"It requires so much time, we know, so much patience, 'skill,' memory, to be initiated into the classical Chinese language and to venture into its immense forest of texts and commentaries."[361]

It would benefit the reader to take to heart the manner in which Jullien abides by ecological metaphor in pointing out the vastness of the terrain spread out before us. The present volume represents nothing short of several decades of conjoint devotion to this medicine and its ecological worldview.

For my part, the opportunity to delve into the source material and to participate in the near-daily dialogues informing this book has been a particularly significant process of personal transformation. For this content cannot simply be read, but must be brought into active embodiment within one's very being. Working alongside the two authors instilled a deeper understanding of the *praxis* contained not only within the original texts, but also within the intimacies of collegial exchange, offering up a critical pedagogy rooted in the ebb and flow of daily life.

---

[361] Jullien,"*The Book of Beginnings*," pg. 3

In the weeks leading up to the Year of the Wood Dragon, I had the distinct pleasure of working with Stephen on his New Year's divination poem, offered up to a cohort of students of the Chinese scholar-physician and legendary *tàijí* master Cheng Man-ching. The characters revealed themselves in the following order:

癸不向日
忠赤傾心
大開月
兇兇兇有了
梅花便不

Celestial Stems
don't grow towards the Sun.
Red-blooded devotion pours from their Heart.
Their greatness begins with the Moon.
All the violence and misfortune these days,
I've got a solution:
Plum blossoms bloom!
Are they not opportune?

The poem offers up a multiplication of the latent power contained within each character as it enters into a broader mythopoetic and semantic field. It is presented here as a homage to the diligent effort of its two authors in seeing this book come to fruition. I conclude with the following remarks by Richard Tarnas in his landmark work *Cosmos and Psyche: Intimations of a New World View*:

Striving to combine the intellectual rigor of scientific observation with the intuitive insight of the poetic and spiritual imagination, depth psychology attempted to bring the light of reason to the deep mysteries of human interiority, yet often witnessed the converse: the light of reason reevaluated, transformed, and deepened by the very mysteries it sought to illuminate.

A continuity extends from the interior world of the human to the world outside. In the primal experience, what we would call the "outer" world possesses an interior aspect that is continuous with human subjectivity. Creative and responsive intelligence, spirit and soul, meaning and purpose are everywhere. The human being is a microcosm within the macrocosm of the world, participating in its interior reality and united with the whole in ways that are both tangible and invisible.[362]

Doctors' Rosenberg and Cowan gift us with an original, imaginative and rigorous exegesis on a difficult subject, one which promises to support its readers in their own inquiries into this ancient and ever evolving medicine. Perhaps the modern age is providing the necessary preconditions, by way of the profound disequilibriums occurring at the planetary scale, for the true potential and flourishing of this medicine to take place. The present volume suggests just that sort of possibility.

Brian S. Kirbis
Jǐngmǎi 景买 Mountains, Yunnan Province
Year of the Wood Dragon

---

[362] Tarnas, *"Cosmos and Psyche: Intimations of a New World View,"* pg. 43-47.

Appendix I: Case Histories: *Branching (Divergent) Channels, Extraordinary Vessel, Five Transporting Points and Developing Fāngfǎ 方法 Methodology*

Z'ev Rosenberg

Often when feeling pulses / palpating vessels on patients with autoimmune or neurological disorders, I will detect what Wáng Shūhē 王叔和 (180-270) calls a "spinning bean" pulse.[363] Rather than the positions (*cùn* 寸 / *guān* 關 / *chǐ* 尺) beating in unison, specific positions will 'spin in their own orbits' with a lack of coordination with other positions. A visiting patient whose pulse I checked years ago in a La Jolla hotel had that "spinning bean" (*zhuàn dòu mài* 轉豆脈) quality in the *chǐ* position on both wrists, indicating that her diagnosed Parkinson's disease[364] was mainly situated in the lower burner, kidney *jīng* 精, therefore it was a "core" disorder.

Another "Parkinson's" case that I've followed more closely with regular treatments has manifested with the "spinning bean" pulse in the *cùn* / *guān* positions, specifically on the left side. This pulse will vary according to dosage of Ldopa and lexipro (5 mg., very small dose), with a wiry core and slippery periphery. Each position (*cùn* / *guān*) seems on certain occasions to "spin in its own orbit," which means the Gall Bladder and Heart channels, upper and middle burners are not communicating. When the channel system is balanced, these pulses smooth out and flow into one another. The right wrist vessel / pulse almost never manifest these qualities and tend to be slightly soggy *tàiyīn* 太陰

---

[363] Rosenberg, *"Ripples in the Flow: Reflections on Vessel Dynamics in the Nàn Jīng,"* pg. 95.

[364] Stephen and I want to emphasize that biomedical disease names / entities often obscure as much as define patients' symptom patterns, as they lump all cases, stages and unique symptom qualities into fixed quantities and definitions. In the case of disorders affecting the central nervous system and brain, this is even more evident, as brain / CNS networks are as yet poorly understood in terms of diagnostics and therapeutics, and neuroscience is still a relatively young science.

pulses. The *chǐ* pulses on both sides sometimes feel rooted, other times noticeably thin and week.

With a patient like this, I often will choose to treat paired extraordinary vessel master/couple points such as *hòu xī* 後谿/back stream (SI 3)/*shēn mài* 申脈/extended vessel (BL 62) for the *yáng qiāo mài* 陽蹺脈. *Gōng sūn* 公孫/grandfather grandson (Sp 4)/*nèi guān* 內關/inner pass (PC 6) for the *chòng mài* 衝脈. Or *zhào hǎi* 照海/shining sea (Ki 6) with *liè quē* 列缺/broken sequence (LU 7) and *tōng lǐ* 通里/penetrating the interior (Ht 5) for the *yīn qiāo mài* 陰蹺脈.

I will also use the liver/gall bladder divergents, including *tóng zǐ liáo* 瞳子髎/pupil crevice (GB 1), *yáng líng quán* 陽陵泉/yang mound spring (GB 34), *qū quán* 曲泉/spring at the crook (Liv 8), *tài chōng* 太沖/great rushing (Liv 3) and *qiū xū* 丘墟/mound of ruins (GB 40), with powerful changes to pulse, abdominal palpation (softening and warming) and general qì flow.

I will sometimes alternate with the KI/BL divergents on the back, using *dà zhù* 大杼/great shuttle (BL 11) (meeting point of the bones), *shèn shū* 腎俞/kidney shu (Bl 23), *yīn gǔ* 阴谷 /yin valley (Ki 10) and *tài xī* 太溪 /supreme stream (Ki 3). I find this treatment in general to be powerfully boosting to the kidney *yáng* and essence. Note that both of these treatments include *yuán xué* 原穴 (source points) of the kidney and liver. In addition, I will use scalp acupuncture points, abdominal points along the *chòng mài* and *rén mài* 任脈, and "open orifice" (my words) points around the head such as *sī zhú kōng* 絲竹空/silken bamboo hollow (TB 23), *fēng chí* 風池/wind pool (GB 20), *fēng fǔ* 風府/palace of wind (Du 16), *bǎi huì* 百會/one hundred meeting (Du 20), *shén tíng* 神庭/courtyard of the spirit (Du 24).

Another patient who has been diagnosed with multiple sclerosis in 1996. Originally he was prescribed copaxone and betaserone, which made him feel horrible. He suffered a steady decline, couldn't write, and was limping on his right leg, with intense pain in the left thigh and arm, and his balance was way off. He was forced to retire, and suffered from deep seated fear and anxiety. Once he started regular acupuncture treatments, he was able to stop all the medications, and recovered much of his poise and balance. He also practices qigong regularly. He has improved his diet, sleep has improved and he hasn't needed to see a Western physician for several years. His circulatory problems in his legs has been alleviated by the use of Tibetan herbal foot soaks. His pulses which had been generally weak, deep thin, forceless and rough, have gradually gotten stronger. His tongue originally was very pale and floppy, but has returned to a normal color and body since supplementing his blood and kidney qi with herbs and moxibustion during treatments. I treat him every two weeks, and often will use the kidney and liver divergent treatments, and extraordinary vessel master/couple treatments to great effect. He also has taken the following formulas over time: *zhēn wǔ tāng* 真武湯 / true warrior decoction, *dāng guī sì nì jiā wú zhū yú shēng jiāng tāng* 當歸四逆加吳茱萸生薑 湯 / tangkuei decoction for frigid extremities plus evodia and fresh ginger, and *shèn qì wán* 腎氣丸 / kindey qi pill with *tiān xióng sàn* 天雄散 / tian xiong powder.

When treating patients with chronic disorders, whether neurological or immunological, the goal is to continually repair damage to the channel system, and access from *yáng* / outside to *yīn* / inside, as these chronic disorders are of a yin nature. While the original perverse qi may have invaded from the outside, and been stirred by emotional / constitutional internal changes, these are all disorders which damage and / or influence *jīng* and its circulation through the organism. In order to restore / stimulate / repair *jīng* and associated viscera and tissues we need to "program" the channel system to access *yuán qì* 原氣 / source qì and the body / mind's self repair mechanisms. The results will often be efficacious.

Additionally, hormones such as melatonin are produced in all cells, saving to regulate circadian rhythm clocks. In Chinese medicine, consciousness is thought to be distributed throughout the organism through the five *zàng* 臟 / viscera. Each viscus is associated with an aspect of personality, mind and spirit, the *hún* 魂, the *shén* 神 , the *pò* 魄, the *zhì* 志 and the *yì* 意.[365] By working on these channel systems, and their associated viscera, we are able to treat these kind of illnesses without necessarily having to only focus on treating the brain and central nervous system. Restoring communication between the *zàngfǔ* 臟腑 using the five phase transporting holes, *bié mài* 別脈 / branching channels and the eight extraordinary vessels allows for a global, holistic approach to these disorders.

---

[365] See *"Nàn Jīng* 難經 *34: Constructing a Clinical Mandala,"* pg. 93-105.

Appendix II: Blueprints and Charts from Z'ev's Notebook

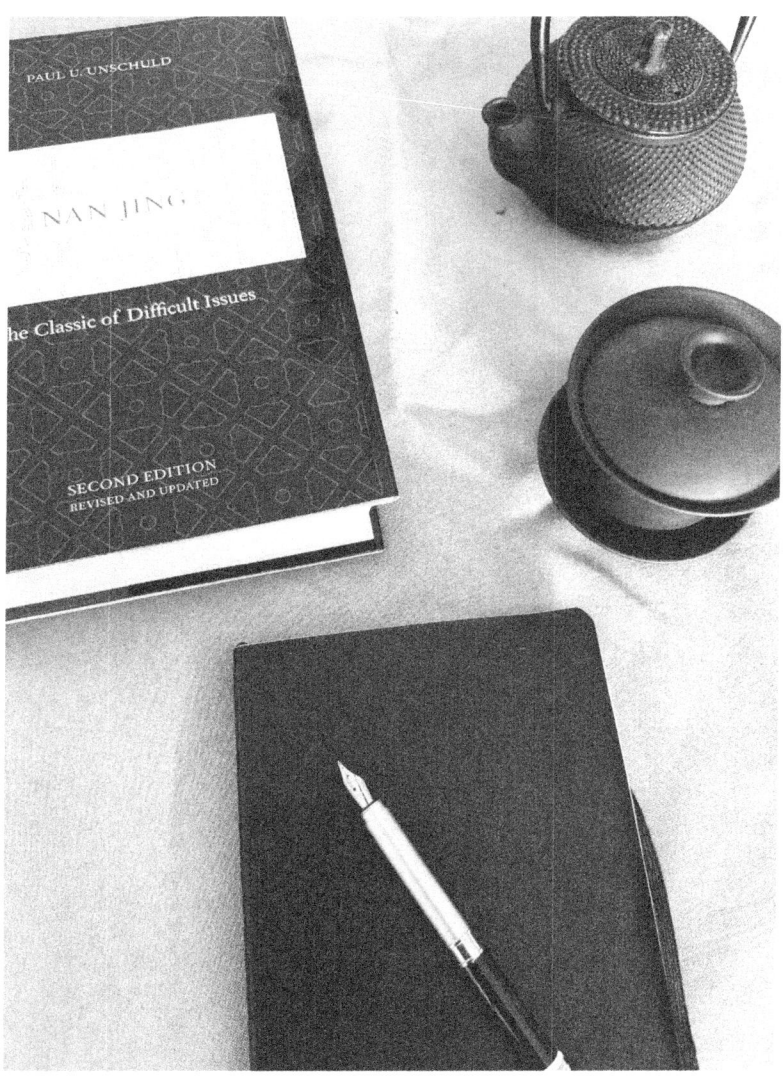

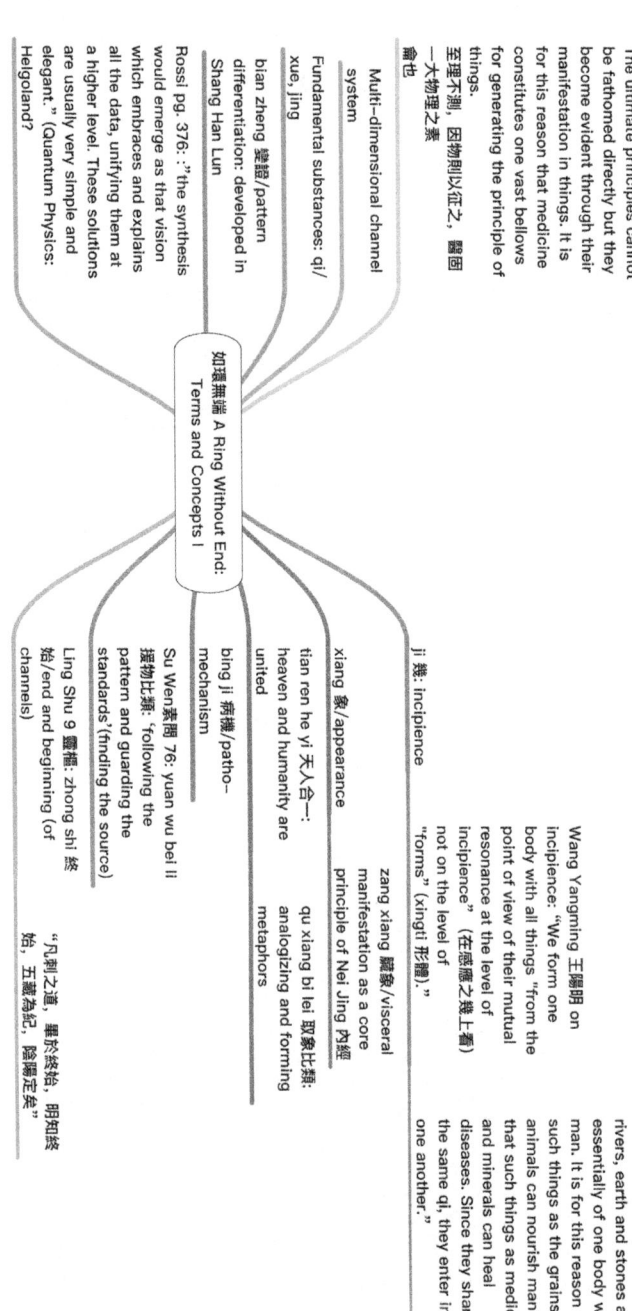

如環無端 A Ring Without End: Terms and Concepts I

The ultimate principles cannot be fathomed directly but they become evident through their manifestation in things. It is for this reason that medicine constitutes one vast bellows for generating the principle of things.
至理不測，因物則以征之，醫固一大物理之橐籥也

Multi-dimensional channel system

Fundamental substances: qi/ xue, jing

bian zheng 變證/pattern differentiation: developed in Shang Han Lun

Rossi pg. 376: :"the synthesis would emerge as that vision which embraces and explains all the data, unifying them at a higher level. These solutions are usually very simple and elegant." (Quantum Physics: Heigoland?

ji 幾: incipience

xiang 象/appearance

tian ren he yi 天人合一: heaven and humanity are united

bing ji 病機/patho–mechanism

Su Wen 素問 76: yuan wu bi li 提物比類: "following the pattern and guarding the standards"(finding the source)

Ling Shu 9 靈樞: zhong shi 終始/end and beginning (of channels)

zang xiang 臟象/visceral manifestation as a core principle of Nei Jing 內經

qu xiang bi lei 取象比類: analogizing and forming metaphors

Wang Yangming 王陽明 on incipience: "We form one body with all things "from the point of view of their mutual resonance at the level of incipience" (在感應之幾上看) not on the level of "forms" (xingti 形體)."

"Wind, rain, dew, thunder, sun and moon, stars, animals and plants, mountains and rivers, earth and stones are essentially of one body with man. It is for this reason that such things as the grains and animals can nourish man and that such things as medicines and minerals can heal diseases. Since they share the same qi, they enter into one another."

"凡刺之道，畢於終始，明知終始，五藏為紀，陰陽定矣"

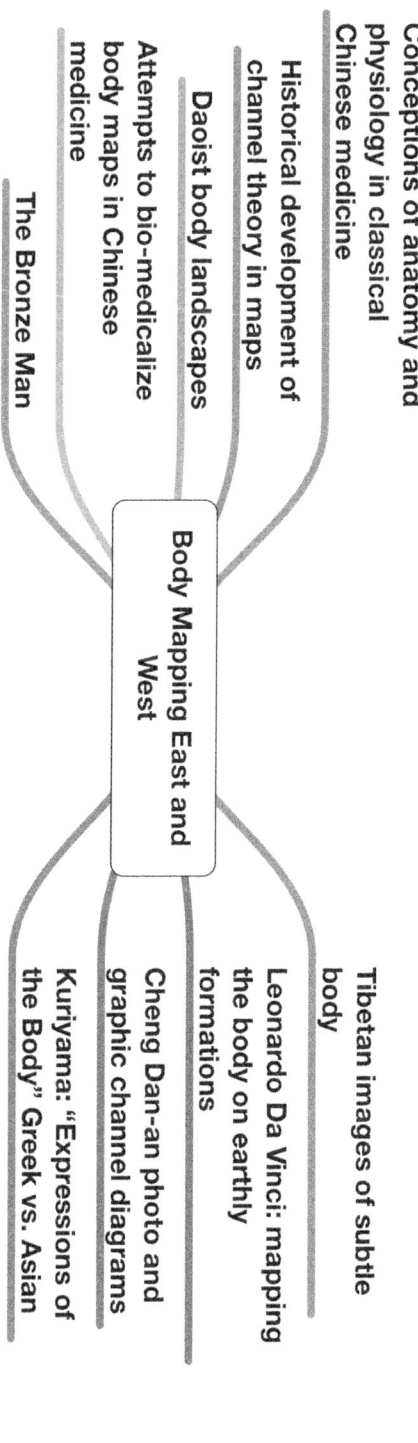

Conceptions of anatomy and physiology in classical Chinese medicine

Historical development of channel theory in maps

Daoist body landscapes

Attempts to bio-medicalize body maps in Chinese medicine

The Bronze Man

Body Mapping East and West

Tibetan images of subtle body

Leonardo Da Vinci: mapping the body on earthly formations

Cheng Dan-an photo and graphic channel diagrams

Kuriyama: "Expressions of the Body" Greek vs. Asian

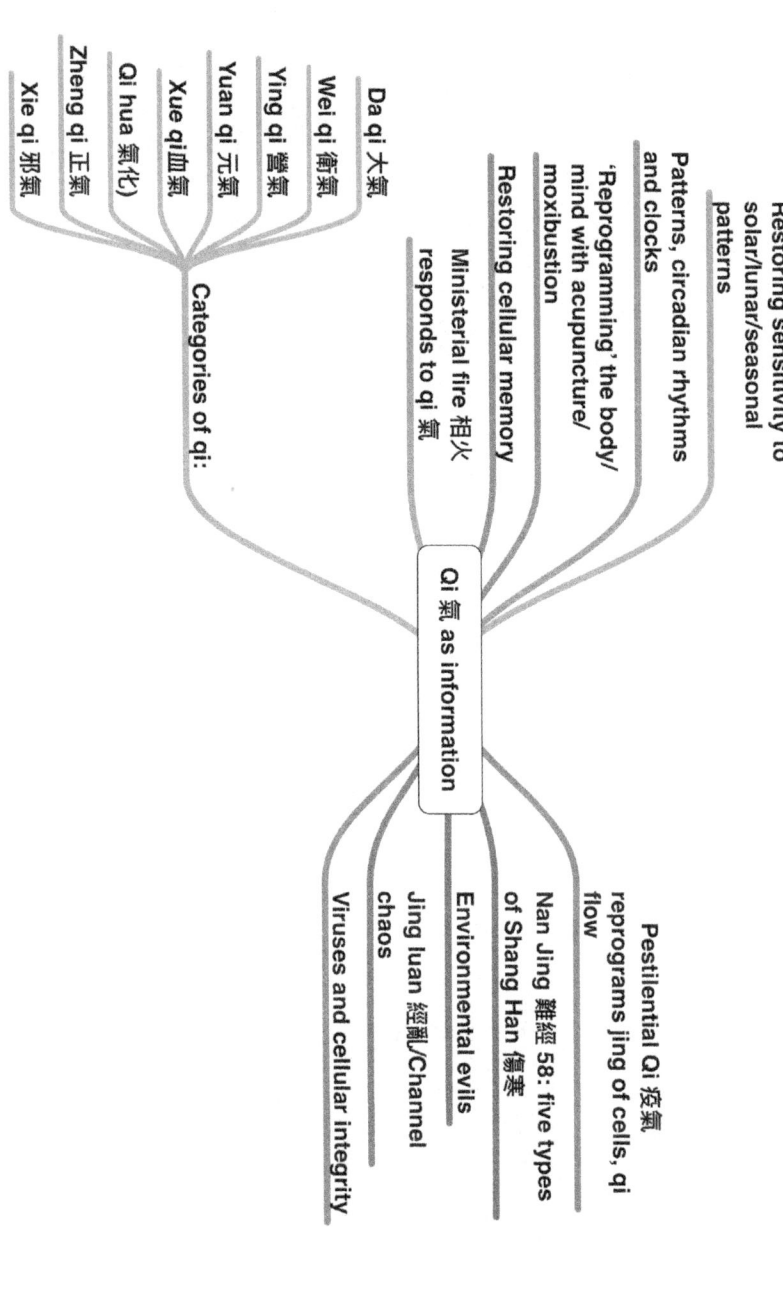

Qi 氣 as information

Restoring sensitivity to solar/lunar/seasonal patterns

Patterns, circadian rhythms and clocks

'Reprogramming' the body/mind with acupuncture/moxibustion

Restoring cellular memory

Ministerial fire 相火 responds to qi 氣

Pestilential Qi 疫氣, reprograms jing of cells, qi flow

Nan Jing 難經 58: five types of Shang Han 傷寒

Environmental evils

Jing luan 經亂/Channel chaos

Viruses and cellular integrity

Categories of qi:

Da qi 大氣

Wei qi 衛氣

Ying qi 營氣

Yuan qi 元氣

Xue qi 血氣

Qi hua 氣化

Zheng qi 正氣

Xie qi 邪氣

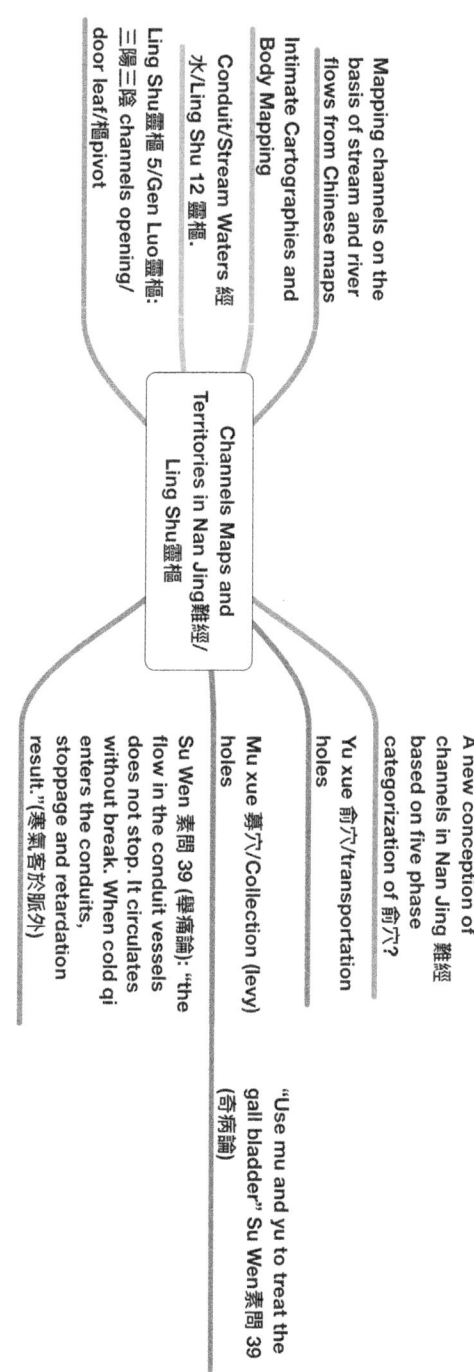

Mapping channels on the basis of stream and river flows from Chinese maps

Intimate Cartographies and Body Mapping

Conduit/Stream Waters 經水/Ling Shu 靈樞 12 靈樞.

Ling Shu 靈樞 5/Gen Luo 靈樞: 三陽三陰 channels opening/door leaf/樞pivot

Channels Maps and Territories in Nan Jing 難經/Ling Shu 靈樞

A new conception of channels in Nan Jing 難經 based on five phase categorization of 前穴?

Yu xue 前穴/transportation holes

Mu xue 募穴/Collection (levy) holes

Su Wen 素問 39 (舉痛論): "the flow in the conduit vessels does not stop. It circulates without break. When cold qi enters the conduits, stoppage and retardation result."(塞氣客於脈外)

"Use mu and yu to treat the gall bladder" Su Wen素問 39 (奇病論)

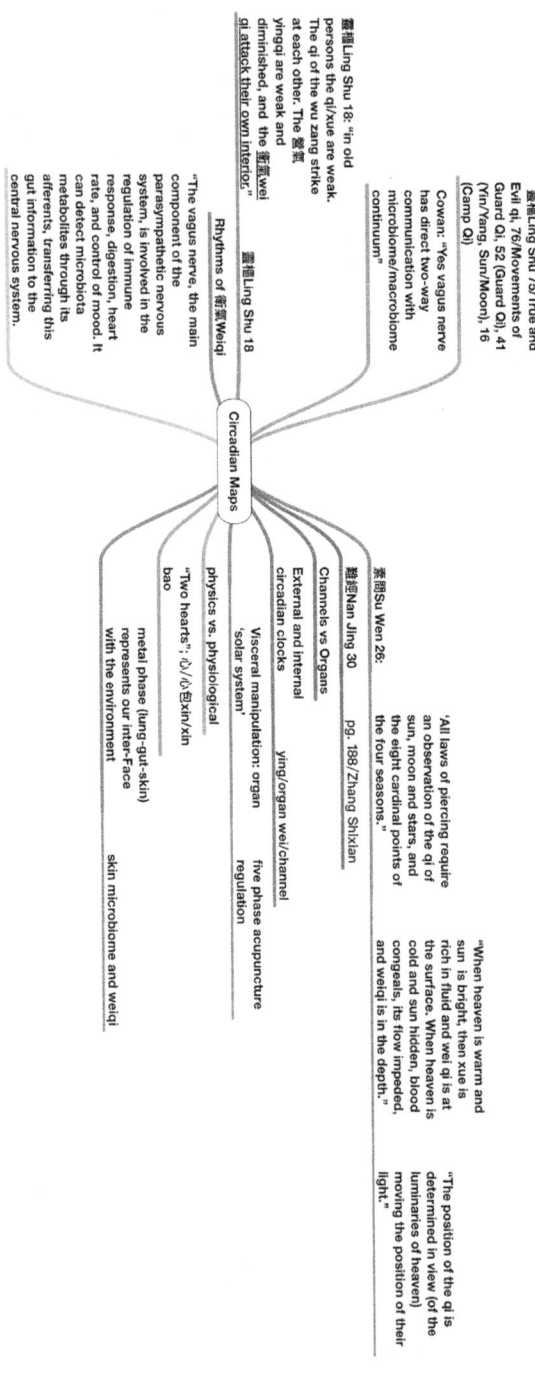

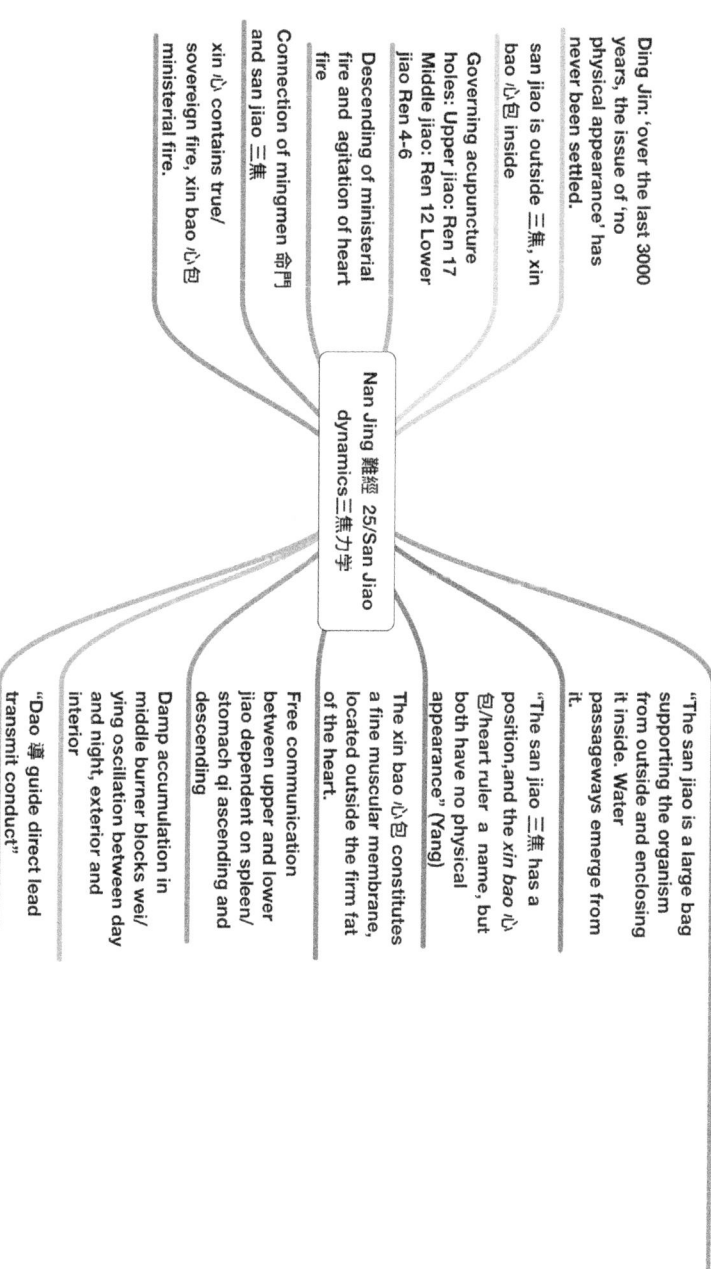

Nan Jing 難經 25/San Jiao dynamics 三焦力学

Ding Jin: 'over the last 3000 years, the issue of 'no physical appearance' has never been settled.

san jiao is outside 三焦, xin bao 心包 inside

Governing acupuncture holes: Upper jiao: Ren 17 Middle jiao: Ren 12 Lower jiao Ren 4-6

Descending of ministerial fire and agitation of heart fire

Connection of mingmen 命門 and san jiao 三集

xin 心 contains true/ sovereign fire, xin bao 心包 ministerial fire.

"Dao 導 guide direct lead transmit conduct"

Damp accumulation in middle burner blocks wei/ ying oscillation between day and night, exterior and interior

Free communication between upper and lower jiao dependent on spleen/ stomach qi ascending and descending

The xin bao 心包 constitutes a fine muscular membrane, located outside the firm fat of the heart.

"The san jiao 三焦 has a position, and the xin bao 心 包/heart ruler a name, but both have no physical appearance" (Yang)

"The san jiao is a large bag supporting the organism from outside and enclosing it inside. Water passageways emerge from it.

as long as the heart is firm and stable, it will not accept evil qi

Whenever evil qi is present in the heart, it is always in the xin tao

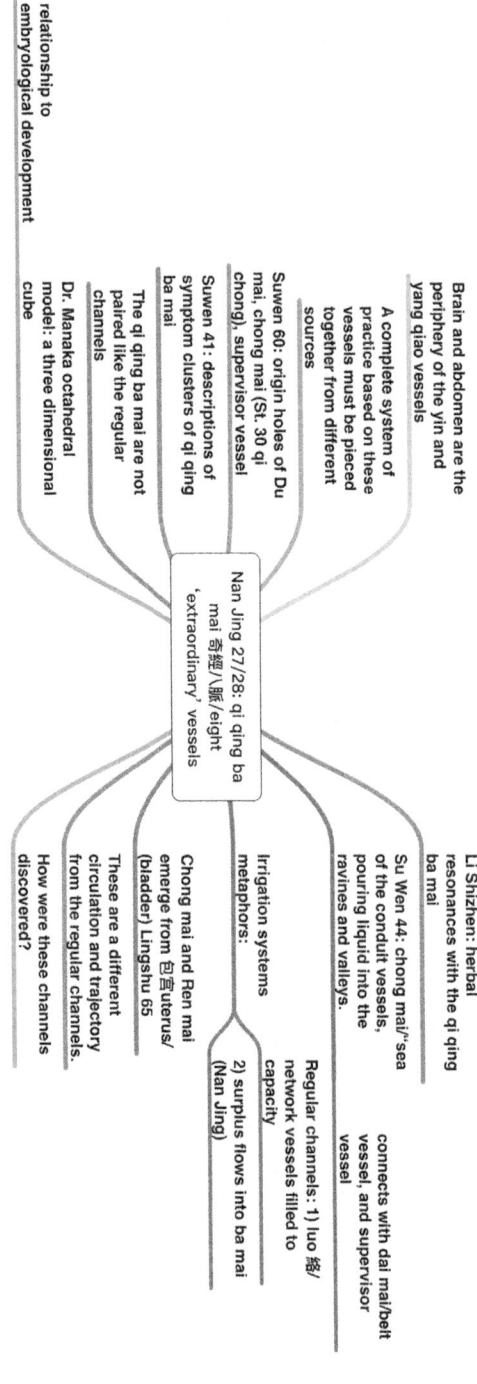

Nan Jing 27/28: qi qing ba mai 奇經/脈/eight 'extraordinary' vessels

Brain and abdomen are the periphery of the yin and yang qiao vessels

A complete system of practice based on these vessels must be pieced together from different sources

Suwen 60: origin holes of Du mai, chong mai (St. 30 qi chong), supervisor vessel

Suwen 41: descriptions of symptom clusters of qi qing ba mai

The qi qing ba mai are not paired like the regular channels

Dr. Manaka octahedral model: a three dimensional cube

relationship to embryological development

Li Shizhen: herbal resonances with the qi qing ba mai

Su Wen 44: chong mai/"sea of the conduit vessels, pouring liquid into the ravines and valleys.

connects with dai mai/belt vessel, and supervisor vessel

Regular channels: 1) luo 絡/network vessels filled to capacity

2) surplus flows into ba mai (Nan Jing)

Irrigation systems metaphors:

Chong mai and Ren mai emerge from 包宫/uterus/(bladder) Lingshu 65

These are a different circulation and trajectory from the regular channels.

How were these channels discovered?

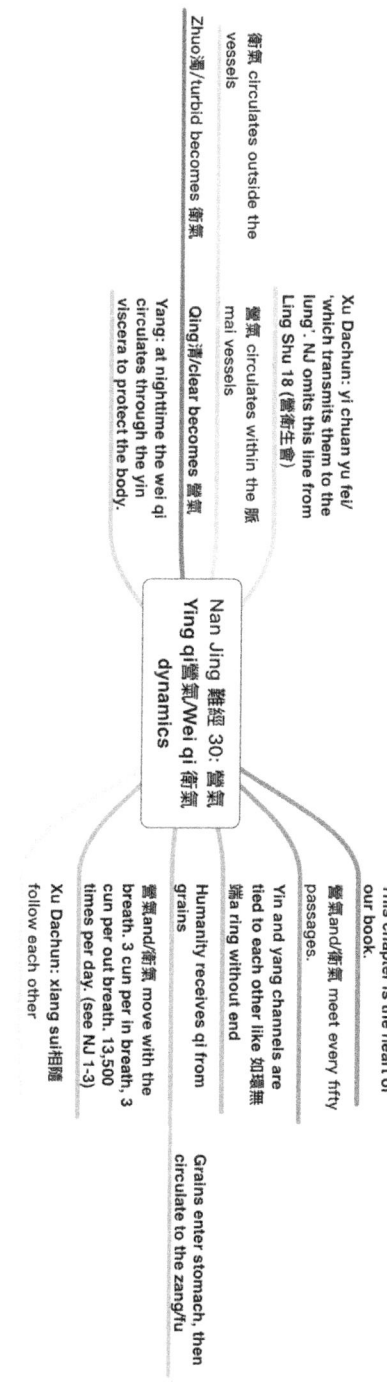

Zhuo濁/turbid becomes 衛氣

衛氣 circulates outside the vessels

Xu Dachun: yí chuan yu fei/ 'which transmits them to the lung : NJ omits this line from Ling Shu 18 (營衛生會)

營氣 circulates within the 脈 mai vessels

Qing清/clear becomes 營氣

Yang: at nighttime the wei qi circulates through the yin viscera to protect the body.

Nan Jing 難經 30: Ying qi營氣/Wei qi 衛氣, dynamics

This chapter is the heart of our book.

營氣 and/衛氣 meet every fifty passages.

Yin and yang channels are tied to each other like 如環無 端 a ring without end

Humanity receives qi from grains

營氣 and/衛氣 move with the breath, 3 cun per in breath, 3 cun per out breath, 13,500 times per day. (see NJ 1-3)

Grains enter stomach, then circulate to the zang/fu

Xu Dachun: xiang sui相隨 follow each other

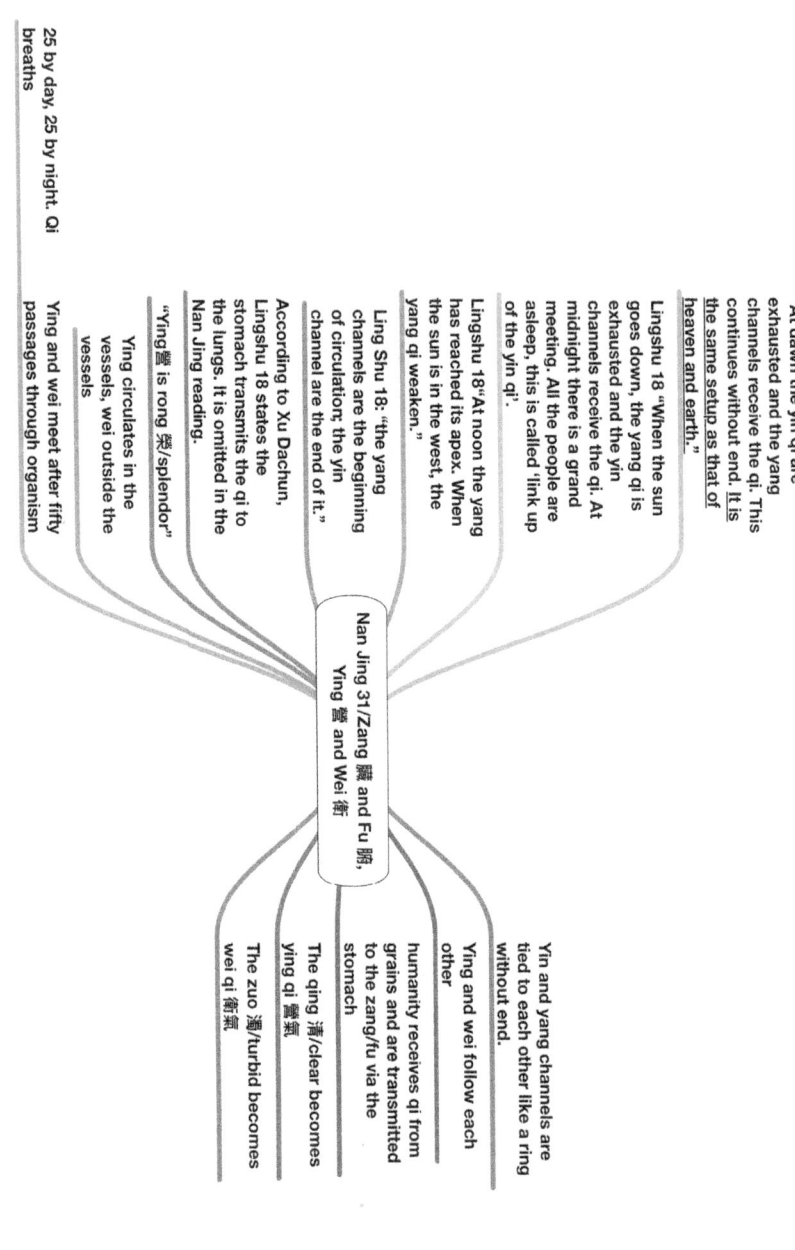

Nan Jing 31/Zang 臟 and Fu 腑, Ying 營 and Wei 衛

"At dawn the yin qi are exhausted and the yang channels receive the qi. This continues without end. It is the same setup as that of heaven and earth."

Lingshu 18 "When the sun goes down, the yang qi is exhausted and the yin channels receive the qi. At midnight there is a grand meeting. All the people are asleep, this is called 'link up of the yin qi'.

Lingshu 18 "At noon the yang has reached its apex. When the sun is in the west, the yang qi weaken."

Ling Shu 18: "the yang channels are the beginning of circulation; the yin channel are the end of it."

According to Xu Dachun, Lingshu 18 states the stomach transmits the qi to the lungs. It is omitted in the Nan Jing reading.

"Ying 營 is rong 榮/splendor"

Ying circulates in the vessels, wei outside the vessels

Ying and wei meet after fifty passages through organism

25 by day, 25 by night. Qi breaths

Yin and yang channels are tied to each other like a ring without end.

Ying and wei follow each other

humanity receives qi from grains and are transmitted to the zang/fu via the stomach

The qing 清/clear becomes ying qi 營氣

The zuo 濁/turbid becomes wei qi 衛氣

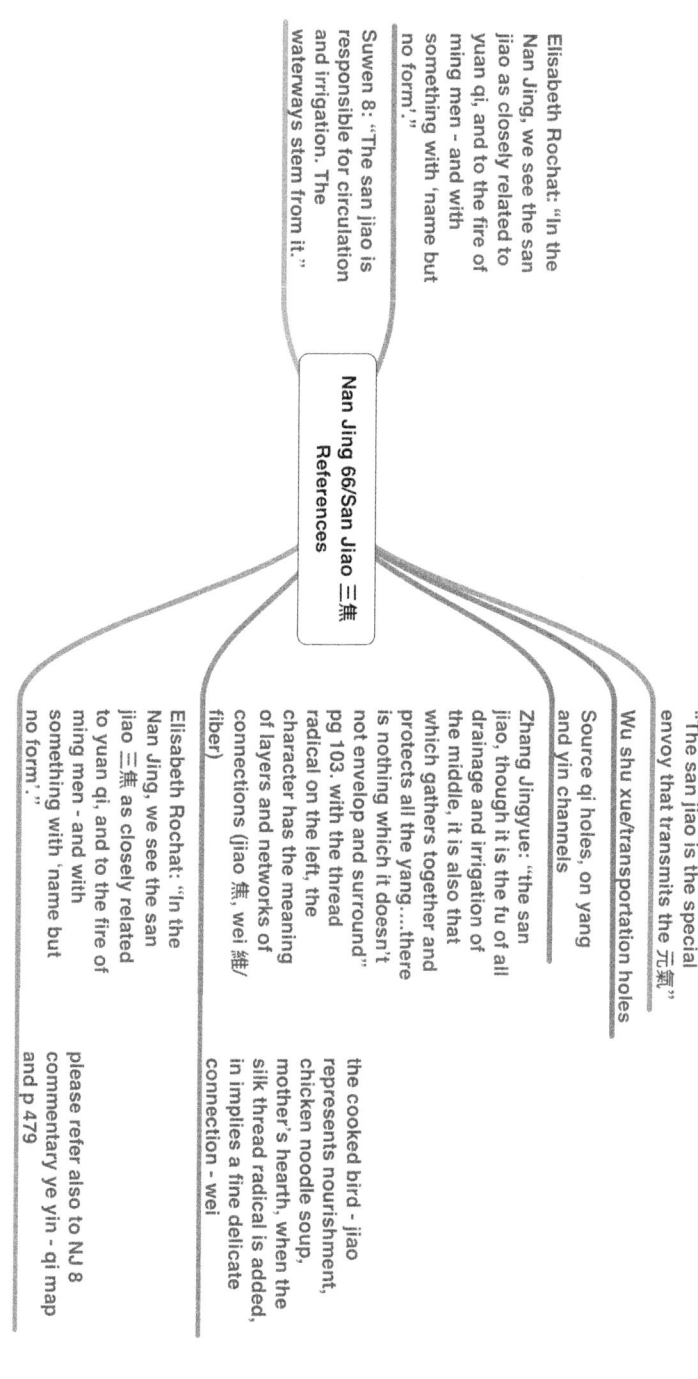

Nan Jing 66/San Jiao 三焦 References

Elisabeth Rochat: "In the Nan Jing, we see the san jiao as closely related to yuan qi, and to the fire of ming men - and with something with 'name but no form'."

Suwen 8: "The san jiao is responsible for circulation and irrigation. The waterways stem from it."

"The san jiao is the special envoy that transmits the 元氣"

Wu shu xue/transportation holes

Source qi holes, on yang and yin channels

Zhang Jingyue: "the san jiao, though it is the fu of all drainage and irrigation of the middle, it is also that which gathers together and protects all the yang....there is nothing which it doesn't not envelop and surround" pg 103. with the thread radical on the left, the character has the meaning of layers and networks of connections (jiao 焦, wei 維/ fiber)

the cooked bird - jiao represents nourishment, chicken noodle soup, mother's hearth, when the silk thread radical is added, in implies a fine delicate connection - wei

Elisabeth Rochat: "In the Nan Jing, we see the san jiao 三焦 as closely related to yuan qi, and to the fire of ming men - and with something with 'name but no form'."

please refer also to NJ 8 commentary ye yin - qi map and p 479

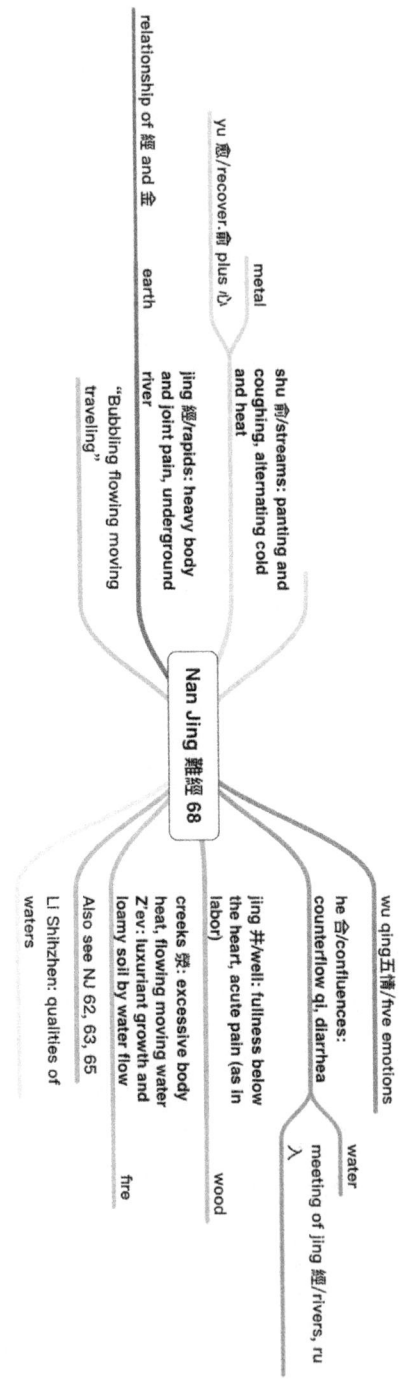

relationship of 經 and 金

yu 愈/recover.前 plus 心

metal

shu 劑/streams: panting and
coughing, alternating cold
and heat

jing 經/rapids: heavy body
and joint pain, underground
river

earth

"Bubbling flowing moving
traveling"

Nan Jing 難經 68

wu qing五情/five emotions

he 合/confluences:
counterflow qi, diarrhea

jing 井/well: fullness below
the heart, acute pain (as in
labor)

creeks 滎:
heat, flowing moving water

Z ev: luxuriant growth and
loamy soil by water flow

Also see NJ 62, 63, 65

LI Shizhen: qualities of
waters

water

meeting of jing 經/rivers, ru
入

wood

fire

References

Adler, Joseph Alan. *Reconstructing the Confucian dao: Zhu Xi's appropriation of Zhou Dunyi.* Albany, NY: State University of New York Press, 2014.

Ames, Roger. T. (1989). *Putting the Te Back into Taoism.* In C. J. Baird, & A. R. T. Albany (Eds.), Nature in Asian Traditions of Thought: Essays in Environmental Philosophy (pp. 113-44). New York: State University of New York Press.

Ames, Roger T. *"The Great Commentary (Dazhuan 大傳) and Chinese Natural Cosmology." International Communication of Chinese Culture* 2, no. 1 (March 5, 2015): 1–18. https://doi.org/10.1007/s40636-015-0013-2.

Ames, Roger T. *Confucian role ethics: A vocabulary.* Albany, NY: State University of New York Press, 2020.

Ames, Roger T., and David L. Hall. *Dao De Jing: Making this life significant: A philosophical translation.* New York, NY: Ballantine Books, 2003.

Bateson, Gregory. *Mind and nature: A necessary unity.* Cresskill, NJ: Hampton Press, 1979.

Bray, Francesca, Vera Dorofeeva-Lichtmann, and Georges Métailie. *Graphics and text in the production of technical knowledge in China: The warp and the weft.* Leiden: Brill, 2007.

Buell, Paul D., and Eugene Newton Anderson. *Arabic medicine in China: Tradition, innovation, and change.* Leiden: Brill, 2021.

Camazine, Scott, Jean-Louis Deneubourg, Nigel Franks, James Sneyd, Guy Theraulaz, and Eric Bonabeau. *Self-organization in Biological Systems .* Princeton, NJ: Princeton University Press, 2001.

Capra, Fritjof. "What We Can Learn from Leonardo." ecoliteracy.org, November 10, 2010. https://www.ecoliteracy.org/article/what-we-can-learn-leonardo.

Ceurvels, Will. An archaeology of the Qiao vessels. Purple Cloud Press, 2021.

Chace, Charles, Miki Shima, and Shizhen Li. *An exposition on the Eight extraordinary vessels: Acupuncture, Alchemy, and Herbal Medicine.* Seattle, WA: Eastland Press, 2010.

Chan, Alan Kam-leung, and Yuet Keung Lo. *Philosophy and religion in early medieval China.* Albany, NY: State University of New York Press, 2010.

Cheng, Man-Ch'ing. *T'ai chi ch'uan: A simplified method of calisthenics for Health and self-defense.* Taipei, Taiwan: Shih Chung Tai-chi Chuan Center, 1961.

Chipps, Bradley E. "Randomized Trial of Peanut Consumption in Infants at Risk for Peanut Allergy." *Pediatrics* 136, no. Supplement_3 (December 1, 2015). https://doi.org/10.1542/peds.2015-2776ff.

Cooper, K. E. "Some Historical Perspectives on Thermoregulation." *Journal of Applied Physiology* 92, no. 4 (April 1, 2002): 1717–24. https://doi.org/10.1152/japplphysiol.01051.2001.

Damasio, Antonio R. The Strange Order of Things: Life, feeling, and the making of Cultures. New York, NY: Random House Audio, 2018.

Danchin, Antoine. *The delphic boat: What genomes tell us*. Cambridge, MA: Harvard University Press, 2003.

"Do My Cells Really Change Every 7 Years?" Quest Diagnostics, February 21, 2023. https://www.questdiagnostics.com/patients/blog/articles/do-my-cells-really-change-every-7-years.

Dweck, Carol S. *Mindset: The New Psychology of Success*. New York, NY: Ballantine Books, 2007.

Foucault, Michael. *The Birth of the Clinic: An Archaeology of Medical Perception*. New York, NY: Vintage Books, 1975.

Farquhar, Judith. *A way of life: Things, thought, and action in Chinese medicine*. New Haven, CT: Yale University Press, 2020.

Friedman, Danielle. "Your Medical Test Results Are Available. but Do You Want to View Them?" The New York Times, October 3, 2022. https://www.nytimes.com/2022/10/03/well/live/medical-test-results-cures-act.html.

Garner, Andrew, and Michael Yogman. "Preventing Childhood Toxic Stress: Partnering with Families and Communities to Promote Relational Health." *Pediatrics* 148, no. 2 (August 1, 2021). https://doi.org/10.1542/peds.2021-052582.

Gregory, Richard L. *Even odder perceptions*. London: Routledge, 1994.

Gregory, Richard. "DNA in the Mind's Eye." *Nature* VOL 368, no. Spring, March 21, 1994.

Guidi, Jenny, Marcella Lucente, Nicoletta Sonino, and Giovanni A. Fava. "Allostatic Load and Its Impact on Health: A Systematic Review." *Psychotherapy and Psychosomatics* 90, no. 1 (August 14, 2020): 11–27. https://doi.org/10.1159/000510696.

Gyatso, Janet. *Being human in a Buddhist world: An intellectual history of medicine in early modern tibet*. New York, NY: Columbia University Press, 2017.

Hablitz, Lauren M., and Maiken Nedergaard. "The Glymphatic System: A Novel Component of Fundamental Neurobiology." *The Journal of Neuroscience* 41, no. 37 (September 15, 2021): 7698–7711. https://doi.org/10.1523/jneurosci.0619-21.2021.

Hall, David L., and Roger T. Ames. *Thinking from the Han: Self, truth, and transcendence in Chinese and Western culture*. Albany, NY: State University of New York Press, 1998.

"The Healthy Human Microbiome." National Institutes of Health, November 28, 2018. https://www.nih.gov/news-events/nih-research-matters/healthy-human-microbiome.

Hilton, M.F., M.U. Umali, C.A. Czeisler, J.K. Wyatt, and S.A. Shea. "Endogenous Circadian Control of the Human Autonomic Nervous System." *Computers in Cardiology* Vol.27 (2000): 197–200. https://doi.org/10.1109/cic.2000.898490.

Hinton, David, and Zhuangzi. *Chuang Tzu. the inner chapters*. Berkeley, CA: Counterpoint, 1997.

Hippocrates. "The Internet Classics Archive: On Airs, Waters, and Places by Hippocrates." The Internet Classics Archive | On Airs, Waters, and Places by Hippocrates. Accessed December 23, 2024. http://classics.mit.edu/Hippocrates/airwatpl.html.

Hsu, Elisabeth. *The transmission of Chinese medicine*. Cambridge, UK: Cambridge University Press, 2004.

Hsu, Elisabeth. "A Hybrid Body Technique: Does the Pulse Diagnostic Cun Guan Chi Method Have Chinese-Tibetan Origins?" *Gesnerus* 65, no. 1–2 (November 11, 2008): 5–29. https://doi.org/10.1163/22977953-0650102001.

Hsu, Elisabeth. *Pulse diagnosis in early chinese medicine: The telling touch*. Cambridge, United Kingdom: Cambridge University Press, 2010.

Huang, Shih-shan Susan. Picturing the true form: Daoist visual culture in traditional China. Cambridge, MA: Harvard University Asia Center, 2015.

Hughes, Patrick A, Heddy Zola, Irmeli A Penttila, Ashley L Blackshaw, Jane M Andrews, and Doreen Krumbiegel. "Immune Activation in Irritable Bowel Syndrome: Can Neuroimmune Interactions Explain Symptoms?" *American Journal of Gastroenterology* 108, no. 7 (July 2013): 1066–74. https://doi.org/10.1038/ajg.2013.120.

Imada, Toshie, Stephanie M. Carlson, and Shoji Itakura. "East–West Cultural Differences in Context-sensitivity Are Evident in Early Childhood." *Developmental Science* 16, no. 2 (December 20, 2012): 198–208. https://doi.org/10.1111/desc.12016.

Jacob, François. *The possible and the actual*. Seattle, WA: University of Washington Press, 1982.

Jacobsen, Rowan. "Against Sunscreen Absolutism." The Atlantic, May 29, 2024. https://www.theatlantic.com/magazine/archive/2024/06/sun-exposure-health-benefits/678205/.

Jullien, François. *The book of beginnings*. Translated by Jody Gladding. New Haven, CT: Yale University Press, 2015.

Jullien, François. *The propensity of things: Toward a history of efficacy in China*. New York, NY: Zone Books ; MIT Press (distributor), 1999.

Kaibara, Ekiken, and Mary Evelyn Tucker. *The Philosophy of Qi: The Record of great doubts*. New York, NY: Columbia University Press, 2007

Kaptchuk, Ted J. *The web that has no weaver: Understanding chinese medicine*. Chicago, IL: Contemporary Books, 2000.

KC, Ashish, Nisha Rana, Mats Målqvist, Linda Jarawka Ranneberg, Kalpana Subedi, and Ola Andersson. "Effects of Delayed Umbilical Cord Clamping vs Early Clamping on Anemia in Infants at 8 and 12 Months." *JAMA Pediatrics* 171, no. 3 (March 1, 2017): 264. https://doi.org/10.1001/jamapediatrics.2016.3971.

Kemp, Martin. *Leonardo da Vinci: Experience, experiment and Design*. London: V & A Publications, 2006.

Kleidon, Axel. "How Does the Earth System Generate and Maintain Thermodynamic Disequilibrium and What Does It Imply for the Future of the

Planet?" *Philosophical Transactions of the Royal Society A: Mathematical, Physical and Engineering Sciences* 370, no. 1962 (March 13, 2012): 1012–40. https://doi.org/10.1098/rsta.2011.0316.

Köhle, Natalie, and Shigehisa Kuriyama. "Fluid Matter(s): Flow and Transformation in the History of Medicine. Edited by Natalie Köhle and Shigehisa Kuriyama. Introduction." ANU Press. https://press-files.anu.edu.au/downloads/press/n7034/html/02-introduction/index.html#group-1-What-is-a-Body-xH1E6VjLtd.

Komjathy, Louis. *The Daoist tradition.* New York, NY: Bloomsbury Publishing, 2013.

Komjathy, Louis. Traces of a Daoist immortal: Chén tuán 陳摶 of the western marchmount. Leiden: Brill, 2024.

Komjathy, Louis. "Electronic Supplement to Traces of a Daoist Immortal." ALTERNATE HOMEPAGE OF DR. LOUIS KOMJATHY. https://louiskomjathy.com/wp-content/uploads/2024/05/DaoistTimeMachineBlueprints_Komjathy.pdf.

Korzybski, Alfred. *Science and sanity: An introduction to non-Aristotelian Systems and general semantics. introduction to the second edition.* Chicago, IL: Institute of General Semantics, 1941.

Kuriyama, Shigehisa. *The expressiveness of the body and the divergence of Greek and chinese medicine.* New York, NY: Zone Books, 1999.

Kuriyama, Shigehisa. *"The Imagination of the Body and the History of Embodied Experience: Chinese Views of the Viscera." Shigehisa Kuriyama Ed., The Imagination of the Body and the History of Bodily Experience (Kyoto: International Research Center for Japanese Studies, 2001), 17-29. , 2001.*

Kwok, Man-Ho. *Complete Chinese horoscopes.* London, UK: Sunburst Books, 1995.

Lackner, Michael. "4. Diagrams as an Architecture by Means of Words: The Yanji Tu." *Graphics and Text in the Production of Technical Knowledge in China,* January 1, 2007, 341–77. https://doi.org/10.1163/ej.9789004160637.i-772.50.

Lan, Fengli, and Friedrich Wallner. *Metaphor the weaver of Chinese medicine.* Nordhausen: Verlag Traugott Bautz GmbH, 2015.

Larre, Claude, Elisabeth Rochat de la Vallée, and Caroline Root. *Essence, spirit, blood and qi.* Cambridge, England: Monkey Press, 1999.

Lehrer, Jonah. "Trials and Errors: Why Science Is Failing Us." Wired, December 16, 2011. https://www.wired.com/2011/12/ff-causation/.

Li, Gao, and Bob Flaws. *Li Dong-Yuan's treatise on the Spleen & Stomach: A translation of the Pi Wei Lun.* Boulder, CO: Blue Poppy Press, 2004.

Liu, Lihong. *Classical Chinese medicine.* Edited by Heiner Fruehauf. Translated by Sabine Wilms, Henry Buchtel, and Gabriel Weiss. Hong Kong: The Chinese University Press, 2019.

"Liver: Anatomy and Functions." Johns Hopkins Medicine, November 19, 2019. https://www.hopkinsmedicine.org/health/conditions-and-diseases/liver-anatomy-and-functions.

Lo, Vivienne, and Penelope Barrett. *Imagining chinese medicine.* Leiden: Brill, 2018.

Loewenstein, Werner R. *The Touchstone of Life: Molecular Information, cell communication, and the foundations of life*. New York, NY: Oxford University Press, 2000.

Marco-Gracia, Francisco J. "The Influence of the Lunar Cycle on Spontaneous Deliveries in Historical Rural Environments." *European Journal of Obstetrics & Gynecology and Reproductive Biology* 236 (May 2019): 22–25. https://doi.org/10.1016/j.ejogrb.2019.02.020.

Masuda, Takahiko, and Richard E. Nisbett. "Attending Holistically versus Analytically: Comparing the Context Sensitivity of Japanese and Americans." *Journal of Personality and Social Psychology* 81, no. 5 (2001): 922–34. https://doi.org/10.1037//0022-3514.81.5.922.

Matsumoto, Shin-ichiro, and Kiyohiko Shirahashi. "Novel Perspectives on the Influence of the Lunar Cycle on the Timing of Full-Term Human Births." *Chronobiology International* 37, no. 7 (July 2, 2020): 1082–89. https://doi.org/10.1080/07420528.2020.1785485.

McMahon, Bryan. "Circular Dynamics of Ancient Chinese Medicine I." The Wandering Cloud ACM, January 24, 2020. https://www.thewanderingcloud.com/the-archives/circulardynamics1?rq=Circular+dynamics+of+ancient+Chinese+Medicine+I.

Nakayama, Shigeru. Academic and scientific traditions in China, Japan, and the West. Tokyo, Japan: University of Tokyo Press, 1984.

Needham, Joseph. *Science and civilisation in China: Vol. Physics and Physical Technology: Part III: Civil Engineering and Nautics*. Cambridge: Cambridge University Press, 1971.

Neumann, Gabriele, and Yoshihiro Kawaoka. "Seasonality of Influenza and Other Respiratory Viruses." *EMBO Molecular Medicine* 14, no. 4 (February 14, 2022). https://doi.org/10.15252/emmm.202115352.

Nield, David. "Keeping the Body's Multiple Clocks in Sync Could Be the Secret to Slowing Aging." ScienceAlert, May 6, 2024. https://www.sciencealert.com/keeping-the-bodys-multiple-clocks-in-sync-could-be-the-secret-to-slowing-aging.

Ortega, Marcus V., Michael K. Hidrue, Sara R. Lehrhoff, Dan B. Ellis, Rachel C. Sisodia, William T. Curry, Marcela G. del Carmen, and Jason H. Wasfy. "Patterns in Physician Burnout in a Stable-Linked Cohort." *JAMA Network Open* 6, no. 10 (October 6, 2023). https://doi.org/10.1001/jamanetworkopen.2023.36745.

Peng Ziyi 彭子益. 2007. Yuandong de gu zhongyi xue 圓動的古中醫學, p.1. Translated by Bryan McMahon,2019, as "Circular dynamics of ancient Chinese Medicine I" and available at https://www.thewanderingcloud.com/

Porter, Bill. Road to heaven: Encounters with chinese hermits. San Francisco , VA: Mercury House, 1993.

Rochat de la Vallée, Elisabeth. *The double aspect of the heart*. Cambridge, UK: Monkey Press, 2012.

Rogers, Carl R. *On becoming a person: A therapist's view of psychotherapy*. Boston, MA: Houghton Mifflin, 1961.

Rosenberg, Z'ev. *Returning to the source: Han Dynasty Medical Classics in modern clinical practice*. London, UK: Singing Dragon, 2018.

Rosenberg, Z'ev. *Ripples in the flow: Reflections on vessel dynamics in the nàn jīng*. London, UK: Singing Dragon, 2019.

Rosenberg, Z'ev. *Afterglow: Ministerial fire and Chinese Ecological Medicine*. London, UK: Singing Dragon, 2023.

Rosenberg, Z'ev. "Meditations on Dìng Zhì Wán 定志丸 (Settle the Emotions Pill)." Journal of Chinese Medicine, no. Issue 135 (June 2024): 48–51.

Roshi, Susan Murphy. "Earth as Koan, Earth as Self – with Susan Murphy Roshi." Emergence Magazine, October 3, 2024. https://emergencemagazine.org/interview/earth-as-koan-earth-as-self/.

Rovelli, Carlo, Simon Carnell, and Erica Segre. *Reality is not what it seems: The journey to quantum gravity*. New York, NY: Riverhead Books, 2018.

Schatz, Jean, Claude Larre, and Elisabeth Rochat de la Vallée. *Survey of traditional chinese medicine*. Columbia, MD: L'Institut Ricci ; Traditional Acupuncture Foundation, 1986.

Scheid , Volker, and Tieqiao Yun. "Yun Tieqiao and the Disappearance of the Body from Chinese Medicine." Volkerscheid.net, October 21, 2020. https://www.volkerscheid.net/post/yun-tieqiao-and-the-disappearance-of-the-body-from-chinese-medicine.

Schipper, Kristofer. *The Taoist body*. Berkeley, CA: University of California Press, 1993.

Schroën, Jan H.T. "Non-Linear Dynamics and Chinese Medicine: An Essay on Research Models, TCM, and Recent Changes in Modern Scientific Philosophy." *Clinical Acupuncture and Oriental Medicine* 3, no. 2 (June 2002): 92–98. https://doi.org/10.1054/caom.2002.0004.

Shaffer, Fred, and J. P. Ginsberg. "An Overview of Heart Rate Variability Metrics and Norms." *Frontiers in Public Health*, 5:258 (September 28, 2017). https://doi.org/10.3389/fpubh.2017.00258.

Shi, Yunli. "The Astronomical Meaning of Some Jade Artifacts Unearthed at the Lingjiatan Site. 2: The Jade Pigs." *Journal of Astronomical History and Heritage* 27, no. 3 (September 1, 2024): 503–20. https://doi.org/10.3724/sp.j.1440-2807.2024.03.05.

Shima, Miki, and Charles Chace. *The channel divergences: Deeper pathways of the web*. Boulder, CO: Blue Poppy Press, 2005.

Shoja, Mohammadali M., R. Shane Tubbs, Ghaffar Shokouhi, and Marios Loukas. "Wang Qingren and the 19th Century Chinese Doctrine of the Bloodless Heart." *International Journal of Cardiology* 145, no. 2 (November 2010): 305–6. https://doi.org/10.1016/j.ijcard.2009.10.042.

Shubin, Neil. *The universe within: Discovering the common history of rocks, planets, and people*. New York, New York: Pantheon Books, 2013.

Simon, Paul. *Mother and child reunion*. Vinyl recording. *Paul Simon*. Roy Halee & Paul Simon, n.d. 1972

Smets, Hugo, Lars Stumpp, Javier Chavez, Joaquin Cury, Louis Vande Perre, Pascal Doguet, Anne Vanhoestenberghe, Jean Delbeke, Riëm El Tahry, and Antoine Nonclercq. "Chronic Recording of the Vagus Nerve to Analyze Modulations by the Light–Dark Cycle." *Journal of Neural Engineering* 19, no. 4 (July 8, 2022): 046008. https://doi.org/10.1088/1741-2552/ac7c8f.

Snyder, Gary, and Robert Hass. *The practice of the wild: Essays*. Berkeley, CA: Counterpoint, 2020.

Strachan, D. P. "Hay Fever, Hygiene, and Household Size." *BMJ* 299, no. 6710 (November 18, 1989): 1259–60. https://doi.org/10.1136/bmj.299.6710.1259.

莊蕙芷，〈得「意」忘「形」- 漢墓壁畫中天象圖的轉變過程研究〉，《南藝學報》8：1-42 (2014)

Sun, Bin, D. C. Lau, and Roger T. Ames. *Sun Pin: The art of warfare*. New York, NY: Ballantine Books, 1996.

Tarnas, Richard. Cosmos and psyche: Intimations of a new world view. New York, NY: Plume, 2014.

"Tensegrity." Wikipedia, July 3, 2024. https://en.wikipedia.org/wiki/Tensegrity.

Theise, Neil. *Notes on complexity: A scientific theory of connection, consciousness, and being*. New York, NY: Spiegel & Grau, 2023.

Thompson, J. Michael, and Jan Sieber. "Climate Predictions: The Influence of Nonlinearity and Randomness." *Philosophical Transactions of the Royal Society A. Mathematical, Physical and Engineering Sciences* 370, no. 1962 (March 13, 2012): 1007–11. https://doi.org/10.1098/rsta.2011.0423.

Trungpa, Chögyam, and Sherab Chödzin. *Orderly chaos: The mandala principle*. Boston, MA: Shambhala Publications, 1991.

Unschuld, Paul U. *Nan-ching: The classic of difficult issues*. Berkley, CA: University of California Press, 1986.

Unschuld, Paul U. *Medicine in China: Historical artifacts and images*. Munich, Germany: Prestel, 2000.

Unschuld, Paul U. *What is medicine?: Western and eastern approaches to healing*. Berkeley, CA: University of California Press, 2009.

Unschuld, Paul U. *Medicine in China: A history of ideas*. Berkeley, CA: University of California Press, 2010.

Unschuld, Paul U. *Huang Di Nei Jing Ling Shu: The ancient classic on needle therapy*. Berkeley, CA: University of California Press, 2016.

Unschuld, Paul U. *Nan Jing: The classic of difficult issues*. Berkeley, CA: University of California Press, 2016.

Unschuld, Paul U., Hermann Tessenow, and Jinsheng Zheng. *Huang Di Nei Jing Su Wen: An annotated translation of Huang Di's inner classic - basic questions, 2 volumes*. Berkeley, CA: University of California Press, 2011.

Van Drunen, Rachel, and Kristin Eckel-Mahan. "Circadian Rhythms as Modulators of Brain Health during Development and throughout Aging." *Frontiers in Neural Circuits* 16 (January 19, 2023). https://doi.org/10.3389/fncir.2022.1059229

Varela, Francisco. "Chapter 12 'The Emergent Self.'" Edge.org. Accessed December 21, 2024. https://www.edge.org/conversation/francisco_varela-chapter-12-the-emergent-self.

Vesalius, Andreas. *De humani corporis fabrica libri septem*. Basileae: Ex officina Joannis Oporini, 1543.

Walters, Derek. The Complete Guide to Chinese astrology. London, UK: Watkins, 2005.

Wang, Fangyu, Suzanne Graham Storer, Mary de G. White, and Wei Wang. *Walking to where the river ends*. Hamden, CT: Archon/The Shoe String Press, 1980.

Wang, Ju-Yi, and Jason D. Robertson. *Applied Channel Theory in chinese medicine: Wang Ju-Yi's lectures on Channel Therapeutics*. Seattle, WA: Eastland Press, 2008.

Watson, Burton. *Basic writings of Mo Tzu, Hsün Tzu, and Han Fei Tzu*. New York, NY: Columbia University Press, 1967.

Watson, Burton. *The Complete Works of Chuang Tzu*. New York, NY: Columbia University Press, 1968.

Welden, John. "To Bring Order out of Chaos: Literati Medicine of the Jin Dynasty (1115-1234)." *To Bring Order out of Chaos: Literati Medicine of the Jin Dynasty (1115-1234)*. Dissertation, University of Hawai'i at Mānoa, 2015.

Wieger, Léon, and L. Davrout. *Chinese characters, their origin, etymology, history, classification and signification: A thorough study from Chinese documents*. New York, NY: Dover Publications, 1965.

Wilms, Sabine. *Venerating the root: Part 1*. Corbett, OR: Happy Goat Productions, 2013.

Wilms, Sabine. *Humming with elephants: The great treatise on the resonant manifestations of yin and Yang: A translation and discussion of chapter five of the yellow emperor's inner classic plain questions*. Whidbey Island, WA: Happy Goat Productions, 2018.

Wu, Rusong, Duanzhi She, and Yanjuan Wang. *Sun Zi's " Art of war" and Health Care: Military Science and Medical Science*. Beijing: New World Press, 1997.

Wilhelm, Richard, C. G. Jung, and Huayang Liu. *The secret of the golden flower, a chinese book of life*. New York, NY: Harcourt, Brace & World, 1967.

White, David (instituteofneijingresearch), '*Observing the natural divisions and geographical*,' Instagram, April 8, 2024, https://www.instituteofneijingresearch.com/

Yoke, HoPeng. Chinese mathematical astrology: Reaching out to the stars. New York, NY: Routledge, 2013.

Zielinski, Mark R., and Allison J. Gibbons. "Neuroinflammation, Sleep, and Circadian Rhythms." *Frontiers in Cellular and Infection Microbiology* 12 (March 22, 2022). https://doi.org/10.3389/fcimb.2022.853096.

Zhang, Zhongjing, Nigel Wiseman, and Sabine Wilms. *Jin Gui Yao Lue Essential Prescriptions of the Golden Cabinet: Translation and Commentaries*. Taos, NM: Paradigm Publications ; Distributed by Redwing Books, 2013.

Zhuangzi, and Angus Charles Graham. *Chuang-Tzu: The seven inner chapters and other writings from the book chuang-tzu*. London, UK: G. Allen & Unwin, 1981.

Index

About the Authors

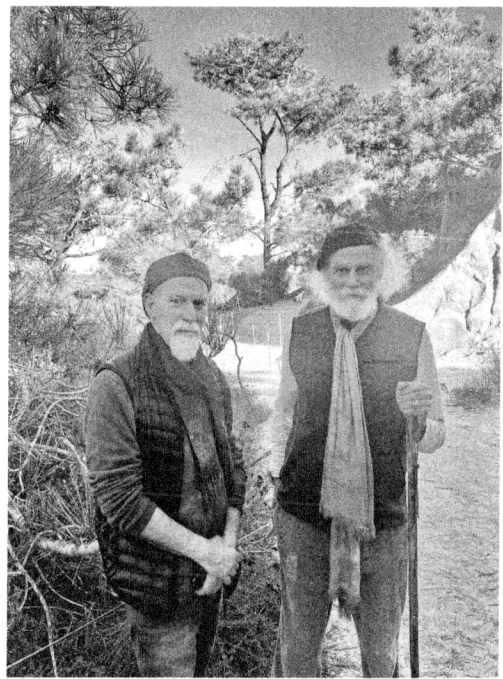

Stephen Cowan is a board-certified pediatrician with 35 years of clinical experience working with children. He sub-specializes in developmental pediatrics and is New York state certified in Medical Acupuncture. Dr. Cowan is a fellow in the American Academy of Pediatrics, and a member of both the AAP Committee on Children with Disabilities and the American Academy of Medical Acupuncture. He is a long-time student of Chinese medicine and *tàijí*. Dr. Cowan is the author of *Fire Child, Water Child* and has contributed chapters to several books about holistic approaches to childhood conditions.

Z'ev Rosenberg is recognized as one of the first generation of practitioners of traditional Chinese medicine in America. In private practice since 1983 and professor/department chair emeritus at Pacific College of Oriental Medicine, where he taught for 23 years, he has lectured widely around the United States, and has written many articles published in all of the professional English-language journals of the Chinese/East Asian Medical profession. He is the author of *Returning to the Source: Han Dynasty Classics in Modern Clinical Practice; Ripples in the Flow: Reflections on Vessel Dynamics in the Nàn Jīng*, and *Afterglow: Ministerial Fire and Ecological Chinese Medicine*.

About the Contributors

Brian Kirbis is a tea practitioner and an independent scholar trained in environmental and medical anthropology. He is the co-founder of Theasophie, a tea organization dedicated to preserving ancestral tea traditions and transmitting The Story of Tea.

Daniel Schrier is a practitioner of East Asian Medicine and licensed acupuncturist in Maryland and is an ordained 23rd generation Daoist priest in the *Quánzhēn Lóngmén* 全眞 龍門 lineage. He holds a Doctorate in Oriental Medicine (DOM) and is a professor at the Virginia University of Integrative Health (VUIM) and Yo San University. He previously served as the Director of Experiential Learning and adjunct faculty at the Maryland University of Integrative Health (MUIH).

Anne Shelton Crute is a Doctor of Acupuncture and Oriental Medicine, licensed acupuncturist, and Chinese Polestar astrology practitioner. She is the founder and director of Ritual Health clinic in the San Francisco Bay Area. There, she practices acupuncture, Chinese medicine, Ayurvedic, and Tibetan herbalism. Anne teaches local and international online coursework in astrology and Chinese medicine, guiding people towards living the worldview of natural medicine.

Printed in Great Britain
by Amazon